Body Systems Review III: Nervous, Skin/Connective Tissue, Musculoskeletal

2nd edition

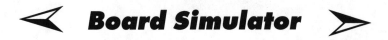

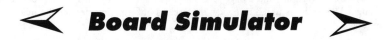

Body Systems Review III: Nervous, Skin/Connective Tissue, Musculoskeletal

2nd edition

≼ *Board Simulator* ≽

DEVELOPED BY

NATIONAL MEDICAL SCHOOL REVIEW®

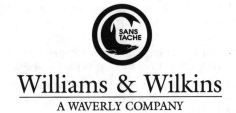

Williams & Wilkins
A WAVERLY COMPANY

BALTIMORE • PHILADELPHIA • LONDON • PARIS • BANGKOK
BUENOS AIRES • HONG KONG • MUNICH • SYDNEY • TOKYO • WROCLAW

Editor: Elizabeth A. Nieginski
Managing Editors: Amy G. Dinkel, Darrin Kiessling
Development Editors: Melanie Cann, Beth Goldner, Carol Loyd
Manager, Development Editing: Julie Scardiglia
Editorial Assistant: Lisa Kiesel
Marketing Manager: Rebecca Himmelheber
Production Coordinator: Danielle Hagan
Text/Cover Designer: Cotter Visual Communications
Typesetter: Port City Press
Printer/Binder: Port City Press

Copyright © 1997 Williams & Wilkins

351 West Camden Street
Baltimore, Maryland 21201-2436 USA

Rose Tree Corporate Center
1400 North Providence Road
Building II, Suite 5025
Media, Pennsylvania 19063-2043 USA

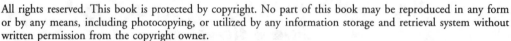

Accurate indications, adverse reactions, and dosage schedules for drugs are provided in this book, but it is possible that they may change. The reader is urged to review the package information data of the manufacturers of the medications mentioned.

Printed in the United States of America

First Edition,

Library of Congress Cataloging-in-Publication Data
Body systems review III : nervous skin / connective tissue,
   musculoskeletal / National Medical School Review. — 2nd ed.
       p.   cm. — (Board simulator)
   Edited by Victor Gruber.
   ISBN 0-683-30300-7
   1. Nervous system—Pathophysiology—Examinations, questions, etc.
2. Connective tissues—Pathophysiology—Examinations, questions,
etc.   3. Musculoskeletal system—Pathophysiology—Examinations,
questions, etc.   4. Nervous system—Physiology—Examinations,
questions, etc.   5. Connective tissues—Physiology—Examinations,
questions, etc.   6. Musculoskeletal system—Physiology
—Examinations, questions, etc.   I. Victor Gruber.   II. National
Medical School Review (Firm)   III. Series.
   [DNLM: 1. Nervous System—examination questions.   2. Connective
Tissue—examination questions.   3. Musculoskeletal System
—examination questions.   WL 18.2 B668 1997]
RC347.B63   1997
616′.0076—dc21
DNLM/DLC
for Library of Congress   97-8375
                                                                    CIP

The publishers have made every effort to trace the copyright holders for borrowed material. If they have inadvertently overlooked any, they will be pleased to make the necessary arrangements at the first opportunity.

To purchase additional copies of this book, call our customer service department at **(800) 638-0672** or fax orders to **(800) 447-8438.** For other book services, including chapter reprints and large-quantity sales, ask for the Special Sales department.

Canadian customers should call **(800) 665-1148,** or fax **(800) 665-0103.** For all other calls originating outside of the United States, please call **(410) 528-4223** or fax us at **(410) 528-8550.**

Visit Williams & Wilkins on the Internet: http://www.wwilkins.com or contact our customer service department at **custserv@wwilkins.com.** Williams & Wilkins customer service representatives are available from 8:30 am to 6:00 pm, EST, Monday through Friday, for telephone access.

                                                                    97 98 99 00
                                                        1 2 3 4 5 6 7 8 9 10

DEDICATION

This book is dedicated to the loving memory of Dr. Richard Swanson: 1954–1996. Rick was an inspiration as an author, teacher, and physician. Rick led by example, and his death is a loss to all of us whose lives he touched.

Rick is survived by his wife Stella, daughter Heidi, and sons Eric and Jason.

CONTENTS

EDITORS AND CONTRIBUTORS

GERALD D. BARRY, Ph.D.
Professor of Physiology and Director of the MA/MD
  Biomedical Program
Touro College School of Health Sciences

GRACE BINGHAM, Ed.D.
President and Educational Consultant
Bingham Associates, Inc.
Toms River, NJ
Coordinator of Cognitive Skills
National Medical School Review

GEORGE M. BRENNER, Ph.D.
Professor and Chairman
Department of Pharmacology
Oklahoma State University
College of Osteopathic Medicine

BARBARA FADEM, Ph.D.
Professor, Department of Psychiatry
University of Medicine and Dentistry
New Jersey Medical School

EDWARD F. GOLJAN, M.D.
Associate Professor and Chairman of Pathology
Oklahoma State University
College of Osteopathic Medicine

DAILA S. GRIDLEY, Ph.D.
Professor
Department of Microbiology and Molecular Genetics
Department of Radiation Medicine
Loma Linda University
School of Medicine

KENNETH H. IBSEN, Ph.D.
Professor, Emeritus
Department of Biochemistry
University of California at Irvine
Director of Academic Development
National Medical School Review

KIRBY L. JAROLIM, Ph.D.
Professor and Chairman
Department of Anatomy
Oklahoma State University
College of Osteopathic Medicine

KATHLEEN KEEF, Ph.D.
Professor
Department of Physiology and Cell Biology
University of Nevada
School of Medicine

JAMES KETTERING, Ph.D.
Professor and Assistant Chairman
Department of Microbiology and Molecular Genetics
Loma Linda University
School of Medicine

RICHARD M. KRIEBEL, Ph.D.
Professor
Department of Anatomy
Philadelphia College of Osteopathic Medicine

WILLIAM D. MEEK, Ph.D.
Professor
Department of Anatomy
Oklahoma State University
College of Osteopathic Medicine

STANLEY PASSO, Ph.D.
Associate Professor
Department of Physiology
New York Medical College

JAMES P. PORTER, Ph.D.
Associate Professor
Department of Physiology and Biophysics
University of Louisville
School of Medicine

VERNON REICHENBECHER, Ph.D.
Associate Professor
Department of Biochemistry and Molecular Biology
Marshall University
School of Medicine

DAVID SEIDEN, Ph.D.
Professor
Department of Neuroscience and Cell Biology
University of Medicine and Dentistry
Robert Wood Johnson Medical School

PREFACE

Since its establishment in 1988, the goal of National Medical School Review® (NMSR) has been to provide medical students and physicians with the information they need to know to pass their national licensing examinations. During this period, NMSR has developed a national reputation for high-quality programs delivered by the best teaching faculty available in United States and Canadian medical schools. Nearly 12,000 participants in NMSR programs have had access to outstanding faculty lectures as well as diagnostic and practice examinations and high-yield notes that can be kept as learning tools. As a result, NMSR students have achieved an impressive level of success on the United States Medical Licensing Examination (USMLE) Steps 1, 2, and 3.

With the development and publication of the *Board Simulator Series* (BSS), NMSR ushered in a truly innovative new educational experience for medical students and physicians preparing for Step 1 of the USMLE. This five-volume series' unique format was designed to follow the content guidelines published by the National Board of Medical Examiners (NBME) for the USMLE, Step 1, rather than being organized strictly by isolated basic science discipline (for example, volumes dealing only with biochemistry or anatomy). Therefore, just as they appear on the real Step 1 examination, many questions in this series are preceded by a clinical vignette that often integrates two or more disciplines and can require the student to perform a multi-step reasoning process to arrive at a correct answer. Thus, students are challenged not only to recall a particular fact or principle, but to analyze and apply that information to the situation defined by the clinical vignette.

One proven way to increase the likelihood of answering these questions correctly is to practice with questions that are at a similar level of difficulty and that have a similar emphasis. The BSS series provides students with just such an experience. In fact, it is NMSR's belief that this series gives most second-year medical students attending a United States medical school the essential information and test-taking experience required to pass the USMLE, Step 1. This series could also serve as an adjunct to students who feel they would benefit from attending a structured review program.

Furthermore, the BSS series provides far more than simulated Step 1 examinations, because each question is answered with a full and detailed explanation. A student can use these explanations to clarify why the right answers are correct choices and the wrong answers are incorrect choices. In the process of doing this evaluation the student will have performed a comprehensive review of the material covered on the Step 1 examination.

To make this process even more effective, this second edition of the BSS contains 770 questions in each volume, 120 more than in the first edition. Each of the tests in each volume, with the exception of the introductory 50-question diagnostic test, contains 180 questions, which reflects the new USMLE examination booklet's length. This edition also includes a subject item index, allowing students who wish to use these books in a subject-based fashion to do so with greater ease. NMSR believes that as an educational tool this series can help maximize a student's opportunity to make reviewing for the USMLE, Step 1 both a successful and rewarding experience.

Victor Gruber, M.D.
Founder and Executive Director
National Medical School Review®

ACKNOWLEDGMENT

NMSR would like to recognize Edward F. Goljan, M.D., for his valuable contribution to the development and unique organization of topics in this series.

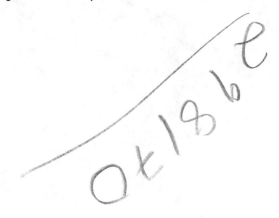

GUIDE TO USING THIS BOOK

During the past 10 years, a number of changes in curriculum organization have occurred in many U.S. and Canadian medical schools, particularly within the first 2 years of education. A number of meaningful innovations have been implemented, such as more self-directed learning, de-emphasis of lectures as the dominant instructional mode, earlier introduction of clinical experiences, and increases in the proportion of problem-based learning.

Today, regardless of which curriculum a medical school adopts, one trend exists even in those schools that have maintained a traditional stance: a loosening of the boundaries that organized basic science material into large territorial "subject" courses. The move is toward synthesizing domains of medical knowledge into more flexible cross-disciplinary patterns believed to approximate interactions that characterize medical practice today.

From a student's perspective, all the attention given to the number and variety of medical school curriculum reforms may have highlighted only the differences among the curricula and neglected to underscore the important similarities remaining. Regardless of the specific curriculum followed at any school, medical students are still expected to:

1. Read and understand large quantities of material. Whether the access mode is texts, handouts, specialized print materials, or computer modules, the reading demands remain significant.

2. Organize information in meaningful ways. No matter how well written a concept may appear in a text, or how well explained in a lecture, the students should *generate* the pattern of meaning that makes the most sense to them.

3. Develop relationships among experiences. All medical students are expected to engage in higher order thinking processes. New information about a topic will need to be *encoded* and *synthesized* with prior knowledge; *compared* with a lab experiment; *evaluated* through discussion with a colleague; or *solved* as a problem.

4. Store, retrieve, and remember information dependably. Historically, the demands on memory for medical personnel have been exceptional. The rapidity with which new technological advances in diagnosis and increases in treatment options are becoming available makes it more difficult than ever to learn and stay up to date in the field. Distinguishing between what needs to be mastered and recalled readily and what does not is a professional decision with which medical practitioners will struggle for the rest of their careers.

5. Demonstrate achievement through various forms of evaluation. Regardless of their curriculum model, all medical schools still require high levels of performance of their students. Evaluators can choose from a large range of methods to assess students, from the traditional instructor-designed examinations to oral evaluations, on-site observations, behavioral checklists,and product evaluations (e.g., written reports, research papers, problem solutions). Whatever the method, students will need to give evidence of competency.

6. Demonstrate competency on national standardized examinations. To qualify for licensure, students need to be successful on Steps 1, 2, and 3 of the USMLE. After further graduate training, students need to demonstrate success on specialty examinations to qualify for Board certification.

Series Design

Some of the more positive changes that characterize medical learning today are already reflected in the design of current instructional materials. One such change is the design of the five books in this series. The organization differs from the traditional subject-oriented subdivisions of basic science in that it conforms more closely to the content outline of USMLE Step 1 as presented in the *General Instructions* booklet. In Step 1, basic science material is organized along two dimensions: system (consisting of general principles and individual organ systems) and processes, which divide each organ system into normal development, abnormal processes, therapeutics, and psychosocial and other considerations.

Book I: General Principles in the Basic Sciences
Book II: Normal and Abnormal Processes in the Basic Sciences
Book III: Body Systems Review I: Hematopoietic/Lymphoreticular, Respiratory, Cardiovascular
Book IV: Body Systems Review II: Gastrointestinal, Renal, Reproductive, Endocrine
Book V: Body Systems Review III: Nervous, Skin/Connective Tissue, Musculoskeletal

Each book contains five examinations: a condensed 50-question diagnostic test and four tests containing 180 questions each, for a total of 770 questions per book. The distribution of questions within each test in books III, IV, and V approximates subcategory percentages as follows: normal development,10%–20%; normal processes,20%–30%; abnormal processes, 30%–40%; principles of therapeutics,10%–20%; psychosocial, cultural, and environmental considerations,10%–20%. By comparing your performance on the diagnostic test in each volume, you will be able to prioritize your use of the books.

Questions in each test are presented using the two multiple-choice formats that appear in USMLE Step 1: One Best Answer (including negatively phrased items) and Matching Sets, with the largest number of questions of the One Best Answer type.

Who Can Use These Questions?

The group likely to use the questions in this series of books most frequently is students preparing for USMLE Step 1. However, other student groups who can benefit from these questions are medical students in years I, II, III, and IV. These students may turn to individual books in the series or use the entire set of books as a supplemental self-testing resource.

Students Preparing for USMLE Step 1
Students preparing for the Step 1 exam will use these books as a **diagnostic tool,** as a **guide to focus further study,** and as a **self-evaluation device.**

Specific instructions about how to use the question sets for each purpose will be described in the next section.

Students in Years I and II
Students in years I and II will use these books for **periodic self-testing.** Students in the first 2 years of medical school take a large number of examinations that evaluate their performance on material covered in their courses or other learning experiences. Those tests are usually compiled by the instructors and reflect the intructors' choice of emphasis. The questions in the five books in this series provide a sampling of the wide range of material typically taught in the first 2 years of medical school. For students who want to practice with questions that go beyond the scope of their specific school's course, these question sets provide another level of testing, one that approximates more closely the expectations of the Step 1 exam. These questions also offer opportunities for practice to those students in medical school courses that use Board shelf exams as one of their required evaluations. The section How to Use These Practice Exams provides guidance on their use.

Students in Years III and IV

Students in years III and IV will use these books for **reactivating and assessing prior learning.** During their third and fourth years, students may find during clinical situations that they have forgotten some material they learned during the first 2 years. One way to stimulate, reactivate, and supplement that knowledge is by responding to questions. The content and organization of the questions in each book of the series make it possible for students in the clinical years to select and use specific segments for review.

How to Use These Practice Exams

The practice questions in this book assess knowledge of both normal and abnormal processes associated with each of the systems addressed (Nervous, Skin/Connective Tissue, Musculoskeletal). Whereas the specific content of questions in each system differs, certain categories of knowledge organization recur. Questions in this book relate to:

— Normal processes
  Development and structure
  Metabolic, physiologic, and regulatory processes
  Repair and regeneration
— Abnormal processes
  Disorders arising from a variety of origins:
    Traumatic
    Mechanical
    Metabolic, physiologic, or regulatory
    Neoplastic
    Idiopathic
    Vascular
— Therapeutic processes
  Uses of drugs to treat disorders, and their mechanisms of action
  Adverse effects of drug treatment
— Psychosocial, cultural, and environmental factors affecting disease processes

These question sets may be used in a number of ways: (1) as a diagnostic tool (pretest), (2) to guide and focus further study, and (3) for self-evaluation. The least effective use of these questions is to "study" them by reading them one at at time, and then looking at the correct response. Although the questions have been compiled to be representative of the domains of information found in USMLE Step 1, simply knowing the answers to these particular 770 questions does not ensure a passing grade on the exam. The questions are intended to be an integral part of a well-planned review, rather than an isolated resource. If used appropriately, the four sets can provide self-assessment information beyond a numeric score.

As a diagnostic tool. It is possible to use each set of questions as a screening device to gather diagnostic information about relative performance across the 10 large topics presented in this book. For those who have been away from basic science study for awhile and have no other recent performance data, using a practice exam in this manner provides a form of feedback before beginning review. This method also allows students to respond to Board-type questions similar to those on the examination so they can experience the structure and complexity of such questions and acquire a sense of what the questions "feel" like.

1. Select any one of the four complete tests in this book. It does not matter which one you choose, since they are all approximately equal in terms of topics represented and question difficulty.

2. Allow yourself the same amount of time as will be allowed on the Board exam (approximately 60 seconds per question).

3. Use a separate sheet of paper for your answers (instead of writing in the book). This will make it easier for you to score, analyze, and interpret the results.

4. Score your responses (but do not read the correct answer to the question or record the correct response next to your incorrect one). Compute an accuracy level by counting the number of correct responses and dividing by the total number of questions to get the percent correct. Note your score, but be careful not to overreact to this initial score. Remember that this type of sampling provides only a rough indication of how familiar or remote this basic science material seems to you before review. Not reading the correct answer to these questions may seem a bit strange at first, but by not doing so now, you will be able to use these questions again later in your review as a posttest to check progress.

5. Know your distribution of errors across the topics. To find out, categorize each error (e.g., biochemistry, cell biology, genetics; tissue biology, pharmacokinetics, multisystem processes). If in doubt about how to categorize a particular question, check the reference listed in the answer and use that to make your decision.

6. Arrange topics in a hierarchy from relatively strong (few errors) to relatively weak (many errors). Did you do well in those topics you thought you would do well in, and vice versa, or were there some unexpected highs or lows?

To guide further study. After reviewing the material of the major areas noted previously and giving the information a complete "first pass," it is time to test yourself using another question set in this book. Your purpose is to check your estimates of which topics and subtopics have been learned well, which are still shaky, and which are quite weak. To do that:

1. Follow the first five steps described previously.

2. Analyze errors using the guidelines described in the section "Monitoring Functions for Consolidating Information."

3. Focus your follow-up study on the content areas or specific subtopics noted to still be weak. Pay particular attention to whether a pattern of errors has emerged (e.g., questions requiring understanding of genetic principles; questions requiring knowledge of repair and regenerative processes; or questions requiring knowledge of metabolic pathways and associated diseases).

There is another possible use for these questions. If you already know from experience the two or three major topics in this book that cause you the greatest concern, you can:

1. Select from *two* question sets only those questions that deal with those specific topics. (You can identify them easily because each answer is topically keyed.)

2. If the number of questions is large, you may want to divide the number in half and reserve one half for a later test.

3. Follow steps 2 to 4 from the diagnostic testing section.

4. In conducting error analysis, try to pin down more specifically your within-topic errors, so that in follow-up study you can concentrate on strengthening weaknesses that remain.

5. When you feel you have firmed up your information base, test yourself with the other half of the questions and note your progress, as well as any remaining subtopics for follow-up study. The questions not used in the first two sets of questions, as well as the two full sets, can be used as your review progresses.

For self-evaluation. As the last few weeks before the exam approach, some students begin to experience feelings of "approach/avoidance"; they would like to know if they are close to, or even beyond, the minimum needed to pass, but they also fear that if they find a large discrepancy, it may deplete their efforts during the final phase of their review. This situation is less likely to occur with students who have engaged in self-testing throughout their preparation. These students have been collecting and analyzing test data all along and adjusting their study agenda accordingly. The last level of evaluation is not likely to give them any surprises about strengths and weaknesses, but will identify areas in which they can continue to fine-tune.

There are a few different ways to handle the last round of self-testing. Some students feel less anxious if they do the final round of self-evaluation in the first few days of the last week and reserve the rest of the time for last-minute follow-up study. Other students prefer to start the week with a composite test, continue with further study, and then take another practice test 2 or 3 days before the exam.

1. If you have used one full question set as a pretest, it would now be informative to start with those questions as a posttest. Follow the steps described previously and compare performance (both total score and the score across each large basic science topic).

2. The four remaining tests can be used as individual question sets, or they can be combined into one large composite set.

3. If none of the tests has been used for pretesting, you might take every other question from all five tests (385 questions) and follow up later with the remaining 385 questions.

4. If you are using other books in this series, you can select a set from each of the other four books to form a comprehensive final evaluation.

Score Interpretation

Keeping in mind that the percentage of items needed to pass the USMLE Step 1 is between 55% and 65% should help you interpret accuracy levels from your self-testing. The practice test samples suggested here (usually 180 questions) provide useful feedback to chart your progress. On your tests, percentages between 55% and 60% are minimal, but encouraging. Percentages between 60% and 75% show you are moving beyond the bare minimum needed for passing. Scores of 75% and above are indicators of substantial strength.

EXAM PREPARATION GUIDE

USMLE Step 1: What to Expect

USMLE Step 1 is the first examination of the three-step sequence required for medical licensure, so it is not surprising that its approach engenders apprehension in many students. Successful performance is particularly consequential in those medical schools that require successful passage of Step 1 before permitting students to proceed to third year. The "new" Step 1 has been in effect since 1991, and although most people are now familiar with its general contours, some "myths" still circulate.

The sources that contain the most complete and specific information about the examination are those distributed to students when they register to take Step 1: *Bulletin of Information* and *USMLE Step 1—General Instructions, Content Outline, and Sample Items.* **Both books should be read in their entirety before taking the examination.** What follows is a brief summary of what can be found in much more detail in those materials.

Description. The purpose of the Step 1 exam is to assess students' understanding and application of important concepts in the basic biomedical sciences: anatomy, behavioral science, biochemistry, microbiology, pathology, pharmacology, and physiology. Emphasis is placed on **principles and mechanisms underlying health, disease, and modes of therapy.**

A "blueprint" in the Guidelines booklet shows how basic science material is organized for the examination. Two dimensions are used: system and process. The first dimension includes a section on General Principles and ten Individual Organ Systems. The second dimension is divided into normal development; normal processes; abnormal processes; principles of therapeutics; and psychosocial, cultural, and environmental considerations. Also shown are the percentages of questions across categories of the two dimensions. The percentages are rather close between General Principles, 40%- -50%, and Individual Organ Systems, 50%–60%. Of the categories in dimension 2, abnormal processes has the largest percentage (30%–40%). A more detailed breakdown of content can be found in the *Step 1 Content Outline*, but not all the topics listed are included in each test administration.

Students are expected to respond to some questions that require straightforward basic science knowledge, but the majority of questions require application of basic science principles to clinical situations. There are also questions that require interpretation of graphic and tabular data and identification of gross and microscopic specimens. There seems to be more coverage of content typically taught in the second year, but interdisciplinary topics such as Immunology, which is usually taught in the first year, receive quite a bit of attention.

Format. The 2-day examination consists of four books with approximately 180 items in each book (total, 720 questions). Two books are given on each of the days. Three hours are allowed to complete each book, or approximately 60 seconds per question.

Question types. Two types of questions are on the exam: single best answer and matching sets, which begin with a list of a certain number of response options used for all items in the set.

Scores. Passing is based on the total score. Raw scores are converted to a standard score scale with a mean of 200 and a standard deviation of 20. A score of 176, or 1.2 standard deviations below the mean, is needed to pass.

Examinees will receive a total test score, a pass/fail designation, and a graphic performance "profile" depicting strengths and weaknesses by discipline and organ system. No individual subscores are reported. A two-digit score is also reported, in which a score of 75 corresponds to the minimum passing score and 82 is equivalent to the mean of 200.

A Framework for Successful Preparation

By the time you reach medical school, you have been a student for most of your life. You have learned in a variety of settings and have achieved a number of personal goals. There is probably little that you have not observed about your own learning. Despite this, you may still approach medical studies with some degree of apprehension and have questions about the effectiveness of your study strategies, specific skills, and attitudes.

After experiencing medical courses during their first year or two, most students accommodate well and, if necessary, make whatever adjustments in their study patterns seem warranted. But, even the most competent student, given the pressure of frequent and demanding examinations, will have occasional doubts regarding the efficiency of a particular study method. For those planning to take USMLE Step 1, many questions occur about how best to proceed. "How much time is adequate for review?" "What materials should I use?" "What should I study and in what order?" In discussions with other students, you will hear about approaches they took and what worked for them. But, eventually, you will need to make important decisions for yourself about how to *initiate* and *sustain* a preparation plan that results in success on the exam.

This preparatory guide selects and summarizes, from many different areas of cognitive and educational psychology, those findings that have most applicability to a medical learning context. Strategies, skills, and functions are organized according to their potential utility for students as they move progressively from initial encounter with new learning at stage I, acquiring information, to stage II, consolidating information, and finally to the goal of self-confident achievement, stage III, reaching mastery. In the sections that follow, the conceptual framework shown in Figure 1 will be used to discuss specific suggestions and activities.

FIGURE 1. Medical learning framework.

Cognitive Learning Strategies

Stage I. Acquiring Information

Stage II. Consolidating Information

Stage III. Reaching Mastery

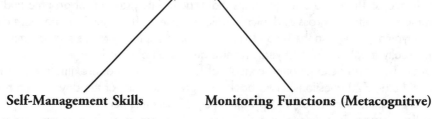

Self-Management Skills	Monitoring Functions (Metacognitive)
Time allocation	Study progress
Effort expenditure	Feelings/stress
Study resources	Self-evaluation

Three main subdivisions are represented in this Medical Learning Framework: cognitive learning strategies, self-management skills, and monitoring functions.

Cognitive learning strategies. These strategies can be used to acquire, retain, and master a massive amount of information in the basic sciences. The strategies will be arranged according to which ones are appropriate at each stage in the learning sequence.

Self-management skills. At each stage of learning noted previously, there are skills that can help students allocate time efficiently, expend effort productively, and use study resources effectively.

Monitoring functions. In addition to the cognitive dimensions, medical learning requires metacognitive functions— the ongoing self-regulation that helps students track their progress and decide whether they need to modify or fine-tune any behaviors. Students also need to monitor and try to control potentially interfering negative feelings and stress.

Cognitive Learning Strategies

Any learning experience a student engages in, whether listening to a lecture, reading a text, observing a demonstration, or viewing a video presentation can be said to move through three stages as the learner proceeds from initial enounter to eventual mastery. Many factors influence the progression from one stage to another, among them the characteristics of the student, such as ability, motivation, attitudes, and interests. Also influential are the characteristics of the material, its conceptual difficulty, its organization, and its relationship to the learner's prior knowledge. The specific study activities the student uses also will have an effect. Whether you are trying to learn medical material for the first time, or reviewing information you learned before and need to reactivate and strengthen, the three-stage concept of how learning takes place offers a handy scheme for deciding which study strategies to use when.

Strategies for Acquiring Information

In this first stage, as you read or listen to a lecture, the main task is consciously and intentionally to generate as much *meaning* (understanding) as you can. Because studies have shown that strong initial *encoding* influences to a large extent what will be stored in long-term memory, there is a payoff for being *active* at this stage. The ongoing task is to decide if what you are reading or hearing is unfamiliar information, somewhat familiar, or already part of your fund of knowledge. Rarely will you encounter something that is completely new, but some topics will seem more remote than others if your previous experience with them has been limited. As you move through the information, do so at as brisk a pace as you can without sacrificing meaning. Following are some productive strategies that can be used at this stage:

1. Preview. Before starting to read, notice how a topic or other chunk of material has been organized. Use external arrangements such as titles and subheadings to get an idea of how the topic has been segmented. One technique is to convert these subdivisions into questions. Study any pictorial material such as figures and diagrams. Read the introduction, summary, and questions, if available. Read anything that is printed in different type, such as italic, or highlighted. Notice unfamiliar terms and look them up. Remember that the purpose of previewing is to give you a preliminary cognitive "map" that should help you extract more meaning from your subsequent reading.

2. Read actively. When reading a text, handouts, and notes, some parts will trigger recollection from your previous learning. When you encounter familiarity, try *prompting*: Pause and look away from the page, anticipate what will be coming, and try to bring forth from your memory whatever you can recall about that topic. Also, try to read as if on a *search*. Having looked at the subheading of a section and raised

questions in your mind about what to expect, read to see if you can find responses to your questions.

3. Link information. Many medical students acknowledge that this is an important and useful strategy for enhancing understanding, yet few actually implement it. As you read, stop periodically and (a) summarize in your own words, (b) draw relationships to other knowledge by comparing and contrasting, (c) make an educated guess (inference), and (d) raise questions (What would happen if. . .?). If you are wondering whether you have time to think about the material given the usual pressures, remind yourself that these are the very thinking processes that are built into the questions of the Step 1 exam.

4. Construct notes. You probably have been taking notes in class since your earliest school days, and you may have developed a system for reducing and compacting lecture information that has served you well in the past. If so, continue using it. If, however, you are still trying to listen and write as much as you can, and as fast as you can, then perhaps you want to try a different method. When an instructor has provided a handout or other type of script before a lecture, preview it ahead and "cue" the sections that are obscure and need more elaboration. Then, you can limit note taking to what is essential to make sense of that script. Use whatever symbols you wish as cues (e.g., stars, circles, triangles) and assign a particular meaning to each. When you return to that handout after the lecture, you can translate your cues into further study activities (e.g., rewrite a particular section, supplement from a text, memorize a procedure).

One activity you might find helpful to institute fairly early is a last-minute study list consisting of those topics, mechanisms, procedures, and details that you find particularly problematic. Record either a brief explanation or the page and reference source where the information can be found. This list is particularly useful toward the end of your exam preparation sequence when you will want to make the most effective use of whatever time remains.

Self-Management Skills

At this early stage there are certain activities related to time, effort, and resources that are appropriate to carry out.

Time
Form a realistic study plan. Before plunging in, give some thought to how you want to organize your plan of study and which factors you need to consider. What is the amount of time you can reasonably allocate to preparation for the exam? If you are preparing for Step 1, it might be 3 or 4 months. If your experience with basic science material goes back a number of years, you will be doing more than simply activating former learning. There will be chunks of recent scientific knowledge that will require more intensive processing and more study time to reach a level of familiarity.

There are a few principles worth observing regardless of the total time actually allocated: (a) Use whatever diagnostic information you have (data-based, if possible) to assign time on the basis of relative strengths and weaknesses. Your review should be comprehensive, but some topics should be given more time than others. (b) Draft a long-range, tentative plan across the time you have available and estimate approximately how much you want to assign to each segment of content. Even a rough plan written down will reduce concern about whether you can fit everything in. You will be able to observe whether you underestimated the number of hours needed and increase them as you implement your plan. (c) Leave the last 2 weeks unscheduled so that you can return to areas that need a second pass. (d) At the end of each week, look at your plan and make changes based on your experiences during that week.

Effort
Get started. Perhaps what takes the most effort at this stage is just "lifting off" and getting into some type of study routine. You may find yourself putting off the actual start until you can finish other "essential" things, but you are probably procrastinating. It may help if you begin by studying something that you are strong in because a feeling of success will encourage you to continue. Gradually, shift to a topic that is less familiar and requires a little more intentional effort.

Select conditions conducive to study. Find a place where you can sustain a study block with few or no distractions. Put yourself in an active study posture, sitting upright, not lying on a couch or bed. Make yourself go to your study place as part of your routine. Staying in your apartment may be convenient, but it also makes it tempting to give in to other distractions.

Establish a reasonable, steady pace. If you are highly motivated, you may be tempted to work for exceptionally lengthy stretches, particularly during the early days of your review. Try, instead, to establish a reasonable routine that allows you to get a return from each study block. Know what your peak work periods are and do your most difficult studying at those times. Pay attention to whether you are getting fatigued and losing your ability to concentrate. Build in breaks that will reenergize you and help you feel refreshed when you return to studying.

Resources

Select effective study materials. Whether you are studying for a class exam or USMLE Step 1, finding just the right study material often can prove frustrating. Although quite a number of study resources are available in bookstores, each differs in purpose, format, depth, and comprehensiveness of coverage. For review, your own notes, charts, and handouts are good sources if you still have them available. They are familiar and have personal associations helpful for recalling information. To initiate review, look for publications that summarize or "compact" information, are not excessively wordy, but still provide enough narrative for you to make sense of the topic. The purpose of such books (e.g., Williams & Wilkins' *Board Review Series*) is to stimulate recall of material learned previously. Finally, have a reliable text available in each of the basic sciences so that you can use them selectively as a supplemental resource, if needed.

Monitoring Functions

Since you are just beginning to get into your study routine, this is the time to:

Initiate self-observations. These are the "informal" impressions, thoughts, and reactions that you form as you experience certain learning activities. For example, as you listen to a lecture, everything is making sense and fitting in with what you already know. Or, you feel some discomfort because the lecture is moving at too rapid a pace for you to process material meaningfully. Your reactions may be telling you that all is going well, and you should continue without change, or they may be signaling the need for some attention and possible adjustment in your study strategies.

Monitor emerging negative thoughts. If in reviewing you are reactivating without difficulty material you studied previously, you will feel productive and have a sense of accomplishment. But, there will be times when the proportion of understanding will seem relatively meager, and some discouragement will be felt. Try to confine your discouragement to the specific event that prompted the feeling without letting it generalize to *all* study activities.

Strategies for Consolidating Information

After you have listened to lectures or have read sections of material, you probably have acquired a reasonable percentage of the meaning. But, you also know that to *retain* what you understood, you will need to engage in other study activities. Of the multitude of activities from which you could choose, the following have been found to be effective to *maintain, consolidate, integrate,* and *synthesize* your knowledge.

1. Fill in gaps in your understanding. As soon after a lecture as is practical, follow up any of the "cued" sections in your notes or handouts by filling in what was unclear or incomplete. You can use another reference book, discuss the lecture with a peer, or ask for clarification from the instructor. Whatever action you take will make your learning stronger and move the information to long-term memory.

2. Reorganize for recall. Most students are familiar with the devices that can be used to reorganize information for better retrieval and recall: outlines, charts, index cards, concept maps, tree diagrams, and so forth. Following are guidelines for whether you should bother restructuring information and, if so, when it should be done.

If the material being used for study is already well organized, little if any restructuring may be needed. Sometimes, however, a different schematic format may make even well-organized material easier to recall.

If you reorganize, arrange the information so that *meaning* is emphasized. Note prototypes such as the most common and least common disease for a category, and the most frequent and least frequent treatment. In a set of diseases sharing similar symptoms, note particularly the differentiating feature(s).

If you decide to use one or more of the preceding devices, remember to do so during this stage, rather than close to the exam deadline, so you will have sufficient time to incorporate what you have restructured into your memory.

3. Synthesize from multiple sources. Avoid studying the same topic in three or four different sources. Use one substantive source as your "road map" and check other sources if you think yours is not comprehensive enough. Notice what needs to be added to make yours more complete, but end up with one dependable "script" that you can use for any subsequent study.

4. Rehearse to strengthen recall. Many students read things over and over. Rereading alone is not likely to be effective. The following habits could lead to more durable learning because they involve more active processing:

Use visual imaging. Visualize what you are trying to learn by "seeing" it in the form you will use when you want to retrieve it later (e.g., an anatomic structure as you saw it in lab, or as a schematic representation from the text, or as the instructor detailed it on a transparency).

Form analogies. Wherever possible, try to associate a new concept to a similar and simpler one that is already familiar to you.

Elaborate verbally. Talk about what you want to remember. Say it either to yourself or to others, but in your own words. "Stretch" beyond the script in the book or handout and develop inferences (make reasonable guesses about other relationships or applications).

Use mnemonics. These mental cues can be used to associate a wide range of medical information. Many can be found in student resources, or you can construct your own. Although you can be creative and even bizarre, avoid complexities that make the mnemonic harder to remember than the material itself. Using the first letter of each word to **form acronyms** is a common mnemonic device. For example, the causes of coma are AEIOU TIPS, which means *a*lcoholism, *e*ncephalopathy, *i*nsulin excess or deficiency, *o*piates, *u*remia, *t*rauma, *i*nfection, *p*sychosis, *s*yncope. **Method of loci** is one of the oldest mnemonic devices. You "place" mentally what you want to remember in certain familiar locations, such as rooms in your house, or locations within a room.

5. Establish patterns of practice. Certain "essentials" may need to be memorized and recalled almost verbatim. For such learning, **distribute the practice** so that you rehearse for a number of short periods, with breaks and other activities interspersed, rather than trying to sustain one lengthy period. Try **cumulative practice** by learning a few "chunks" at one session; then at a subsequent session, review those and add a few more. Continue the same pattern until all you want to memorize has been incorporated.

6. Study with others. This can be an effective study activity if used properly. An initial exploration of material by each student in the group will make group discussion more valuable. Discussion can then focus on clarifiying material and confirming and extending understanding. Studying with others works best if the group is small so everyone participates, and if some ground rules are established about how the sessions will be conducted.

7. Self-test periodically. The purpose of self-testing at this stage is **to guide further study.** Self-testing can help you decide which topics need more intense study, which are fairly close to being learned, and which have been learned well. Resources to use for this purpose and the sequence to follow will be described in later sections.

Applying Effective Testing Skills

Following are suggestions that will increase the likelihood that what you have learned and can recall from your study will translate into correct responses on multiple-choice examinations.

General test-taking skills

Read carefully for comprehension, not speed and respond to questions in sequence. Mark every item on your answer sheet as you go along, even if you are not completely sure of your choice. Cue the questions to which you want to return if there is time.

Be positive. Suppose the first question you see as you open the test book is a particularly difficult one, and you can feel yourself getting anxious. After giving it a try, go to the second question and respond to that one, which in all likelihood will feel more manageable.

Avoid mechanical errors. At the end of each page of questions, before going to the next page, check to make sure the **number of the question** you just finished **matches the number on your answer sheet.**

Be alert to key terms in the question stem such as "most," "least," "primarily," "frequently," "most often," and "most likely." Notice transition words that signal a change in meaning, such as "but," "although," and "however."

Let your original response stand unless you have thought of additional information.

Pace yourself. You will have approximately 60 seconds per question. Avoid dwelling on any one question, or rushing to finish. Set up checkpoints in your test booklet of where you want to be at the end of the first hour, second hour, and so on. You will know before you get close to the end whether you need to adjust your pace.

Analyzing questions

When you first read a question and look at the options, the answer may not be immediately apparent. Although you may be uncertain, don't just pick an answer arbitrarily. You can apply systematic skills of logic and deduction to narrow the five options to two or three possibilities.

Search for key information. As you read the question stem, notice key information (e.g., age, symptoms, lab results, chronic or acute condition, history). Highlight the key information by underlining or circling. **Notice particularly the request of the question** in phrases such as "the most likely diagnosis is," "the most appropriate initial step in management is," "which initial diagnostic evaluation is most appropriate." Take a quick look at the last line of the stem before reading the specific information in the remainder of the stem, especially if it is lengthy.

Analyze options. As you read each option, **try to eliminate** those that are inconsistent with the information you highlighted in the stem. For example, if a question concerns a 65-year-old woman, you would eliminate a procedure that you know applies only to children.

Cue each option. As you consider each option, mark down your initial reaction. In a "one best answer" question there are four "false" options and one "true" answer. For negative one best answer questions, the reverse applies. As you read each option, cue those you are sure of with a symbol such as "F," "N," or a minus sign. Cue true responses with a "T," "Y," or a plus sign. Cue those options you are uncertain about with the symbol you are using and a question mark.

Analyze structural clues in words. Pay attention to the meaning of prefixes, suffixes, and root words, which can sometimes help you decide whether to eliminate an option.

Approaching questions strategically. The following examples show how you might approach questions found in the books of this series.

Example: A 52-year-old woman has a radiographic report indicating a brain tumor located in the falx cerebri of the longitudinal fissure in the vicinity of the precentral and postcentral gyri. Which of the following indications would most likely occur first in this patient?
A. Decreasing pain and temperature in shoulder areas

B. Diminishing strength in forearm flexors
C. Tremor in lower extremities
D. Diminishing sensation and strength in leg and foot
E. Diminishing affect in response to social situations.

Analysis: What I need to recall is which areas of functioning are affected by this mass. As the mass grows, which brain tissue in its vicinity is likely to be affected with consequent neurologic dysfunction? I can eliminate E, since behavioral changes or social skills would be related to dysfunctions of the frontal cortex. Precentral and postcentral gyri are primary motor and primary sensory cortex, so there is likely to be diminished sensory perception and decreased motor activity. If I am correct about that, then I can eliminate A, which deals with pain and temperature. I think tremor involves cerebellar neurons, so C is probably not correct. I am left with options B and D, and although I am not sure if the location of the mass would affect lower extremeties, since D includes the word *sensation* , as well as *strength,* I am inclined to choose that one.

Comment: This question assesses the student's knowledge of relationships between injuries or abnormalities in particular sites in the brain and their consequent dysfunctional manifestations in motor, sensation, or behavior. The possibility for error is confusion in recalling which brain areas are somatotopically related to which parts of the body.

Example: Which of the following is the only commonality characterizing both degenerative joint disease and rheumatoid arthritis?
A. Inflammation is present in both
B. Both are autoimmune diseases
C. Both result in ankylosis
D. Cartilage is destroyed in both
E. Both affect mainly weight-bearing joints

Analysis: What do I know about these two musculoskeletal disorders? I know rheumatoid arthritis is an autoimmune disorder and degenerative joint disease is not; therefore, I can eliminate B. Although ankylosis is not *always* one of the results of rheumatoid arthritis, it does not occur in degenerative joint disease; therefore, C is not correct. I think it possible that both diseases can affect some weight-bearing joints, but in rheumatoid arthritis, the effects are *mainly* in the small joints of the hands and feet, so E is incorrect. I think A, inflammation, does not occur in degenerative joint disease, although I am not absolutely certain. However, if I have to choose between cartilage destruction and inflammation, I feel more confident that cartilage destruction is common to both disorders.

Comment: This question is typical of many that ask the student to recall differentiating features of disorders. In this respect, it represents one kind of knowledge expectation prevalent in medical learning, that of similarities and contrasts. Early in their training students learn that categories of drugs, organisms, and diseases have features in common that qualify them for inclusion in a particular grouping; however, each one also has discriminating characteristics that make possible specific identification for diagnositic or treatment purposes.

Relying on test question cues

The ability to use the characteristics or the formats of the test itself to increase your score is sometimes referred to as "test wiseness." It is possible to make use of idiosyncrasies in the way the questions are constructed to decide on the correct choice. This technique should be used only if you are unable to answer the question based on direct knowledge or reasoning. The following are examples of the principles of test wiseness, but you may have little opportunity to use them on USMLE Step 1, because the experts who construct the questions eliminate these cues.

Length of an option. If an option is much longer or much shorter than the others, it is more likely to be correct.

Grammatical consistency. Options that are not grammatically aligned with the stem are probably false.

Specific determiners. Options that contain words such as "all," "always," and "never" overqualify an option and are likely to be false.

Overuse of the same words or expressions. Some test makers have a tendency to repeat words or phrases in the options. If you are unsure of an answer, select from the options with the repeated words or phrases. Another variation of this principle is to select an option in which a key word from the stem is repeated.

Numeric midrange. When all options can be listed in numeric order (e.g., percentages), the correct choice will most often be one of the two middle values.

Guessing

The following are "last resort" strategies, but you should be aware of them.

1. If you have eliminated one or two options, but have no idea about the remaining ones, choose the first in the list.

2. If you are unable to eliminate any options, choose A, B, or C.

3. If you have a number of questions left to do and time is running out, **do not leave blanks.** Choose A, B, or C, and fill in the same letter for all remaining questions.

Self-Management Skills

Time

Study in blocks. Assuming you plan to study 4 to 5 hours each night, you might consider dividing those hours into two study blocks. This allows you to study two areas, one that is weaker and therefore requires more time, and another that is relatively strong and can be allocated less time. The advantage of studying two sciences concurrently is that you will move through your strong science with ease and feel a sense of accomplishment, even if the weaker science does not reach the same level of confidence.

Set goals for each study block. Begin by identifying a few goals you think can be accomplished within that block of time. The goals need not be elaborately stated. Identifying what you think is important to study increases the chances that you will study *actively* (with heightened awareness) since you are controlling the purpose, direction, and rate of the studying.

Set realistic deadlines. Although your accuracy in estimating how long it takes you to complete a study agenda will vary, observe whether you habitually overestimate. Arbitrary deadlines are self-defeating if you have little or no chance of meeting them. Set more realistic targets and attempt to meet them most of the time.

Use record-keeping devices. Calendars and appointment books will help you schedule your study agenda and permit you to look ahead and adjust plans to meet deadlines.

Control distractions. There are many kinds of distractions, some of which are self-imposed. Others, such as telephone calls, can interrupt concentration and make it harder to get back to work. If a call is not urgent, decide on a response within the first 30 seconds (e.g., "I'll call you back later. I'm in the middle of something important."). When you do call later, use it as a reward for having worked well, and enjoy It. Also, learn to say "No" to requests that take time and distract you from your schedule.

Effort

Avoid activities that dissipate effort. Be aware of whether there are things you do each day that reduce your total energy, and particularly the energy you want to give to studying.

Think about which of the "nonessential" tasks you can delegate to other family members, or to friends who want to be helpful. Give them some direction about what kind of help you would appreciate most.

Try to anticipate crises. There are disruptive life events that happen to all of us that we cannot anticipate but must deal with as best we can. But, there are other events of a less traumatic nature that, if they occur, can interrrupt the flow of a study plan and throw you off course (e.g., the car breaking down and needing immediate repair, a relative who wants to come and stay with you, or a friend who needs your advice on a troublesome problem). Anticipate crises that may happen during the span of your preparation and have alternative plans ready that permit you to be a part of what is going on but do not derail you completely.

Reward yourself for good effort. After having sustained a stretch of "heavy duty" studying, reward yourself by doing something that for you is pleasurable. A phone call to or from a friend that might be a distraction if it happens when you are trying to study can be a source of pleasure if you can defer it until you have completed your agenda for that day.

Resources
The following testing materials are appropriate for self-testing to guide further study. Their use is described in the next section.

Instructor content tests. These tests consist of questions prepared by the instructor who taught a particular segment of content. Some medical schools retain former course exams on file for student practice. Although the questions may not be structured as they appear on the Step 1 exam, they are good for pinpointing specific gaps or confusions in your knowledge base. Keep records of each practice test result and note relative performance across sciences and across topics in each science. For example, in pathology, note if one system (e.g., respiratory, cardiovascular, endocrine) is notably weaker than another. Cue topics that will need more sustained study. Take advantage of the instructor's presence to seek help, if needed.

Published books of practice questions. The books in this series arrange basic science content into "principles" (one book), "normal and abnormal processes" (one book), and "body systems" (three books).

Monitoring Functions

Monitor study progress
During this phase, when you are strengthening your learning, you will want to get **data-based feedback** using numeric scores to chart your progress.

Use questions to monitor progress
The pattern that works best is study, test, follow-up. Although there are times when it is appropriate to use questions before study to stimulate motivation or trigger recall, at this stage the best use of questions is after preliminary study. When you believe you have learned a segment of material, try a batch of questions. If time permits, you might want to test yourself on each major topic after completing its study, and before testing yourself on a mixed batch of topics in a science. However, if time is limited, select those topics about which you feel the most uncertainty, and use the feedback to guide additional study.

Select a representative sample of questions and complete them using the same time limits as will be used on your class exam or Board exam (approximately 60 seconds per question). Record your answers on a sheet of paper rather than in the question book or on the class practice exam. A separate sheet will allow you to do error analysis (described later) and keeps the book "clean" for future question retakes.

Do not do questions one at a time and then read the answer. The purpose is not to learn a particular question, but to find out which topics require follow-up.

Score your responses, but do not read answers immediately since you may want to give some questions a second try. After performing error analysis, decide which topics need further study and the type of study needed.

Compute an accuracy percentage by dividing the number correct by the total number of questions. Keep a record of your scores and note whether your accuracy level is approaching the percentage required for passing (for Board exams, between 55% and 65%). For class exams, the percentage may be higher.

Analyze for errors. It is important to analyze more specific aspects of your study and test-taking behavior to direct further study and make it more focused and productive.

1. Were patterns of errors noted (e.g., questions related to DNA principles, or questions about immune responses, or questions regarding quantatitive methods)?
2. Did you misread or misinterpret the question?
3. Were questions missed because, although you understood the concept, you forgot important details?
4. Did you note errors in addressing the *decision* required by the question? For example, although you knew much about the disease process described, you could not differentiate a likely diagnosis, or you were unable to form a judgment about a mechanism involved, draw an inference about the appropriate next step in management, or make a prediction about which drug would cause an adverse effect. In other words, you were unable to transform your conceptual and factual knowledge to meet the request of the question.

Monitor test anxiety
One aspect of self-testing that you should be monitoring is whether you are experiencing *inordinate* anxiety when dealing with test questions. It is not unusual to feel some elevation in anxiety when facing a comprehensive and consequential examination such as Step 1. But, if the amount of worry and the physiologic aspects (rapid breathing, sweaty palms, increased heartbeat) become so preoccupying that they interfere with productive studying, then some professional attention may be needed. If, however, test anxiety is of reasonable proportion, then remember what many studies have found. The best defense against test anxiety is a combination of strong review of subject matter, practice on tests similar to the target test, and positive self-reinforcement throughout the preparation process.

Combat negative self-statements
Part of your monitoring should include awareness of your moods and general state of being. Be sensitive to when you are about to give yourself a negative self-evaluation and combat it with an accurate, but positive one. "What if I don't. . ." statements will intrude periodically and, if permitted, can change your mood and distract you from your study. Start practicing self-talk by having a positive statement ready to use to redirect yourself back to your agenda ("I've been studying well and my scores show I'm making progress. . . I just need to keep going!" or "I can't afford the time to worry now; maybe late tonight; back to the topic now").

Strategies for Reaching Mastery
By the time you reach this stage you should feel more confident that your knowledge is firmer and that you can retrieve information dependably. The tasks of this stage deal with refining, or fine-tuning, for increased accuracy.

1. Focus on follow-up study. Your study agenda at this stage should be based on findings from your error analysis of questions you practiced, as well as any behavioral observations you noted from monitoring your performance.

If there are topics you need to reinforce, check your resources to note if those explanations are adequate, or if confusions still remain that may need to be clarifed through use of another text or discussion with a peer.

If details are eluding you, engage in some of the memory strengthening activities noted in the previous stage, particularly use of mnemonics, and cumulative practice.

If you misread information in questions, remember to highlight pertinent cues as you read, to focus on comprehension and avoid regressions, and to vary your rate to emphasize meaning.

If one of the patterns you noted is that errors were made on questions with very long stems, practice by first reading the "request" at the end of the question stem. You may then be able to interpret the direction and relevance of the information in the question more quickly and accurately.

If you found that you were unable to translate your knowledge to the specific *thinking* requirement of the question (form a judgment, integrate information to form a conclusion, draw an inference), first check to make sure you know the principles or mechanisms the question assumes you know (e.g., biosynthesis and degradation, dose–effect relationships, alterations in immunologic function). Then, analyze the question through a "think aloud" procedure, with a peer if possible, and try to identify why your thinking is inaccurate.

2. Engage in comprehensive self-evaluation. If you have practiced questions topically, and through a systems approach, as in this series, and followed up with focused review, you should be ready to test yourself with comprehensive question sets. These sets will contain questions that sample most of the domains of information represented on the target exam. The procedure in using those questions, scoring them, and analyzing errors is the same as described previously. Since the question sets are likely to be longer (approximately 150–200 questions), schedule them during the last 2 or 3 weeks, with time between each to benefit from the feedback. Some students end self-evaluation before the last week because further testing too close to the exam date heightens their anxiety.

3. Deal with interfering test-taking behaviors and attitudes. If your self-observations have noted any test-taking behaviors that need improvement, this is the time to correct them.

Impulsive responding. Do you find yourself getting annoyed if the answer to a question is not immediately apparent, and simply choose an option impulsively? Try to curb your impatience, and remind yourself that some questions are designed to engage you in an internal dialogue before deciding on a response.

Inability to move on. Are you unable to disengage from a particularly troublesome question and move on to the next one? This is especially bothersome when you have that tip-of-the-tongue feeling that the answer is something you know, but seems just a little out of reach. Difficult as it seems, try not to allow yourself to become irritated and get "stuck" to that question. Choose an answer and move on. It is likely that if you return to it later on, something may trigger recall.

Carrying over previous unsuccessful testing experiences. If comprehensive multiple-choice exams have been problematic for you in the past, and particularly if a recent attempt has not been successful, you may be tempted to see yourself as a "poor test-taker" and allow a defeatist attitude to permeate your self-testing activities. It would be better to start by asking yourself, "Why do I not do as well as I would like on multiple-choice exams?" Then, through your self-observations and data-based assessments, note any interfering behaviors you would like to change and implement activities that are more effective and can lead to success on such exams.

Self-Management Skills

Time

Set and maintain study priorities. One of the biggest problems experienced by some medical students at any level of training is approaching an exam deadline realizing that there is still so much to learn that they will not reach the stage of "mastery." After some last minute cramming they may even "pass," but the feeling of personal accomplishment eludes them. Although this has happened to all of us at one time or another, if it occurs as an ongoing pattern, then some change is needed. Make a list at the beginning of the week of all the study activities you want to accomplish and rank them in order of *importance* and *urgency*. At the beginning of the next week look at any low-priority items left undone and decide where to arrange them in that week's list. Make a record of each time you procrastinated or gave in to other distractions. Also note how often you kept to your schedule—it can motivate and encourage you to stay with it.

Schedule time for self-testing. Avoid deferring your first self-testing until just before an exam deadline. Build it into your schedule as part of your ongoing study activities and benefit from the feedback. You can then do "last minute" testing to aim for greater accuracy.

Effort

Avoid excessive fatigue. It is expected that you will work hard to be ready for an exam, but allowing yourself to get excessively tired and sleep deprived sabotages your goal. Respond to your body's need for rest instead of pushing for another hour's study with little to show for it. Try to pace yourself so that you have energy left to think clearly when you take the exam.

Keep motivation high. One of the possible pitfalls toward the end of your review is a reduction in your level of attention and concentration, because either of fatigue or emerging apprehension about the imminence of the exam. If you have done some record keeping during the preparation sequence, it is now helpful to look back and acknowledge how far you have come from the point where you started. Reward yourself for progress by planning a pleasurable activity following a block of concentrated study, and enjoy it without guilt.

Resources

Comprehensive question sets. For USMLE Step 1, materials such as Williams & Wilkins' *Review for USMLE Step 1* (NMS series), which provides five practice exams with approximately 200 questions in each exam, will be useful for comprehensive evaluation.

Monitoring Functions

As the exam deadline approaches, you may find that you are experiencing frequent mood shifts. When things are going well, your spirits may be high, but after a disappointing day you may feel blue, gloomy, or even angry. Recent research has found that some techniques work better than others to escape from a bad mood:

1. Take some action. If possible, do something to solve the problem that is causing the bad mood.
2. Spend time with other people, particularly to shake sadness. Focus on something other than what is getting you down.
3. Exercise. The biggest boost comes to people who are usually sedentary, rather than the already aerobically fit.
4. Pick a sensual pleasure, such as taking a hot bath or listening to a favorite piece of music. Be careful of using eating for this purpose; it may work in the short run, but may backfire, leaving you feeling guilty. Drinking and drugs are to be avoided for obvious reasons.
5. Try a mental maneuver such as reminding yourself of previous successes to help bolster your self-esteem.
6. Take a walk. Cool down before confronting whatever gave rise to your negative feelings.
7. Try to see the situation from the other person's point of view—why someone might have done whatever provoked your anger.
8. Lend a helping hand to someone in need. If you are studying, offer to help someone understand a science topic in which you feel very competent.
9. Use stress reduction techniques. Among the most effective are progressive relaxation, which uses tension and tension release in the body's muscle groups; mental imagery, which is putting yourself mentally in a location that evokes feelings of calm and peacefulness; and meditation, which aims for a state of relaxed alertness.

Grace Bingham, Ed.D.

◄ Diagnostic Test ►

QUESTIONS

DIRECTIONS:

Each of the numbered items or incomplete statements in this section is followed by answers or by completions of the statement. Select the ONE lettered answer or completion that is BEST in each case.

1. A newborn girl is noted to have decreased abduction of the right hip associated with a palpable click when the thumb is pressed into the hip socket. This disorder is best described as

(A) a sprain
(B) a ligament tear
(C) a slipped capital femoral epiphysis
(D) a dislocation
(E) an injury associated with delivery

2. A 24-year-old upper middle-class female patient with a history of drug abuse is brought into the emergency room. One of her major complaints is that she feels as though bugs are crawling on her skin. Of the following choices, the symptoms of this patient are most likely due to

(A) heroin overdose
(B) alcohol overdose   C
(C) cocaine overdose
(D) heroin withdrawal
(E) alcohol withdrawal

3. Arrange the following bone diseases in the chronological order reflecting earliest to latest onset.

1. Osteogenic sarcoma
2. Chondrosarcoma
3. Ewing sarcoma
4. Metastasis to bone

(A) 3-4-1-2   C
(B) 1-2-3-4
(C) 3-1-2-4
(D) 1-3-4-2
(E) 1-4-3-2

4. Which of the following findings is characteristic of drug-induced lupus erythematosus rather than systemic lupus erythematosus?

(A) Positive anti–double-stranded DNA antibody
(B) Low incidence of renal and central nervous system involvement
(C) Positive anti-Smith antibody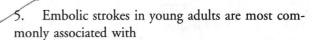
(D) Negative antihistone antibodies
(E) Low complement levels

5. Embolic strokes in young adults are most commonly associated with

(A) infective endocarditis in intravenous drug abusers
(B) Libman-Sacks endocarditis   A
(C) rheumatic valvular disease
(D) mitral valve prolapse
(E) atherosclerosis involving the carotid artery

6. A calf muscle biopsy in a young boy with muscle weakness since birth shows muscle atrophy and increased adipose. His serum creatine kinase is markedly elevated. This patient most likely has an abnormality in

(A) porphyrin synthesis
(B) dystrophin
(C) myoglobin
(D) thyroid function
(E) the mitochondria

7. Which of the following lesions associated with increased pigmentation of skin is related more to the presence of hemosiderin than to increased melanin pigment?

(A) Stasis dermatitis in the legs
(B) Peutz-Jeghers syndrome
(C) Hemochromatosis
(D) Nevocellular nevi
(E) Addison's disease

Questions 8-11

A twenty-five-year-old man presents to the ER with a severe contusion to the right side of the forehead. On examination he has diminished sensation to the forehead and cannot raise the upper eyelid. On further examination it is discovered that he cannot move the eye upward or in a lateral direction. Radiographic studies show some displacement of the bony structure of the orbit.

8. Which is the site into which the bone has been displaced, resulting in all of the described symptoms?

(A) Mental foramen
(B) Supraorbital foramen
(C) Infraorbital foramen
(D) Superior orbital fissue
(E) Inferior orbital fissure

9. Which nerve is involved in the patient's inability to look upward or raise the upper eyelid?

(A) Trochlear
(B) Oculomotor
(C) Abducens
(D) Frontal
(E) Ophthalmic division of the trigeminal (V_1)

10. Which nerve is involved in the patient's inability to move the eye in a lateral direction?

(A) Trochlear
(B) Oculomotor
(C) Abducens
(D) Supratrochlear
(E) Infraorbital

11. Sensory deficit is a result of injury to which nerve?

(A) Zygomaticofacial
(B) Zygomaticotemporal
(C) First cervical spinal nerve (C1)
(D) Maxillary division of trigeminal (V2)
(E) Ophthalmic division of trigeminal (V1)

12. A 42-year-old woman presents with Raynaud phenomenon and dysphagia for liquids and solids. Her fingers are tapered and exhibit focal areas of dystrophic calcification at the tips as wells as telangiectasias over the skin surface. The results of a serum antinuclear antibody (ANA) study are pending. Which additional test would be MOST useful if the serum ANA returns positive?

(A) Anti–SS-A antibody
(B) Erythrocyte sedimentation rate
(C) Anti-centromere antibody
(D) Anti–double-stranded DNA antibody
(E) Anti-Smith antibody

Questions 13-15

A patient presents with hoarseness, right shoulder drop, and difficulty turning the head to the left against resistance. The patient complains of numbness at the "back" of the tongue. On further examination a mass is palpable anterior and deep to the upper aspect of the sternocleidomastoid muscle.

13. Based on the symptoms presented by the patient, which of the following cranial foramina would MOST likely be involved?

(A) Spinosum
(B) Ovale
(C) Jugular
(D) Carotid canal
(E) Rotundum

14. Which cranial nerves are involved?

(A) Facial / accessory / vagus
(B) Hypoglossal / vagus / facial
(C) Facial / hypoglossal / glossopharyngeal
(D) Accessory / glossopharyngeal / vagus
(E) Hypoglossal / glossopharyngeal / facial

15. Which vascular structure would MOST likely be involved?

(A) Middle meningeal artery
(B) Common carotid artery
(C) Vertebral artery
(D) Internal jugular vein
(E) External jugular vein

16. In which of the following joint diseases would you expect to find in the synovial fluid a normal to slightly elevated neutrophil count and a normal mucin clot study?

(A) Osteoarthritis
(B) Rheumatoid arthritis
(C) Reiter's syndrome
(D) Ankylosing spondylitis
(E) Lyme's disease

Questions 17-19

A patient complains of persistent numbness of the chin, lower lip, and lower teeth. She further indicates that she has difficulty chewing. Radiographic studies of the head demonstrate a small discrete mass in the infratemporal fossa.

17. From the patient's symptoms, which cranial foramen is most involved by the mass?

(A) Ovale
(B) Rotundum
(C) Spinosum
(D) Petrotympanic
(E) Stylomastoid

18. Which nerve has been compromised by the mass?

(A) Buccal
(B) Lingual
(C) Auriculotemporal
(D) Inferior alveolar
(E) Superior alveolar

19. Which artery would be compromised by the mass based on the cranial foramen involved?

(A) Sphenopalatine
(B) Inferior alveolar
(C) Superior alveolar
(D) Middle meningeal
(E) Accessory meningeal

20. Osteomalacia differs from osteoporosis in that osteomalacia

(A) is often associated with renal disease
(B) the bone is osteopenic on routine radiograph
(C) is a problem with matrix mineralization
(D) has an overall decrease in bone mass
(E) predisposes to fractures in adults

21. A 42-year-old male patient with pneumonia has been hospitalized in isolation for three days. On the third day, his pneumonia has resolved, but he seems agitated, shows tachycardia and hypertension, and states that he feels bugs crawling on his skin. The patient's symptoms are most likely caused by which of the following?

(A) Heroin overdose
(B) Alcohol overdose
(C) Cocaine overdose
(D) Heroin withdrawal
(E) Alcohol withdrawal

22. The most common benign soft-tissue tumor and sarcoma in adults, respectively, is

(A) lipoma—liposarcoma
(B) leiomyoma—leiomyosarcoma
(C) leiomyoma—malignant fibrous histiocytoma
(D) rhabdomyoma—rhabdomyosarcoma
(E) dermatofibroma—synovial sarcoma

23. A left homonomous hemianopia was discovered when the examiner evaluated both eyes of a patient. This deficit is MOST likely produced by pathophysiology in which one of the following structures?

(A) Left retina
(B) Right optic nerve
(C) Left optic tract
(D) Right optic tract
(E) Left occipital cortex

24. The inflammatory skin reaction associated with exposure to the resin of poison ivy is most closely related in pathogenesis to

(A) contact dermatitis to nickel
(B) atopic dermatitis
(C) psoriasis
(D) pemphigus
(E) porphyria

25. A 28-year-old secretary who has previously been careful with money begins running up her credit-card bills. She is irritable when her husband criticizes her spending habits and tells him that she needs to buy things to look good for the movie in which she will soon star. This most likely diagnosis for this patient is

(A) schizophrenia
(B) bipolar disorder
(C) dysthymic disorder
(D) cyclothymic disorder
(E) hypomania

26. A cerebral abscess and a cerebral infarct are similar in that both

(A) most often result from a primary lesion located outside the cranial vault
(B) are examples of liquefactive necrosis
(C) are most commonly associated with infectious disease
(D) most commonly develop from embolization from another primary site
(E) have collagen formation as part of the healing process

27. Ischemia of the spinal cord may occur when the radicular arterial blood supply is compromised. Which one of the following spinal cord levels is most predisposed to ischemic damage?

(A) C5–C6
(B) T1–T3
(C) T7–T9
(D) L5–S1
(E) S4–Coccygeal 1

28. What virus is the most likely cause of hemorrhagic necrosis that is localized to the temporal lobe and accompanied by Cowdry type A inclusion bodies?

(A) Rabies virus
(B) Herpes simplex virus
(C) Adenovirus
(D) Rubeola virus
(E) Cytomegalovirus

DIRECTIONS:

Each of the numbered items or incomplete statements in this section is negatively phrased, as indicated by a capitalized word such as NOT, LEAST, or EXCEPT. Select the ONE lettered answer or completion that is BEST in each case.

Questions 29-30

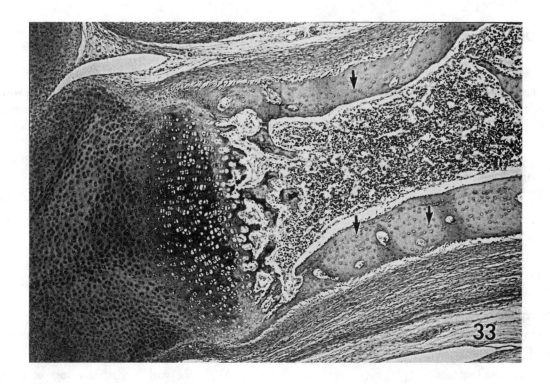

Refer to this figure to answer the questions below.

29. All of the following musculoskeletal elements are present in this figure EXCEPT

(A) bone
(B) periosteum
(C) hyaline cartilage
(D) calcified cartilage
(E) a secondary ossification center

30. Which type of cell is present at the arrows in this figure?

(A) Osteocyte
(B) Osteoblast
(C) Chondrocyte
(D) Chondroblast
(E) Osteoprogenitor

31. Which of the following musculoskeletal disease relationships is NOT CORRECT?

(A) Tennis elbow/tenderness at the medial epicondyle
(B) Idiopathic scoliosis/paraspinous prominence on forward bending
(C) Meniscus tear/positive McMurray test
(D) Cruciate ligament tear/positive draw test
(E) Compartment syndrome/localized increase in tissue pressure commonly seen in the tibia and forearm muscle compartments

DIRECTIONS:

Each set of matching questions in this section consist of a list of four to twenty-six lettered options (some of which may be in figures) followed by several numbered items. For each numbered item, select the ONE lettered option that is most closely associated with it. To avoid spending too much time on matching sets with large number of options, it is generally advisable to begin each set by reading the list of options. Then for each item in the set, try to generate the correct answer and locate it in the option list, rather than evaluating each option individually. Each lettered option may be selected once, more than once, or not at all.

Questions 32-36

Match the clinical correlation with the most closely associated neurotransmitter.

(A) γ-Aminobutyric acid (GABA)
(B) Acetylcholine
(C) Dopamine
(D) Norepinephrine
(E) Endogenous opioid

32. The placebo response

33. Alzheimer disease

34. Schizophrenia

35. Pheochromocytoma

36. Epilepsy

Questions 37-41

Select the drug that would be most beneficial for the signs and symptoms of the patients described.

(A) Carbamazepine
(B) Pergolide
(C) Alprazolam
(D) Tacrine
(E) Risperidone

37. A patient with progressive loss of short-term memory over the past year is brought to the clinic by family members. The patient is subsequently found to have a low score on the mini-mental state exam and activities of daily living scale, but the neurologic exam is otherwise normal.

38. A 62-year-old man presents with resting tremor, cogwheel rigidity, and difficulty initiating purposeful movements.

39. A 27-year-old patient reports episodes of severe anxiety accompanied by sweating, tachycardia, and shortness of breath. These episodes are associated with her fear of going out to buy groceries.

40. A 19-year-old woman is brought to the clinic for evaluation. She reports hearing voices that instruct her to move out of her apartment, and she has become increasingly fearful that her landlady is trying to poison her. Her brother reports that she has become progressively withdrawn and unresponsive to family members.

41. After a head injury in an automobile accident, a young man experiences an abrupt onset of unilateral clonic contractions of his fingers that progressively involve his hand, then lower and upper arms.

Questions 42-46

Match the patient description with the most closely associated psychoactive agent.

(A) Alprazolam
(B) Fluoxetine
(C) Desipramine
(D) Trazodone
(E) Amoxapine

42. Benzodiazepine with antidepressant activity

43. Heterocyclic antidepressant to be avoided in suicidal patients

44. Useful particularly for overweight patients

45. Associated with priapism

46. Useful for the elderly because it is nonsedating

Questions 47-50

For each patient, select the drug that would be most beneficial.

(A) Indomethacin
(B) Ketorolac
(C) Acetaminophen
(D) Phenylbutazone
(E) Naproxen

47. A young child with an acute and severe viral respiratory infection and an oral temperature of 39.5°C

48. A 20-year-old woman with low, midline, wave-like cramping pelvic pain associated with nausea and headache during menses

49. A newborn infant with a vascular shunt connecting the left pulmonary artery and aorta

50. A patient with a history of drug dependence who must be treated for severe postoperative pain

ANSWER KEY

1. D	10. C	19. E	27. B	35. D	43. E
2. C	11. E	20. C	28. B	36. A	44. B
3. C	12. C	21. E	29. E	37. D	45. D
4. B	13. C	22. C	30. A	38. B	46. C
5. A	14. D	23. D	31. A	39. C	47. C
6. B	15. D	24. A	32. E	40. E	48. E
7. A	16. A	25. B	33. B	41. A	49. A
8. D	17. A	26. B	34. C	42. A	50. B
9. B	18. D				

ANSWERS AND EXPLANATIONS

1. The answer is D. *(Pathology)*
A newborn girl with decreased abduction of the right hip associated with a palpable click when the thumb is pressed into the hip socket has a congenital hip dislocation, which is six times more common in girls than boys. A congenital hip dislocation, which limits abduction of the affected joint, is not associated with injury from delivery and can be unilateral, as in this case, or bilateral. The Ortoloni test involves abducting the affected thigh and feeling for a click as the dislocated femoral head slips back into the acetabulum. The Galeazzi test compares the height of the femoral condyles, with the affected hip being shorter.

Sprains are a complete or partial tear of ligaments associated with swelling and tenderness. Because radiography of a sprain will be normal, the diagnosis must be made by physical examination. A dislocation is a disruption of normal relationships between articular surfaces. A ligament tear results in loss of movement of the affected part. A slipped capital femoral epiphysis most commonly occurs in obese adolescent males from 9 to 15 years old; pain located on the medial aspect of the knee is characteristic of the condition.

2. The answer is C. *(Behavioral science)*
Cocaine overdose is associated with formication (a feeling that bugs are crawling on the skin). Although in alcohol withdrawal after long-term use, formication is also seen, this young, upper middle-class patient is more likely to have abused cocaine than to be in alcohol withdrawal after long-term use. This hallucination is not seen commonly with heroin overdose, heroin withdrawal, or alcohol overdose.

3. The answer is C. *(Pathology)*
The age of the patient, location of the disease in bone, radiographic appearance of the lesion, and biopsy material are essential to making a definitive diagnosis of bone disorders. Generally, osteogenic sarcomas tend to occur during childhood during periods of active skeletal growth, while chondrosarcomas and giant cell tumors more commonly arise in the middle years of life. Chrondroblastomas and giant cell tumors of bone are characteristically located in the epiphyseal ends of long bones. Osteoblastic bone lesions (osteogenic sarcoma, osteoid osteoma) commonly yield radiodensities on radiography. The most common benign primary tumor of bone is an osteochondroma, and the most common malignancy in bone is metastatic carcinoma. Multiple myeloma is the most common overall primary malignancy of bone, while an osteogenic sarcoma is the most common malignant primary tumor arising from bone.

Chondrosarcomas are the most common primary malignant cartilaginous tumors, and normally occur in patients older than 35 years. The most common locations for chondrosarcomas, in descending order, are the pelvic bones and the upper end of both the humerus or femur. Predisposing causes include the presence of multiple enchondromas (Ollier disease) and, to a lesser extent, Paget disease of bone; both of the predisposing factors are low-grade tumors with a 90% 10-year survival rate. The lungs and bone are the primary metastatic sites.

Osteogenic sarcomas are the most common primary malignancy arising from bone proper. Most patients are between 10 and 25 years old. Predisposing factors include exposure to radiation, pre-existing bone disease (Paget disease of the bone), and an association with retinoblastoma. Most osteogenic sarcomas are located in the lower end of the femur (35%) and upper end of the tibia (15%). Osteogenic sarcoma destroys the metaphysis of bone and invades subjacent soft tissue; radiography will subsequently show a Codman triangle, caused by elevation of the periosteum, and a "sunburst" appearance, which is caused by calcifed osteoid extending into the soft tissue. Early hematogenous metastases most commonly occur in the lungs. In some cases, removal of the metastatic disease portends a good prognosis. Overall, there is a 60% 5-year survival rate after amputation.

Ewing sarcoma is a highly malignant primary bone tumor of marrow origin exhibiting a primitive neural phenotype and are associated with an 11;22 translocation. The tumors develop predominantly in boys between 10 and 15 years of age. Ewing sarcoma usually arises in the diaphysis of long tubular bones, like the femur, and flat bones of the pelvis, and extend into the surrounding soft tissue. The resulting reactive new bone formation produces concentric "onion skin" layering, which is visible by radiography. The clinical presentation of Ewing sarcoma often mimics an infection with associated fever, localized heat, anemia, and an increased erythrocyte sedimentation rate. There is a 75% 5-year survival rate.

Metastases are the most common malignancy of bone and are 50 times more frequent than primary malignant tumors of bone. Primary cancers most commonly metastasizing to bone are those originating in the female breast, lungs, kidney, prostate, and intestine. The bones most frequently involved are the vertebra (most common), pelvis, ribs, skull, sternum, and the upper ends of the femur. Most metastases to bone are osteolytic and produce radiographic radiolucencies. Osteoblastic metastases producing radiographic radiodensities are most commonly secondary to prostate and breast cancer, which show increased serum alkaline phosphatase levels.

4. The answer is B. *(Pathology)*
The characteristics of drug-induced lupus differ from those of systemic lupus erythematosus in the following ways:

- a very low incidence of renal and central nervous system involvement
- anti–double-stranded DNA and anti-Smith antibodies are negative
- normal complement levels
- the presence of antihistone antibodies (95%)
- the presence of anti–single-stranded DNA antibodies (80%)

The drug most commonly implicated in producing this syndrome is procainamide; other less frequently implicated drugs include phenytoin, hydralazine, quinidine, methyldopa, isoniazid, and chlorpromazine. Drug-induced lupus erythematosus usually resolves upon discontinuance of the drug.

5. The answer is A. *(Pathology)*
Embolic strokes in young adults are most commonly associated with infective endocarditis in intravenous drug abusers. Half of the lesions are on the tricuspid valve and the other half are on the aortic valve. Most of these strokes are in the distribution of the middle cerebral artery. Embolic strokes produce a hemorrhagic infarction.

Libman-Sacks endocarditis is associated with systemic lupus erythematosus. None of the vegetations that occur on surfaces of the valves embolize. Rheumatic valvular disease with secondary infective endocarditis may be associated with embolic strokes, but vegetations secondary to intravenous drug abuse are more common than those associated with rheumatic valvular disease in this age bracket. Mitral valve prolapse is rarely associated with infective endocarditis. Atherosclerosis involving the carotid artery may result in embolization, but in young adults it is distinctly uncommon.

6. The answer is B. *(Pathology)*
A calf muscle biopsy in a young boy with muscle weakness since birth shows muscle atrophy and increased adipose. The laboratory workup demonstrates a markedly elevated serum creatine kinase (CK). The boy has Duchenne's muscular dystrophy. The term "muscular dystrophy" refers to a progressive, genetically determined primary muscle disease, which most commonly presents in early childhood and involves specific muscle groups. The most common and most severe muscular dystrophy is the Duchenne-type of sex-linked recessive muscular dystrophy (70%). This dystrophy usually manifests itself in the second to fifth years of life as weakness and wasting of the proximal pelvic and shoulder girdle muscles, with progressive disablement by 10 years of age, and death by 20 years of age. There is a defect in formation of dystrophin by a gene on the X chromosome. Normally, dystrophin links the sarcolemmal cytoskeleton through a transmembrane complex to an extracellular glycoprotein that binds laminin. The muscle disease is characterized by (1) progressive degeneration of muscle (equal loss of type I and II fibers), (2) an attempt at repair and regeneration of the lost muscle fibers, and (3) progressive fibrosis and infiltration of muscle tissue by fatty tissue, which is responsible for pseudohypertrophy of the calf muscles. The weakness of muscles in the pelvic girdle causes the patient to have difficulty in rising up from a seated position. It also produces a peculiar waddling gait. The antenatal diagnosis of Duchenne's dystrophy is possible by using recombinant DNA technology. The preclinical diagnosis is secured by measuring the serum CK, which is always increased at birth despite the absence of clinical disease. The enzyme declines as muscle tissue is progressively replaced by

fat and fibrous tissue. Female carriers may sometimes be detected by noting elevated serum CK activity (70% of cases) or by molecular probe studies of their DNA. Becker's dystrophy is a weaker variant of Duchenne's muscular dystrophy.

7. The answer is A.   *(Pathology)*

Stasis dermatitis is commonly located around the ankles and is due to deep venous insufficiency with a backup of blood into the vessels around the ankles, which rupture and deposit hemosiderin in the subcutaneous tissue. Increased melanin in the epidermis is associated with (1) hemochromatosis, where iron increases melanin deposition in the basal cell layer; (2) Peutz-Jeghers syndrome, which is an autosomal dominant polyposis syndrome with increased oral pigmentation and hamartomatous polyps in the small/large bowel; (3) nevocellular nevi, which are composed of modified melanocytes; and (4) Addison's disease, in which destruction of the adrenal gland produces hypocortisolism and a stimulus for an increase in adrenocorticotrophic hormone, which has melanocyte-stimulating properties.

8-11. The answers are: 8-D, 9-B, 10-C, 11-E. *(Anatomy)*

The bone is displaced into the superior orbital fissure. The neural structures that pass through this fissure to enter the orbit are the oculomotor (III), trochlear (IV), and abducens (VI) nerves, and the ophthalmic division of the trigeminal nerve (V). Displacement of bone into the superior orbital fissure could potentially injure any or all of these nerves. Based on the patient's symptoms all are damaged except the trochlear nerve. The superior division of the oculomotor nerve supplies the levator palpebrae superiorius and superior rectus muscles with motor innervation, explaining the deficit in the patient's ability to raise the eyelid and move the eyeball upward. The inability to move the eye in the lateral direction indicates the innervation to the lateral rectus muscle was compromised. This muscle is supplied by the abducens nerve. Based on the presenting symptoms, the trochlear nerve was not involved. This nerve supplies the superior oblique muscle, which moves the cornea downward and outward while medially rotating the entire eyeball. This function is assumed to be intact. The loss of sensation to

the forehead is due to injury to the ophthalmic nerve (V1). This division of the trigeminal nerve supplies sensory innervation to the forehead and the scalp as far as the vertex. The supratrochlear nerve is a branch of the ophthalmic nerve but is not included in the sensory deficit question. The maxillary division of the trigeminal nerve (V2) gives rise to the infraorbital, zygomaticofacial, and zygomaticotemporal nerves. This division is located in the inferior orbital fissure, which is not involved in this injury. These branches do not supply the forehead. The first cervical spinal nerve (C1) does not provide the skin with sensation. The infraorbital foramen transmits the infraorbital nerve, and the mental foramen transmits the mental nerve (V3). These nerves supply sensory innervation to the lower face and chin and are not involved. The ophthalmic division of the trigeminal nerve gives rise to the frontal nerve, and this answer is not a choice in any of the questions in this scenario. However, because the ophthalmic nerve is injured, the frontal nerve would have been compromised as well. The supraorbital foramen transmits the supraorbital nerve. This nerve is a branch of the frontal nerve and would have been involved, but is not a choice in any of the questions.

12. The answer is C.   *(Pathology)*

A 42-year-old woman who presents with Raynaud's phenomenon, dysphagia for liquids and solids, and abnormalities involving her fingers most likely has CREST syndrome, which is a variant of progressive systemic sclerosis. The anti-centromere antibody would be the test of choice if the serum antinuclear antibody test was positive. The CREST syndrome is characterized by (1) **c**alcinosis, or dystrophic calcification at the tips of the finger, (2) **R**aynaud phenomenon, with color changes in the fingers, (3) **e**sophageal motility problems, involving a relaxed lower esophageal sphincter and lack of peristalsis in the esophagus, (4) **s**clerodactyly, which refers to long tapered fingers, and (5) **t**elangiectasia, which are dilated blood vessels under the skin surface. Anti–SS-A antibody is positive in systemic lupus erythematosus and in Sjögren syndrome.

The erythrocyte sedimentation rate is increased in any inflammatory condition, so it is too non-specific to be of any value in this instance. Anti–double-stranded

DNA antibody is specific for systemic lupus erythematosus with renal involvement, and usually produces a rim pattern on a serum antinuclear antibody test. Anti-Smith antibody is 100% specific for only systemic lupus erythematosus.

13-15. The answers are: 13-C, 14-D, 15-D.
(Anatomy)
The listed cranial foramen most closely associated with the mass is the jugular foramen. It is just anterior and medial to the attachment of the sternocleidomastoid muscle. The other listed foramina are further anterior and/or medial to the jugular foramen. The three cranial nerves exiting the posterior cranial fossa through the jugular foramen are the glossopharyngeal (IX), vagus (X), and accessory (XI) nerves. The glossopharyngeal nerve supplies the posterior one-third of the tongue with general sensation as well as taste. This would explain the diminished sensation to the posterior aspect of the tongue. Further, branches from the vagus nerve (superior and inferior laryngeal) supply the muscles and mucosa of the larynx and insult to this nerve results in hoarseness. The accessory nerve supplies motor innervation to the trapezius and sternocleidomastoid muscles; when this nerve is compromised, the results are shoulder drop (trapezius) and difficulty turning the head to the side opposite the lesion (sternocleidomastoid). The internal jugular vein is a continuation of the sigmoid sinus that enters the internal jugular foramen and is the vascular structure that would be involved at the described location of the mass. The middle meningeal artery is found in the foramen spinosum, which is the only structure in this foramen. The common carotid artery is located in the carotid canal. The vertebral artery ascends within the transverse foramina of the cervical vertebrae, turns medially, and enters the foramen magnum. The location of the mass would not involve this artery. The external jugular vein is located superficial to the sternocleidomastoid muscle and ends inferiorly in the subclavian vein. This vessel is located too superficially to be involved by the mass. The structures found in the foramen ovale are the mandibular division of the trigeminal nerve (V1) and, when present, the accessory meningeal artery. The mandibular division of the trigeminal nerve innervates the muscles of mastication and is sensory to the lower teeth and oral mucosa; these are not involved in the described scenario. Foramen rotundum transmits the maxillary division of the trigeminal nerve (V2) and is primarily sensory to the upper teeth and skin in the area of the cheek.

16. The answer is A.   *(Pathology)*
Osteoarthritis and neuropathic arthropathy are the two noninflammatory joint diseases. In the synovial fluid (SF) in osteoarthritis, the neutrophil count is between 200 and 2000 cells/μL, the normal being < 200 cells/μL. The mucin clot is a measure of hyaluronic acid content in the SF. Hyaluronic acid is a glycosaminoglycan and is the joint lubricant secreted by the synovial cells. The mucin clot test is performed by adding a few drops of 5% acetic acid and noting a firm button of material at the bottom of the test tube, if hyaluronic acid is present. Inflammatory joint diseases have a poor mucin clot test. Rheumatoid arthritis, Reiter's syndrome, ankylosing spondylitis, and Lyme's disease are inflammatory joint diseases, where the neutrophil counts in SF may range from 2000 to 100,000 cells/μL.

17-19. The answers are: 17-A, 18-D, 19-E.
(Anatomy)
The mandibular division of the trigeminal nerve (V3) enters the infratemporal fossa through the foramen ovale. This division gives rise to the buccal, auriculotemporal, lingual, inferior alveolar, and meningeal nerves, which are sensory. A smaller motor division supplies innervation to the muscles of mastication, mylohyoid, anterior belly of the digastric, tensor tympani, and tensor palati muscles. Judging from the symptoms presented, foramen ovale and a portion of the mandibular division of the trigeminal nerve are involved. More specifically, the inferior alveolar nerve has been compromised. This nerve carries sensory information from the skin of the lower lip and chin and lower teeth. The portion of the inferior alveolar nerve that supplies the lower lip and chin is the mental nerve. Based on the foramen involved, the only vascular structure that is involved would be the accessory meningeal artery. It is typically a branch of the middle meningeal artery and enters the middle cranial fossa through the foramen ovale to supply the semilunar ganglion and adjacent dura. All of the arteries identified are branches of the maxillary artery and exit the infratemporal fossa through foramina other than the

foramen ovale. The buccal nerve supplies the oral mucosa and gums; the lingual nerve supplies the tongue with general sensation; the auriculotemporal nerve is sensory to the skin of the auricle and scalp as well as to the temporal mandibular joint; and the superior alveolar nerve is sensory to the upper teeth. None of these nerves seem to be compromised in terms of the patient's symptoms. The fact that the patient complained of difficulty in chewing suggests a problem with the motor component of the mandibular division. This aspect was not an option in any of the questions, however. The foramen rotundum transmits the maxillary division of the trigeminal nerve (V2) and is not found in the infratemporal fossa. The foramen spinosum transmits the middle meningeal artery and is not compromised in this case. The petrotympanic fissure transmits the chorda tympani that joins with the lingual nerve. Lack of taste was not a presenting symptom in this patient and would eliminate the petrotympanic fissure as a choice. The stylomastoid foramen contains the facial nerve; and since there was no complaint of facial weakness, this would not be the correct choice.

20. The answer is C. *(Pathology)*
Osteomalacia (soft bone) occurs when the osteoid in bone is not mineralized, whereas osteoporosis is an overall decrease in bone mass. The former disease is called rickets when it occurs in children. The most common cause of osteomalacia/rickets is vitamin D deficiency associated with dietary deficiency, malabsorption (e.g., celiac disease), or renal disease (most common overall cause). Since vitamin D reabsorbs both calcium and phosphorus in the gastrointestinal tract, a deficiency of the vitamin produces hypocalcemia and a normal to low phosphorus level. Since phosphorus is the driving force for pushing calcium into the osteoid, the osteoid is left unmineralized.

Osteoporosis is most commonly seen in postmenopausal women who are estrogen deficient. A drop in estrogen increases the release of interleukin-1 from macrophages, which activates osteoclasts to tear down more bone than is being replaced.
Comparison of the two diseases:

- Both osteomalacia and osteoporosis may be associated with renal disease. Osteoporosis occurs because the kidney is unable to excrete hydrogen ions and

a chronic metabolic acidosis develops. Bone is an excellent buffer and is broken down in the buffering process.
- Both diseases exhibit osteopenia on routine radiograph. However, Looser's lines are present only in osteomalacia/rickets. These linear areas in the metaphysis of bone resemble fracture lines (pseudofractures) and are due to blood vessels pushing aside the soft osteoid.
- Osteoporosis, not osteomalacia, has an overall decrease in bone mass.
- Both diseases predispose to fractures in adults.

21. The answer is E. *(Behavioral science)*
During alcohol withdrawal following excessive long-term use, tactile hallucinations such as formication (a feeling that bugs are crawling on the skin), tachycardia, hypertension, and agitation are seen. Tactile hallucinations characterize delirium tremens (DTs), but are unlikely to accompany heroin overdose, heroin withdrawal, or alcohol overdose. While cocaine overdose also is associated with formication ("cocaine bugs"), this patient has been hospitalized in isolation for three days, and there is no indication that he has used cocaine.

22. The answer is C. *(Pathology)*
The most common benign soft-tissue tumor and sarcoma in adults are a leiomyoma and a malignant fibrous histiocytoma, respectively. The most common location for a leiomyoma, which is derived from smooth muscle, is the uterus. In the gastrointestinal tract, it is most commonly located in the stomach, where it may bleed. The malignant fibrous histiocytoma is a soft-tissue malignancy that has foci of histiocytic differentiation. In addition to being the most adult sarcoma, it is also the most common soft-tissue sarcoma encountered after radiation therapy or in surgical scars. It primarily affects older adults, usually men (70%), and has a predilection for the limbs and retroperitoneum. The prognosis depends on the grade of the sarcoma. The majority of soft-tissue tumors arise "de novo." Soft-tissue tumors are classified according to the adult tissue they resemble. Regarding the other soft-tissue tumors:

- A lipoma is a common benign tumor that is present in subcutaneous tissue, most commonly located around the trunk and neck. It has very little clinical significance and does not progress into liposarcoma. Generalized lipomatosis (Dercum's disease) is characterized by the presence of multiple lipomas in subcutaneous tissue which, on rare occasions, may transform into sarcoma. Liposarcomas primarily occur in men (70%), who are usually over 50 years of age. They are the second most common adult sarcoma. The retroperitoneum and thigh (40%) are the favored locations. The myxoid type is the most common variant. The low-grade cancers are slow to metastasize (75% 5-year survival rate), whereas high-grade cancers are more aggressive (20% 5-year survival rate).

- A leiomyosarcoma differs from a benign leiomyoma predominantly in size, the presence of increased mitotic activity with atypical mitotic spindles, and the presence of necrosis. It most commonly arises from the wall of blood vessels, usually located in the limbs. It is the most common sarcoma of the uterus. The majority of leiomyosarcomas eventually metastasize.
- A rhabdomyoma is a benign tumor of skeletal or cardiac muscle. It is the second most common benign tumor in the heart (cardiac myxoma is the most common). When located in the heart, the tumor is usually associated with tuberous sclerosis, which is an autosomal dominant disease with mental retardation, angiomyolipomas in the kidneys, adnexal tumors, and rhabdomyomas in the heart. Embryonal rhabdomyosarcomas are the most common sarcoma in children, where they are located in the vagina and the genitourinary tract of males. They present as grape-like masses, thus the term botryoid embryonal rhabdomyosarcoma. Alveolar rhabdomyosarcoma occurs between 10 and 25 years of age. It is the most common type of rhabdomyosarcoma, favors the upper and lower extremities, and has the worst prognosis. Pleomorphic rhabdomyosarcomas are the least common form of rhabdomyosarcoma, but have the best prognosis.
- A dermatofibroma is a benign tumor of the dermis that is most commonly located on the lower extremity. It has a nodular, pigmented appearance and is composed of benign histiocytes.
- A synovial sarcoma is a malignant sarcoma arising from synovial epithelial cells. It is commonly located around a joint rather than in a joint. On histologic sections, the sarcoma has a biphasic pattern with a sarcomatous stroma (one pattern) and has gland-like spaces (second pattern) mimicking a synovial membrane as the other pattern. The 5-year survival rate is approximately 50%.

23. The answer is D.   *(Anatomy)*
A left homonomous hemianopia represents a visual field deficit found in both eyes. It is characterized by inability to see in the left halves of the visual fields of both eyes. It should be noted that the visual system follows the same rules as other sensory systems in that afferent information from the left environment is ultimately represented on the right side of the cerebral cortex when brought to consciousness. The partial decussation of the human visual pathway maintains this rule. Therefore, the right optic tract contains all axons carrying information pertaining to the left visual fields and, if lesioned, the right optic tract would produce blindness in the left halves of the visual fields. Note that lesions after the optic chiasm will always be homonymous and affect the same halves of visual fields and opposite to the side of the lesion.

A lesion of the left retina would produce blindness associated with one eye. Depending on the location in the retina, this blindness would be total or partially related to visual fields. A right optic nerve lesion would produce a deficit related to one eye. Again, the extent of the lesion would determine whether blindness would be complete or partially related to vision in that eye. A left optic tract lesion would produce findings associated with right halves of the visual fields, producing a right homonomous hemianopia. A lesion in the occipital cortex would produce right visual field deficits. Because of the large surface representation of the visual fields at the cortex, the deficit is usually partial. Occipital cortex lesions are sometimes only related to peripheral or macular visual field deficits.

24. The answer is A.   *(Pathology)*
The inflammatory skin reaction associated with exposure to the resin of poison ivy is most closely related in pathogenesis to a contact dermatitis to nickel. Both reactions are examples of cellular immunity, which is a type IV hypersensitivity reaction. Contact dermatitis is a common inflammatory disorder of skin that is associated with exposure to various antigens and irritating substances. Four types have been described: (1)

allergic contact dermatitis, (2) irritant contact dermatitis, (3) contact photodermatitis, and (4) contact urticaria. The allergic is a cell-mediated reaction. Three conditions must be present for this reaction to occur, that is, (1) a genetic predisposition, (2) absorption of sufficient antigen through the skin surface, and (3) a competent immune system. Antigenic substances of low molecular weight penetrate the skin, are phagocytized by Langerhans' cells, and are then transported to regional lymph nodes where they are presented to T lymphocytes. The T lymphocytes release cytokines that are responsible for the inflammatory response in the tissue. Antigenic substances include (1) rhus, which is found in poison ivy and poison oak, (2) nickel (earrings), (3) potassium dichromate (household cleaners, leather, cement), (4) formaldehyde (cosmetics, fabrics), (5) ethylenediamine (dyes, medications), (6) mercaptobenzothiazole (rubber products), and (7) paraphenylenediamine (hair dyes, chemicals in photography). The patch test is an excellent way to confirm contact dermatitis caused by the preceding antigens. The material in question is placed on a patch and applied to the skin to see whether a reaction occurs.

Irritant contact dermatitis is not a cell-mediated immune response. It is the most common type of contact dermatitis, but is a local toxic effect of a chemical on the skin, like detergents present in soaps, shampoos, and household cleaners.

Contact photodermatitis is similar to allergic contact dermatitis except that the reaction depends on ultraviolet light. Drugs that are photosensitizing include tetracycline, sulfonamides, and thiazides.

Contact urticaria is a wheal-and-flare reaction that may be secondary to a type I hypersensitivity (IgE-mediated) reaction or a nonimmunologic reaction. The clinical presentation of contact dermatitis, regardless of the mechanism, ranges from localized areas of erythema with vesicle formation to erythematous plaques of thickened skin in chronic disease.

Regarding the other choices, only atopic dermatitis may have been confused with the mechanism of poison ivy. Atopic dermatitis occurs in patients who have an allergic history, so it is an IgE-mediated type I hypersensitivity reaction. The onset occurs in the first year of life in 60% of patients. There is usually a family history of an atopic disease, such as asthma or hay fever. It usually begins on the cheeks in neonates

and then moves to the flexor creases as the child gets older. These patients have a lower itch threshold than normal, thus the phrase, it is the "itch that rashes."

Psoriasis, pemphigus, and porphyria are totally unrelated to the pathogenesis of the contact dermatitis associated with poison ivy.

25. The answer is B. *(Behavioral science)*
The most likely diagnosis for this patient is bipolar disorder. This patient is showing the manic phase of bipolar disorder and has the delusion (false belief) that she will soon star in a movie. Excessive credit-card spending is another symptom of mania. That this woman is married and has a job indicate that she has been relatively normal up to this point; so she probably does not have schizophrenia. Delusions are not seen in dysthymic disorder, cylcothymic disorder, or hypomania.

26. The answer is B. *(Pathology)*
A cerebral abscess and a cerebral infarct are similar in that both are examples of liquefactive necrosis. In the brain, the structural support is mainly supplied by processes extending off of astrocytes. In addition, the neuroglial cells have a great number of lysosomes. When infarction occurs (most commonly the result of atherosclerosis), the brain tissue undergoes liquefaction when the lysosomes release enzymes that autodigest the tissue. The supportive framework is not sufficient to produce the classic coagulation necrosis, which is most often associated with infarction. In this type of necrosis, vague outlines of the tissue are still recognized, because lactic acid denatures the proteins, including the enzymes.

Cerebral infarcts are most commonly caused by thrombosis overlying an atherosclerotic plaque in the internal carotid artery near the bifurcation in the upper neck. Cerebral abscesses are most commonly the result of a primary lesion located in the sinuses or mastoid area that extends out into the brain tissue.

Cerebral infarcts are most commonly associated with atherosclerosis, whereas cerebral abscesses are associated with infectious disease.

Neither of the disorders most often result from embolization from another primary site.

Only a cerebral abscess may have collagen formation as part of the healing process, and this comes from the blood vessels. Infarcts are not associated with collagen, but the "scar" is caused by gliosis, or the proliferation of astrocytes with filling in of the lesion by their cytoplasmic extensions.

27. The answer is B.   *(Anatomy)*
The anterior and posterior spinal arteries are augmented in their longitudinal distribution to the spinal cord by radicular branches from the descending aorta. This segmental distribution may be deficient at certain sites along the spinal cord. One of these sites is between spinal cord segments T1 and T3. Spinal cord lesions localized at this level may be caused by ischemia. The segment from L5 to S1 is the next most likely site for ischemic damage to occur. C5–C6, T7–T9, and S4–Coccygeal 1 are less likely to be affected by ischemia.

28. The answer is B.   *(Pathology)*
This patient most likely has Herpes simplex (HSV) type I encephalitis. The clinical presentation for encephalitis is associated with alterations in mental status and either diffuse or focal neurologic signs. The gold standard for the diagnosis of HSV encephalitis is a brain biopsy and isolation of the virus from the tissue. Histologic sections reveal eosinophilic intranuclear inclusion bodies in neurons and glial cells. The presence of eosinophilic (acidophilic) inclusions defines a Cowdry type A inclusion. A Cowdry type B inclusion is basophilic (e.g., cytomegalovirus, adenovirus). Acyclovir is the treatment of choice. Neurologic sequelae are common. The Herpes type II virus (genitalis) is most commonly associated with meningitis rather than encephalitis; however, in patients with AIDS, it may produce a hemorrhagic necrotizing encephalitis, similar to HSV-1.

None of the other viruses listed localizes to the temporal lobe. The rabies and rubeola virus have Cowdry type A inclusions, whereas adenovirus and cytomegalovirus both have basophilic intranuclear inclusions (Cowdry type B).

29-30. The answers are: 29-E, 30-A.   *(Anatomy)*
A secondary ossification center has not begun in the epiphysis. The primary ossification center is well established in the shaft, as the bone collar is quite thick. Secondary ossification usually begins after birth and continues into early adulthood. The first stage is an invasion of the epiphyseal area by blood vessels. No blood vessels are apparent in the epiphysis of this developing bone.

Bone is present in the diaphysis and bone spicules are present in the metaphysis (cone-shaped region between epiphysis and diaphysis).

The periosteum is the connective tissue surrounding the diaphyseal bone.

Hyaline cartilage is present in the epiphysis. The characteristic isogenous groups of chondrocytes are apparent even at this low magnification. The epiphyseal plate has also formed, with the hypertrophied chondrocytes evident. Hyaline cartilage remains in the epiphyseal plate and articular cartilage. The epiphyseal plate or cartilage disappears at about 18 to 20 years, leaving only the articular cartilage as a hyaline cartilage. Development of a bone from a cartilage model is called endochondral ossification.

Calcified cartilage is present in the epiphyseal plate. Bone is being laid down on calcified cartilage spicules.

The osteocytes are distributed throughout the diaphyseal bone. They reside in lacunae within the bone matrix. Canaliculi that link processes of the osteocytes are not visible at this low magnification. The bone and the cartilage look different from one another, with cells spaced throughout instead of arranged in isogenous groups.

Osteoblasts are seen along the surface of the diaphyseal bone on both the endosteal (marrow) and periosteal surface.

Chondrocytes are present in the cartilage of the epiphysis.

Chondroblasts are cells that differentiate from the inner layer of the perichondrium.

Osteoprogenitor cells are found in the periosteum and give rise to osteoblasts and perhaps osteoblasts.

31. The answer is A.   *(Pathology)*
Tennis elbow refers to pain in the area where the extensor muscle tendons insert near the lateral epicondyle (mnemonic: LET). Pain is reproduced by extending the wrist against resistance with the elbow extended. Golfer's elbow is characterized by pain that is located where the flexors insert near the medial epicondyle (mnemonic: GEM).

Idiopathic scoliosis is most commonly seen in adolescent girls from 10 to 16 years old. Forward bending causes paraspinous prominence caused by a hump in the ribs. Scoliosis is a lateral displacement of vertebra, while kyphosis refers to a forward displacement (hump back). Complications include chest restriction with the potential for respiratory acidosis.

When the knee joint is forced into a valgus position (sideways displacement) with the foot firmly anchored, a number of abnormalities may occur in the joint, such as rupture of the medial collateral ligament or a tear of the medial meniscus. During a McMurray test, where the leg is externally rotated as the knee is extended from the supine position, if a click is felt along the posteromedial margin of the joint, then the medial meniscus is torn; a click on the posterolateral margin indicates a torn lateral meniscus. Rupture of the anterior cruciate is indicated by a positive anterior draw sign: While the foot is planted firmly, the knee moves forward when the lower leg is moved forward. The posterior draw test is performed to diagnose a tear of the posterior cruciate ligament: In this case the leg will move posteriorly as the lower leg is compressed anteriorly.

Compartment syndrome (compartment hypertension) refers to a buildup of pressure in closed muscle compartments resulting in decrease perfusion—venous flow is affected first, followed by arterial flow—and subsequent potential for permanent ischemic contractures of the muscle. The tibial and forearm muscle compartments are prone to this injury. Supracondylar fractures of the humerus in children creates a predisposition toward entrapment of the brachial artery and median nerve. Loss of the brachial artery blood supply due to compartment syndrome can result in the development of Volkmann ischemic contracture of the forearm muscles. Intracompartmental pressure can be measured and, if elevated, must be treated by incision to relieve the pressure.

32-36. The answers are: 32-E, 33-B, 34-C, 35-D, 36-A. *(Physiology)*
The endogenous opioids have been implicated in the placebo response, which may be blocked by prior treatment with naloxone, an opiate receptor blocker. Degeneration of cholinergic neurons has been implicated in Alzheimer disease. A hyperdopaminergic state has been implicated in schizophrenia. Pheochromocytoma, an adrenal tumor, is associated with increased production of adrenal norepinephrine. Decreased activity of γ-aminobutyric acid (GABA) is implicated in the development of epilepsy.

37-41. The answers are: 37-D, 38-B, 39-C, 40-E, 41-A. *(Pharmacology)*
Tacrine is the only drug that is currently approved for Alzheimer disease, which is characterized by loss of short- and long-term memory and other cognitive deficits. Tacrine is a central inhibitor of cholinesterase, thereby increasing acetylcholine at central synapses, including those in the hippocampus, which are believed to be involved in Alzheimer disease. Parkinson disease, which is characterized by resting tremor, rigidity, and akinesia, can be treated with drugs that activate dopamine receptors, for example, pergolide, bromocryptine, and levodopa—the precursor to dopamine. Panic attacks and other forms of severe anxiety may respond to a benzodiazepine such as alprazolam. Risperidone is a new antipsychotic agent that blocks dopamine and serotonin receptors. It is believed to be more effective against negative schizophrenic symptoms than are other traditional antipsychotic agents. Partial seizures can be treated with traditional drugs such as carbamazepine, as well as several new agents, including gabapentin, lamotrigine, and vigabatrin. Carbamazepine is believed to block sodium channel–mediated nerve depolarization and conduction.

42-46. The answers are: 42-A, 43-E, 44-B, 45-D, 46-C. *(Behavioral science)*
Alprazolam is a benzodiazepine with antidepressant activity. Amoxapine should be avoided in suicidal patients because it is the most dangerous in overdose. Fluoxetine is a useful agent for overweight patients because, in contrast to the heterocyclic agents, it is associated with weight loss. Use of trazodone has been associated with priapism, a permanent state of erection, which is often a surgical emergency. Desipramine is useful for the elderly because it is nonsedating.

47-50. The answers are: 47-C, 48-E, 49-A, 50-B. *(Pharmacology)*
Acetaminophen is probably the safest antipyretic for use in a young child with a viral disease. Acetamino-

phen is less likely to cause gastric distress than other antipyretics, and an association between Reye's syndrome and the administration of aspirin in children with viral diseases has caused concern. Phenylbutazone is no longer widely used because of its association with agranulocytosis and aplastic anemia as well as a number of other serious adverse effects.

Naproxen and ibuprofen are usually preferred for the management of dysmenorrhea, which results in part from excessive prostaglandin production in the uterus.

Indomethacin is a potent prostaglandin synthesis inhibitor that is specifically indicated for the treatment of patent ductus arteriosus. In premature infants, the ductus is maintained by prostaglandins, and inhibition of their synthesis leads to closure. Treatment with indomethacin can obviate the need for surgery.

Ketorolac is a novel agent with potent analgesic activity that can be administered parenterally or orally. An ophthalmic preparation is also available for treating ocular inflammation. Ketorolac is limited to the short-term management of postoperative pain.

Test 1

QUESTIONS

DIRECTIONS:

Each of the numbered items or incomplete statements in this section is followed by answers or by completions of the statement. Select the ONE lettered answer or completion that is BEST in each case.

1. Which type of cell is derived from the neural crest?

(A) Oligodendrocytes
(B) Dura mater cells
(C) Postganglionic neurons
(D) Astrocytes
(E) Microglial cells

2. A 32-year-old woman with a history of scanning speech, intention tremor, and nystagmus presents with a sudden loss of vision in her left eye. Physical examination finds pain on movement of the eyes, a poor pupillary light reflex, a swollen optic disc, and flame hemorrhages around the disc margin. The intraocular pressure is normal. Her visual loss is most closely associated with

(A) a demyelinating disease
(B) atherosclerotic carotid artery disease
(C) left heart disease with embolization
(D) a hypercoagulable state
(E) an increase in intracranial pressure

3. A 9-month-old child develops a high fever associated with febrile convulsions. The fever ends abruptly after 3 days and is followed by a maculopapular rash. What is the most likely diagnosis?

(A) Rubella
(B) Rubeola
(C) Roseola
(D) Fifth disease
(E) Varicella

4. A 68-year-old man has the following Weber and Rinne test results:

Test	Left Ear	Right Ear
Weber lateralizes to	Yes	No
Rinne	Bone conduction > air conduction	Air conduction > bone conduction

The patient's clinical findings are most consistent with

(A) presbycusis involving the right ear
(B) presbycusis involving the left ear
(C) otosclerosis involving the right ear
(D) otosclerosis involving the left ear
(E) a normal examination

5. Where would a lesion resulting in a fluent (sensory) Wernicke aphasia most likely be found?

(A) Temporal lobe
(B) Parietal lobe
(C) Frontal lobe
(D) Occipital lobe
(E) Limbic lobe

6. A 31-year-old barber complains of numbness and paresthesias on the palmar aspect of his right thumb, second and third fingers, and the radial side of the fourth finger. The dorsal tips of these fingers exhibit the same findings. Thenar atrophy is noted as well as weakness when apposing his thumb to his fifth digit. Tapping over the transverse carpal ligament and forced flexion of the wrists in a downward direction reproduces the symptoms. These findings are most closely related to the compression of the

(A) radial nerve
(B) musculocutaneous nerve
(C) ulnar nerve
(D) axillary nerve
(E) median nerve

7. A pig farmer in the Midwest complains of generalized aches and pains. The peripheral blood exhibits an increased eosinophil count (35%). Which of the following pathogens is most likely responsible for this patient's disease?

(A) *Strongyloides stercoralis*
(B) *Ascaris lumbricoides*
(C) *Trichinella spiralis*
(D) *Trichuris trichiura*
(E) *Ancylostoma duodenale*

8. Cataracts secondary to an increase in sorbitol production in the lens are most commonly associated with

(A) congenital rubella
(B) myotonic dystrophy
(C) old age
(D) diabetes mellitus
(E) corticosteroid eye drops

9. A patient presents with gait unsteadiness. When standing with his feet together he is slightly unsteady. When he closes his eyes he becomes markedly unsteady and must be held in order to avoid falling. Where is the disease located?

(A) Dorsal columns
(B) Lateral spinothalamic tract
(C) Anterior horn cells
(D) Lateral corticospinal tract
(E) Anterior white commissure

10. An afebrile 15-year-old boy complains of itchy eyes, nasal congestion, and increased lacrimation. Physical examination reveals blue-white, boggy nasal mucosa, bilateral conjunctival redness with no exudate, and puffiness and discoloration of the skin beneath both eyes. It can be expected that

(A) another member in his family recently had a cold
(B) this only occurs at certain times of the year
(C) there is a strong family history for autoimmune disease
(D) a number of students in his school have "pink eye"
(E) these findings are often followed by a pounding headache that lasts for 30 minutes and then subsides

11. Which of the following tests is most useful in determining whether penicillin or cephalosporins will be effective in killing *Staphylococcus aureus, Haemophilus influenzae,* or *Neisseria gonorrhoeae?*

(A) Schlichter test
(B) Quellung test
(C) Gram stain
(D) Kirby-Bauer
(E) Beta lactamase

12. Which of the following is more commonly associated with diabetic rather than hypertensive retinopathy?

(A) Progressive narrowing of the arterioles
(B) Arteriovenous nicking
(C) Papilledema
(D) Microaneurysms
(E) Proliferative retinopathy

13. Sensory information concerning temperature and sharp pain is relayed to the somatosensory cortex via neurons in the

(A) ventrobasal complex, or ventroposterolateral (VPL) and ventroposteromedial (VPM) nuclei
(B) anterior nuclei
(C) geniculate nuclei
(D) ventroanterior (VA) and ventrolateral (VL) nuclei
(E) hypothalamic nuclei

14. An afebrile 35-year-old woman with mitral stenosis and an irregularly irregular pulse has a sudden onset of weakness and anesthesia in her right lower face and right arm. She cannot speak and does not appear to understand the spoken word. No bruits are noted in the carotid arteries. An echocardiogram reveals dilatation of the left atrium but no visible clots. No vegetations are noted on the mitral valve. A computerized tomography scan of the patient's skull 4 hours after the episode is reported as normal. Which of the following best describes the pathogenesis of her clinical condition?

(A) Subarachnoid hemorrhage from a ruptured berry aneurysm
(B) Embolus to the left middle cerebral artery
(C) An intracerebral bleed involving the internal capsule
(D) An atherosclerotic stroke involving the left middle cerebral artery
(E) Embolus to the right middle cerebral artery

15. Which of the following diseases has a pathogenesis that is different from the other diseases listed?

(A) Rheumatic fever
(B) Scarlet fever
(C) Toxic shock syndrome
(D) Diphtheria
(E) Cholera

16. A 32-year-old alcoholic has a 3-month history of progressive blurriness of vision in both eyes. Approximately 6 months ago, he states that he felt very sick after drinking some wine given to him by a person he met outside a bar. He states that it made him feel sick to his stomach and caused him to vomit. Since that time, he has had progressive problems with his vision. Retinal examination reveals pale optic discs bilaterally and a reduced number of disc vessels. This patient's visual problem most closely relates to

(A) toxicity related to ethyl alcohol
(B) a demyelinating disease
(C) an increase in intraocular pressure
(D) toxicity related to methyl alcohol
(E) a vitamin deficiency

17. The homunculus arrangement of the precentral and postcentral gyri locates the area involved in motor and sensory function of the lower extremity closest to the

(A) collateral fissure
(B) calcarine fissure
(C) lateral fissure
(D) longitudinal fissure
(E) primary fissure

18. A 45-year-old woman with a complaint of intermittent dizziness and an unsteady gait now presents with the following abnormality on neurologic examination. When the patient looks to the left, the left eye abducts and exhibits a horizontal jerk nystagmus, but the right eye remains stationary. When she looks to the right, the right eye abducts and exhibits horizontal jerk nystagmus, but the left eye remains stationary. However, the patient is able to converge (adduct) both eyes together. There is no motor weakness in the upper or lower face. The clinical findings in this patient most closely relate to

(A) hypertension
(B) ischemic cerebral disease
(C) a demyelinating disease
(D) a cerebellar tumor
(E) a brain stem glioma

19. A 25-year-old woman presents with fever, painful postauricular, posterior cervical, and postoccipital lymphadenopathy and polyarthritis. This is followed in 24 hours by a confluent maculopapular rash that began on her face and spread over her trunk. She most likely has

(A) rubella
(B) juvenile rheumatoid arthritis
(C) rubeola
(D) infectious mononucleosis
(E) Lyme disease

20. A 2-year-old boy presents with poor vision in the right eye first noticed by his mother when watching him play with his toys. Physical examination shows a white eye reflex in the right eye, strabismus, and pain and tenderness in the eye on gentle compression. An intraocular mass is present on retinal examination. The pathogenesis of this lesion most closely relates to

(A) an intrauterine infection
(B) trauma
(C) inactivation of a suppressor gene
(D) blood in the anterior chamber
(E) cavernous sinus thrombosis

21. A 50-year-old woman presents after 12 months of progressive weakness primarily associated with distal muscles of the upper limb. Examination shows a significant sensory loss related to dermatomes C8 and T_1, and the patient confirms progressive tingling and aching (paresthesia) in this area. Radiographic studies do not show any compression or mass lesions that can account for this presentation. The conclusion is vascular deficiency. Which vessel is most likely to be affected?

(A) Anterior spinal artery
(B) Left posterior spinal artery
(C) Posterior inferior cerebellar artery
(D) Vertebral arteries
(E) Internal carotid arteries

22. A 5-year-old boy does not appear to be listening in class and prefers to stay by himself during recess. A Weber test lateralizes to his right ear. The Rinne test exhibits bone conduction greater than air conduction on the right and air conduction longer than bone conduction on the left. Additional history from the child's mother would reveal that

(A) the child had previous trauma to the head
(B) the mother had rubella during her first trimester of pregnancy
(C) the mother handled cat litter when she was pregnant
(D) the child has a history of repeated ear infections
(E) the mother had gestational diabetes during her pregnancy

23. Which disease has a pathogenesis other than traumatic implantation?

(A) Maduromycosis
(B) Chromoblastomycosis
(C) Herpetic whitlow
(D) Sporotrichosis
(E) Onychomycosis

24. A previously healthy 32-year-old afebrile woman presents with a recent onset of repeated episodes of spinning dizziness. She states that she has a fluctuating loss of hearing in her right ear associated with a low-pitched roaring and sense of fullness behind the ear drum. The attacks are associated with nausea and vomiting. The Weber test lateralizes to her left ear, and air conduction is longer than bone conduction in both ears. The patient most likely has

(A) a demyelinating disease
(B) a glomus jugulare tumor
(C) a brain stem glioma
(D) a cerebellar tumor
(E) an increase in endolymph in the inner ear

25. A 60-year-old man presents with sudden onset of speech arrest and right-sided weakness. Examination shows 0/5 strength in the right arm, 3/5 strength in the right leg. Decreased right-sided sensation is also present. This combination most likely represents

(A) left anterior cerebral artery infarction
(B) left middle cerebral artery infarction
(C) right middle cerebral artery infarction
(D) left lacunar infarction of anterior choroidal artery
(E) subarachnoid hemorrhage of right posterior cerebral artery

26. A patient has been developing progressive, bilateral concentric contraction of the visual fields and loss of central vision. These findings may be associated with

(A) Friedrich ataxia
(B) Werdnig-Hoffmann disease
(C) multiple sclerosis
(D) tabes dorsalis
(E) retrolental fibroplasia

27. Tenosynovitis in a veterinarian would most likely be due to

(A) *Pseudomonas aeruginosa*
(B) *Afipia felis*
(C) *Pasteurella multocida*
(D) *Staphylococcus aureus*
(E) *Pseudomonas mallei*

28. Tuberous sclerosis differs from neurofibromatosis in which of the following ways? Tuberous sclerosis

(A) includes skin abnormalities
(B) is an autosomal dominant inheritance
(C) involves the central nervous system
(D) is associated with hamartomas
(E) is associated with mental retardation

29. A right-leg paralysis characterized as spastic may indicate damage to

(A) the medial aspect of the left precentral gyrus
(B) the lateral aspect of the left precentral gyrus
(C) the lateral aspect of the right precentral gyrus
(D) the anterior horn cell
(E) the right fasciculus gracilis

30. Cognitive abnormalities, cerebellar atrophy, and distal sensorimotor peripheral neuropathy all may be associated with

(A) vitamin B_{12} deficiency
(B) multiple sclerosis
(C) Alzheimer's disease
(D) alcoholism
(E) diabetes mellitus

31. Which of the following organisms would most likely be associated with an HLA-B27–positive reactive arthritis?

(A) *Yersinia enterocolitica*
(B) *Staphylococcus aureus*
(C) *Pseudomonas aeruginosa*
(D) *Haemophilus influenzae*
(E) *Escherichia coli*

32. Chronic hepatitis associated with degeneration of the lenticular nucleus best characterizes a disease associated with

(A) a defect in iron metabolism
(B) a defect in copper metabolism
(C) thiamine deficiency
(D) excess alcohol intake
(E) vitamin B_{12} deficiency

33. Which change occurs in the patellar (knee-jerk) reflex after destruction of α-motor neurons in the lumbar spinal cord?

(A) The γ-motor neuron maintains the reflex unchanged
(B) The extrafusal muscle cells maintain the reflex unchanged
(C) The Ia afferent fibers maintain the reflex unchanged
(D) There is no reflex response
(E) Descending motor systems sprout to innervate other neurons

34. The photograph shows synovial fluid removed from a painful, hot, swollen right knee of a 35-year-old alcoholic. When the slow axis of the compensator is oriented parallel to the long axis of the crystal in the slide, the crystal turns yellow. The mechanism most likely responsible for precipitating this patient's disease is

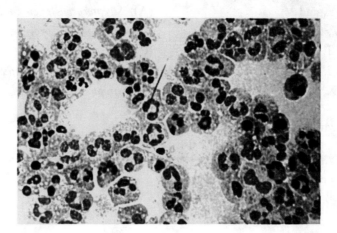

(A) decreased excretion of uric acid in the kidney

(B) defective urea metabolism in the liver

(C) alcohol enhanced synthesis of 5-phosphoribosyl-1-pyrophosphate (PPRP) in purine metabolism

(D) alcohol inhibited hypoxanthine-guanine phosphoribosyltransferase (HGPRT) in purine metabolism

(E) a toxic effect of alcohol on synovial tissue

35. Which of the following would more likely occur in a fish handler than in a veterinarian who specializes in large animals?

(A) Brucellosis

(B) Leptospirosis

(C) Erysipeloid

(D) Q fever

(E) Listeriosis

36. Which of the following autoantibody combinations is associated with disease in the same organ/tissue?

(A) Anti–smooth muscle antibody and antimitochondrial antibody

(B) Antmicrosomal antibody and antineutrophil cytoplasmic antibody

(C) Anticentromere antibody and antigliadin antibody

(D) Anti–parietal cell antibody and antihistone antibody

(E) Antiepithelial antibody and anti–islet cell antibody

37. Which set of cranial nerves is closely related anatomically to the corticospinal tract as it passes longitudinally through the brain stem?

(A) Cranial nerves III, IV, and V
(B) Cranial nerves III, V, and VII
(C) Cranial nerves III, VI, and VIII
(D) Cranial nerves III, VI, and XII
(E) Cranial nerves III, IX, and X

38. A 23-year-old man with a week-long history of chlamydial urethritis now presents with bilateral conjunctivitis, painful swelling of his right knee and ankle, and painless ulcers on his penis. Which of the following tests would most likely be positive or abnormal in this patient?

(A) Rheumatoid factor
(B) Serum antinuclear antibody
(C) Serum uric acid
(D) Gram stain of the penile ulcers
(E) HLA-B27 haplotype

39. A patient with colorectal cancer develops septicemia complicated by endocarditis. The blood culture most likely will show

(A) *Streptococcus pneumoniae*
(B) *Streptococcus pyogenes*
(C) *Streptococcus bovis*
(D) *Streptococcus agalactiae*
(E) *Streptococcus viridans*

40. The figure represents non-polarized (A) and polarized (B) synovial fluid from the left knee of a 65-year-old man who complains of recurrent pain. The knee is warm, crepitant on movement, and contains an effusion, and a radiograph shows calcifications in the articular cartilage. Which of the following best describes this patient's clinical disorder?

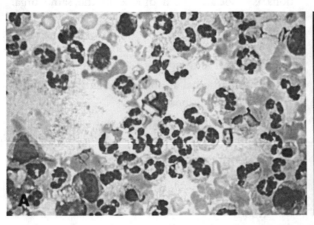 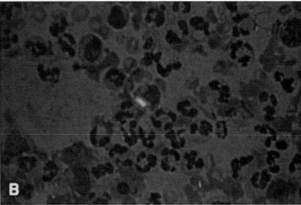

(A) Calcium pyrophosphate dihydrate crystal deposition arthropathy
(B) Osteoarthritis with superimposed chronic gouty arthritis
(C) Chondrocalcinosis associated with gout
(D) Osteoarthritis with a previous joint injection with corticosteroids
(E) Chondrocalcinosis with a previous joint injection with corticosteroids

41. If the electrogenic pump (3 Na⁺:2 K⁺) in a resting nerve cell is changed to a nonelectrogenic pump (1 Na⁺:1 K⁺)

(A) the membrane potential (MP) will hyperpolarize to a value at which the ratio of sodium influx to potassium efflux is 3:2
(B) the MP depolarizes to a value at which the ratio of sodium influx to potassium efflux is 3:2
(C) the MP hyperpolarizes to a value at which the ratio of sodium influx to potassium efflux is 1:1
(D) the MP depolarizes to a value at which the ratio of sodium influx to potassium efflux is 1:1
(E) the MP will not change but the ratio of sodium influx to potassium efflux is 1:1

42. Which of the following joint disease/radiograph finding relationships is correct?

(A) Osteoarthritis/erosions with overhanging margins
(B) Rheumatoid arthritis/ankylosis
(C) Gout/osteophytes
(D) Psoriatic arthritis/"bamboo" spine
(E) Ankylosing spondylitis/"pencil-in-cup" deformity

43. In which of the following diseases is *Escherichia coli* more likely to be the primary pathogen than *Pseudomonas aeruginosa*?

(A) Third-degree burns
(B) Pneumonia in cystic fibrosis
(C) Infections with nail punctures through rubber footwear
(D) Malignant otitis externa
(E) Spontaneous peritonitis in alcoholics

44. Which of the following features is seen more commonly in osteoarthritis than in rheumatoid arthritis?

(A) Pannus formation
(B) Involvement of the metacarpophalangeal joint
(C) Involvement of weight-bearing joints
(D) An IgM antibody against IgG
(E) An HLA-DR4 haplotype

45. In the spinal cord axon, collaterals from sensory neurons for touch are believed to synapse on the axon terminal of sensory neurons for pain. Neurons that synapse on the axon terminal of a second neuron, i.e., axoaxonic synapses, are most likely to

(A) initiate on the postsynaptic neuron an action potential that is propagated in an anterograde direction (orthodromic conduction)
(B) initiate on the postsynaptic neuron an action potential that is propagated in a retrograde direction (antidromic conduction)
(C) initiate on the postsynaptic neuron an action potential that is propagated in both an anterograde and retrograde direction
(D) block the propagation of any action potential
(E) alter the quantity of neurotransmitter released by the postsynaptic neuron in response to an action potential on its axon

46. Which of the following is seen more commonly in rheumatoid arthritis than in ankylosing spondylitis?

(A) An HLA-B27 haplotype
(B) Sacroiliitis
(C) Increased incidence in men
(D) Aortic regurgitation
(E) Autoantibody against IgG

47. Which of the following diseases could potentially be transmitted at the same time as the pathogen responsible for Lyme disease?

(A) Colorado tick bite fever
(B) Babesiosis
(C) Relapsing fever
(D) Ehrlichiosis
(E) Rocky Mountain spotted fever

48. Patients with syringomyelia, diabetes mellitus, and tabes dorsalis have an increased incidence of

(A) osteoarthritis
(B) rheumatoid arthritis
(C) ankylosing spondylitis
(D) Reiter syndrome
(E) Charcot joint

49. Consider a typical resting cell with a membrane potential of -80 mV and an intracellular chloride concentration that is less than one tenth the concentration of chloride in the extracellular fluid. If chloride is in electrochemical equilibrium across the cell membrane, which change should cause a net influx of chloride ions into the cell?

(A) Opening additional chloride channels
(B) Decreasing the concentration of Cl⁻ outside the cell
(C) Increasing the concentration of Cl⁻ inside the cell
(D) A hyperpolarization of the cell membrane potential
(E) A depolarization of the cell membrane potential

50. A 45-year-old woman who is obese complains of bilateral hip pain when walking. Radiographs of both hips reveal narrowing of the joint space and spurs at the margins of the joints. Which of the following results would you expect laboratory tests to show?

(A) Positive rheumatoid factor
(B) Hyperuricemia
(C) Positive HLA-B27 haplotype
(D) Positive serum antinuclear antibody
(E) No laboratory test abnormalities

51. A normal number of eosinophils in the peripheral blood would most likely be associated with

(A) enterobiasis
(B) strongyloidiasis
(C) ascariasis (larval phase)
(D) cutaneous larva migrans
(E) hookworm disease

52. Nodular masses have developed in the periarticular tissue of the proximal and distal interphalangeal joints of the right hand of a 58-year-old man with a 10-year history of gout. Which of the following choices best describes the characteristics of these masses?

(A) Pathognomonic lesion of chronic gout
(B) Histologically similar to a rheumatoid nodule
(C) Contains weakly positive birefringent monosodium urate crystals
(D) Associated with fibrinoid necrosis
(E) Rarely associated with destructive joint disease

53. Poisoning with a "nerve gas" such as the organophosphate Sarin would most likely produce

(A) mydriasis
(B) rhinorrhea
(C) relaxation of the ciliary muscles
(D) bronchodilation
(E) diminished sweating in response to heating

54. A 22-year-old man presents with a 4-month history of morning stiffness in his lower back, which is relieved by exercise. He has diminished anterior flexion of the spine, loss of lumbar lordosis, and paravertebral muscle spasms in his lumbar region. Which of the following tests would most likely be positive or abnormal in this patient?

(A) Serum uric acid
(B) Rheumatoid factor
(C) Serum antinuclear antibody
(D) Radiograph of the sacroiliac joints
(E) Serum alkaline phosphatase

55. The triad of sinus bradycardia, absolute neutropenia, and hepatosplenomegaly is most likely associated with

(A) Chagas disease
(B) typhoid fever
(C) falciparum malaria
(D) AIDS
(E) amebiasis

56. Restrictive lung disease, pleural effusion, absolute neutropenia, and xerostomia would most likely be associated with

(A) sarcoidosis
(B) progressive systemic sclerosis
(C) rheumatoid arthritis
(D) systemic lupus erythematosus
(E) mixed connective tissue disease

57. The history and physical exam of a patient indicate a meningioma within the tentorium cerebelli. You visualize this tumor as residing

(A) between the right and left cerebral hemispheres
(B) within the operculum of the frontal lobe
(C) in the cisterna magna
(D) at the cerebellopontine angle
(E) between the occipital lobe and the cerebellum

58. A child with a constellation of findings including fever, disabling arthritis, rash, and blindness is MOST likely suffering from

(A) rheumatic fever
(B) Lyme disease
(C) juvenile rheumatoid arthritis
(D) Henoch-Schoenlein vasculitis
(E) dermatomyositis

59. Black individuals are protected from developing malaria due to *Plasmodium vivax* because of the

(A) presence of glucose 6-phosphate dehydrogenase deficiency
(B) presence of sickle cell disease
(C) presence of β-thalassemia
(D) absence of Duffy antigen on the surface of red blood cells
(E) absence of D antigen on the surface of red blood cells

60. Which of the following conditions is more likely to involve the epiphysis of a long bone than the vertebral column?

(A) Osteoblastoma
(B) Osteoporosis
(C) Metastatic breast cancer
(D) Pott disease
(E) Giant cell tumor of bone

61. Patients with Huntington disease may benefit from treatment with drugs that antagonize

(A) γ-aminobutryric acid (GABA)
(B) dopamine
(C) acetylcholine
(D) serotonin
(E) histamine

62. A patient with fever of unknown origin has a positive blood culture for coagulase-negative *Staphylococcus* that was drawn from the right arm and a negative culture drawn from the left arm. The patient most likely has

(A) infective endocarditis
(B) pneumonia
(C) osteomyelitis
(D) a prosthetic heart valve
(E) a contaminated blood sample

63. An aneurysm near the bifurcation of the internal carotid artery into the anterior and middle cerebral arteries produces deficits. With which of the following cranial nerves are they most likely to be associated?

(A) Oculomotor
(B) Trigeminal
(C) Trochlear
(D) Optic
(E) Olfactory

64. Which of the following is more likely to be a community-acquired infection rather than a nosocomial infection?

(A) *Staphylococcus aureus* septicemia
(B) *Pseudomonas aeruginosa* pneumonia
(C) *Mycoplasma pneumoniae* pneumonia
(D) *Candida albicans* septicemia
(E) *Escherichia coli* septicemia

65. Benzodiazepines that are metabolized only to inactive glucuronides include

(A) oxazepam
(B) lorazepam
(C) diazepam
(D) oxazepam and lorazepam
(E) lorazepam and diazepam

66. Which of the following infectious diseases most commonly has an admixture of both *Fusobacterium* and *Bacteroides* species, particularly in alcoholics?

(A) Septicemia
(B) Lung abscess
(C) Decubitus ulcer
(D) Peritonitis
(E) Trench mouth

67. A 64-year-old man is diagnosed with a permanent speech disorder described as Broca aphasia. This condition is due to loss of neurons in the left cerebral hemisphere as a result of a cerebrovascular accident that most likely involves the

(A) anterior cerebral artery
(B) middle cerebral artery
(C) lenticulostriate arteries
(D) posterior cerebral artery
(E) posterior communicating arteries

68. Which of the following bacteria is associated with food poisoning and myonecrosis?

(A) *Clostridium difficile*
(B) *Clostridium perfringens*
(C) *Clostridium botulinum*
(D) *Clostridium tetani*
(E) *Bacillus cereus*

69. Which function is shared by neurons in dorsal horn laminae I, II and the spinal nucleus and tract of the trigeminal nerve?

(A) Localization of unconscious proprioception
(B) Visceral sensory perception associated with stretch reception
(C) Relay and execution of deep-tendon extensor reflexes
(D) Reception of nociceptor (pain) afferents
(E) Perception of two-point discriminative touch

70. Which of the following is the single most common infectious cause of death in the world?

(A) AIDS
(B) Tuberculosis
(C) Influenza
(D) *Streptococcus pneumoniae* pneumonia
(E) Cholera

71. A 21-year-old man with a history of spina bifida has recently complained of severe headaches and sensations of pressure in his head, especially behind the eyes. Neurologic examination reveals bilateral deficiency in voluntary motor control of the appendages (particularly toe movement) and diminished sensory perception in all modalities. Magnetic resonance imaging (MRI) shows generalized enlargement of all ventricular components. Given this history and general findings, what do you suspect as the cause of these complaints?

(A) Occlusion of the cerebral aqueduct
(B) Tonsillar herniation
(C) Arteriovenous malformation associated with the anterior cerebral artery
(D) Aneurysm of vertebrobasilar artery
(E) Uncal herniation

72. A 35-year-old woman has been referred to your service with a radiographic report indicating a brain tumor located at the cerebellopontine angle. To determine preoperative impairment from your complete neurologic examination, which cranial nerve should receive special attention?

(A) Trochlear nerve
(B) Oculomotor and abducens nerves
(C) Trigeminal nerve
(D) Facial and vestibulocochlear nerves
(E) Optic nerve

73. An individual with an intelligence quotient (IQ) of 95 is classified as

(A) severely mentally retarded
(B) moderately mentally retarded
(C) mildly mentally retarded
(D) borderline
(E) average

74. Anorexia nervosa

(A) is most common in middle age
(B) is more common in lower socioeconomic groups
(C) has few serious medical consequences
(D) can be treated effectively on an ongoing basis with family therapy
(E) has loss of appetite as its main feature

75. Which nerve is most likely to be injured by a midshaft fracture of the humerus?

(A) Axillary
(B) Median
(C) Ulnar
(D) Musculocutaneous
(E) Radial

76. After falling on her outstretched hand, the patient complains of point tenderness in the space between the tendons of the extensor pollicis longus and the extensor pollicis brevis. Which bone is most likely to be fractured?

(A) Radius
(B) First metacarpal
(C) Trapezium
(D) Scaphoid
(E) Lunate

77. A patient has fallen on her outstretched hand and dislocated a carpal bone. Which bone is most likely to be dislocated?

(A) Scaphoid
(B) Lunate
(C) Hamate
(D) Triquetrum
(E) Capitate

78. When a dislocation of the glenohumeral joint occurs, through which part of the joint capsule does the humeral head pass?

(A) Superior
(B) Inferior
(C) Anterior
(D) Posterior
(E) Medial

79. The most commonly abused substance in the United States is

(A) marijuana
(B) alcohol
(C) cocaine
(D) LSD
(E) heroin

80. Where is the barrier between the blood and brain parenchyma?

(A) Leaky ependyma (epithelial)
(B) Tight ependyma (epithelial)
(C) Capillary endothelium
(D) Neuronal membrane
(E) Fenestrated endothelium

81. Of the following people, which one is most likely to sexually abuse a 9-year-old girl?

(A) Father
(B) Stepfather
(C) Eleven-year-old brother
(D) Uncle
(E) Teacher

82. Which region begins closure of the neural tube?

(A) Cranial end
(B) Caudal end
(C) Cervical region
(D) Lumbar region
(E) Sacral region

83. Which statement is likely to be true about the treatment of unipolar disorder in a 50-year-old female patient?

(A) Lithium is more effective than a tricyclic antidepressant
(B) A selective serotonin reuptake inhibitor (SSRI) is more effective than a tricyclic antidepressant
(C) An SSRI works faster than a tricyclic antidepressant
(D) Psychotherapy increases her compliance with pharmacologic treatment
(E) None of the above are true

84. A patient has suffered a blow to the lateral side of the leg immediately distal to the knee. Which nerve is most likely to be injured?

(A) Tibial
(B) Common peroneal
(C) Obturator
(D) Femoral
(E) Sural

85. Which personality disorder is more common in women than in men?

(A) Antisocial
(B) Schizoid
(C) Dependent
(D) Narcissistic
(E) Obsessive compulsive

86. An attending physician hands the intern a tuning fork and asks him to test the perception of the vibratory modality in the individual that the physician is checking. Which system is tested by using this instrument?

(A) Spinothalamic (anterolateral) system
(B) Posterior spinocerebellar pathway
(C) Dorsal-column-medial lemniscus system
(D) Tectospinal pathway
(E) Rubrospinal pathway

87. The second most common genetic cause of mental retardation in the population is

(A) Down syndrome
(B) cri du chat syndrome
(C) Klinefelter syndrome
(D) fragile X syndrome
(E) Lesch-Nyhan syndrome

88. Which nuclear group in the brain stem is responsible for the reticular activating system norepinephrine input to cerebral structures?

(A) Raphae nuclei
(B) Locus coeruleus
(C) Lateral reticular formation
(D) Nucleus gracilis
(E) Anterior mamillary bodies

89. A 35-year-old male patient who has previously been aggressive and assaultive injures his head in a boating accident. After the accident, the nurses report that although he is very easy to deal with, he constantly masturbates and often makes sexually suggestive gestures toward them. What is the most likely site of his brain injury?

(A) Basal ganglia
(B) Hippocampus
(C) Amygdala
(D) Parietal lobes
(E) Frontal lobes

90. Which structure is the release site of neurohormones synthesized in the paraventricular and supraoptic nuclei that manufacture oxytocin and vasopressin?

(A) Median eminence
(B) Pineal gland
(C) Posterior pituitary
(D) Lamina terminalis
(E) Anterior pituitary

91. Which membrane forms the transverse tubule system of skeletal muscle?

(A) Sarcolemma
(B) Sarcoplasmic reticulum
(C) Junctional or subneural folds
(D) Rough endoplasmic reticulum
(E) Smooth endoplasmic reticulum

92. The second neuron in the pathway carrying pain and temperature in the anterolateral system

(A) crosses to the opposite side within one segment rostrally
(B) crosses randomly along the longitudinal axis of the spinal cord
(C) remains ipsilateral the length of the spinal cord
(D) crosses the midline within a small area of the medulla
(E) is involved only with intersegmental reflexes

93. A 25-year-old schizophrenic patient is brought to the hospital with a temperature of 104.5°F, blood pressure of 190/110, and muscular rigidity. Which drug is most likely to have caused this problem?

(A) Clozapine
(B) Lithium
(C) Thioridazine
(D) Haloperidol
(E) Fluoxetine

94. Hirschsprung disease is marked by the absence of parasympathetic enteric ganglia in the distal gut tube. This disease results from an abnormality in the migration of

(A) endoderm cells
(B) splanchnic mesoderm cells
(C) somatic mesoderm cells
(D) hypomere cells
(E) neural crest cells

95. Intramembranous ossification is the source of

(A) flat bone
(B) long bone
(C) cancellous bone
(D) bone of the diaphysis
(E) bone of the epiphysis

96. The pituitary gland is formed by the fusion of an evagination of the floor of the third ventricle with an evagination of

(A) ectoderm that forms the roof of the stomodeum
(B) endoderm that forms the roof of the pharnyx
(C) endoderm that forms the first branchial pouch
(D) ectoderm that forms the first branchial cleft
(E) mesoderm that forms the first branchial arch

97. Which substance, if used for a long time, is associated with memory loss?

(A) Marijuana
(B) Alcohol
(C) Cocaine
(D) LSD
(E) Heroin

98. In the posterior (dorsal) spinocerebellar tract, where are the cell bodies of origin?

(A) Posterior (dorsal) horn
(B) Dorsal root entry zone (DREZ)
(C) Dorsal nucleus of Clarke
(D) Laminae VIII and IX
(E) γ-Neuron nuclei

99. Methadone is used to treat heroin addiction primarily because

(A) it does not cause physical dependence
(B) its use does not result in tolerance
(C) it does not cause euphoria
(D) it blocks the heroin withdrawal syndrome
(E) it has a shorter duration of action than heroin

100. The oculomotor nerve passes between which pair of arteries?

(A) Superior cerebellar artery and posterior cerebral artery
(B) Posterior inferior cerebellar artery and anterior inferior cerebellar artery
(C) Posterior cerebral artery and middle cerebral artery
(D) Labyrinthine artery and anterior inferior cerebellar artery
(E) Posterior cerebral artery and posterior communicating artery

101. Uncontrolled flailing of an arm is a symptom of

(A) amyotrophic lateral sclerosis
(B) lower motor neuron syndrome
(C) dysdiadochokinesia
(D) hemiballismus
(E) athetosis

102. Which nerve is a branch of a root of the brachial plexus?

(A) Suprascapular nerve
(B) Dorsal scapular nerve
(C) Upper subscapular nerve
(D) Lateral pectoral nerve
(E) Thoracodorsal nerve

103. In schizophrenia, hallucinations are most likely to be

(A) visual
(B) kinesthetic
(C) auditory
(D) olfactory
(E) cenesthetic

104. Which sequence best describes the path that a drop of cerebrospinal fluid follows from the lateral ventricle to the superior sagittal sinus?

(A) Foramen of Magendie → cerebral aqueduct → fourth ventricle → arachnoid villi
(B) Foramen of Monro → foramen of Luschka → fourth ventricle → cisterna magna
(C) Septum pellucidum → third ventricle → fourth ventricle → foramen of Luschka
(D) Arachnoid villi → cisterna magna → foramen of Magendie → foramen of Monro
(E) Foramen of Monro → cerebral aqueduct → foramen of Luschka → arachnoid villi

105. In schizophrenia, clozapine is more effective than haloperidol against

(A) hallucinations
(B) bizarre behavior
(C) delusions
(D) talkativeness
(E) withdrawal

106. Which muscle receives its nerve supply from a direct branch of the ansa cervicalis?

(A) Mylohyoid
(B) Geniohyoid
(C) Sternohyoid
(D) Cricothyroid
(E) Cricoarytenoid

107. Both diazepam and phenobarbital

(A) induce cytochrome P-450 enzymes
(B) suppress rapid eye movement (REM) sleep
(C) can be used as a muscle relaxant
(D) are contraindicated in intermittent porphyria
(E) have analgesic activity

108. Which muscle has the phrenic nerve on its anterior surface?

(A) Sternocleidomastoid
(B) Anterior digastric
(C) Superior belly of the omohyoid
(D) Anterior scalene
(E) Middle scalene

109. Untreated episodes of bipolar disorder commonly last approximately

(A) 1 month
(B) 3 months
(C) 6 months
(D) 12 months
(E) the lifetime of the individual

110. In an experimental nerve–muscle preparation under some resting tension, what reflex responses occur in both the la and lb afferent fibers after an increase in stimulation of the α-motor neurons?

(A) An increase in the number of action potentials on both the la and lb neurons
(B) A decrease in the number of action potentials on both the la and lb neurons
(C) An increase in the number of action potentials on the la but a decrease on the lb
(D) A decrease in the number of action potentials on the la but an increase on the lb
(E) An increase in the number of action potentials on the la but no change on the lb

111. If a nerve membrane is stimulated once per second with a series of 10 stimuli beginning with a stimulus that is 10 times threshold strength, followed by stimuli that are each half as strong as the preceding stimulus

(A) every stimulus produces an equivalent action potential
(B) every stimulus produces an action potential half as strong as the preceding one
(C) only the first stimulus produces an action potential
(D) the first four stimuli produce equivalent action potentials, and the last six produce no action potentials
(E) wave summation of the 10 action potentials occurs

112. Which statement best describes a typical nerve cell, e.g., a motor neuron that has a resting membrane potential of -80 mV and an electrogenic pump (3 Na^+:2 K^+):

(A) The membrane permeability to potassium exceeds the permeability to sodium, and the rate of movement of sodium into the cell exceeds the rate of potassium moving out
(B) The membrane permeability to potassium exceeds the permeability to sodium, and the rate of movement of sodium into the cell is less than the rate of potassium moving out
(C) The membrane permeability to potassium is less than the permeability to sodium, and the rate of movement of sodium into the cell exceeds the rate of potassium moving out
(D) The membrane permeability to potassium is less than the permeability to sodium, and the rate of movement of sodium into the cell is less than the rate of potassium moving out
(E) The membrane permeability to potassium equals the permeability to sodium, and the rate of movement of sodium into the cell equals the rate of potassium moving out

113. Which of the following diseases is only transmitted by a louse?

(A) Relapsing fever
(B) Babesiosis
(C) Rocky Mountain spotted fever
(D) Lyme disease
(E) Epidemic typhus

114. Which nerve is most likely to be damagd by a fracture of the surgical neck of the humerus?

(A) Radial nerve
(B) Musculocutaneous nerve
(C) Axillary nerve
(D) Median nerve
(E) Ulnar nerve

115. A 47-year-old type I insulin–dependent patient with diabetes has a burning sensation around his ankles and on the bottoms of both feet. Neurologic examination reveals depressed achilles and knee-jerk reflexes bilaterally and decreased light touch sensation in both lower extremities. The mechanism for this finding most closely relates to

(A) osmotic damage of the Schwann cells
(B) vitamin deficiency
(C) underlying pernicious anemia
(D) an underlying malignancy
(E) nonenzymatic glycosylation

DIRECTIONS:

Each of the numbered items or incomplete statements in this section is negatively phrased, as indicated by a capitalized word such as NOT, LEAST, or EXCEPT. Select the ONE lettered answer or completion that is BEST in each case.

116. A 24-year-old patient is brought into the emergency room intoxicated with cocaine. Which condition is LEAST likely to characterize the patient?

(A) Stupor
(B) Euphoria
(C) Aggressiveness
(D) Agitation
(E) Hypersexuality

117. Which of the following bone disease/pathogenesis relationships is NOT CORRECT?

(A) Osteogenesis imperfecta: decreased mineralization of bone
(B) Osteopetrosis: osteoclast dysfunction
(C) Achondroplasia: premature closure of the epiphyseal plate of long bones
(D) Postmenopausal osteoporosis: osteoclastic activity predominates over osteoblastic activity
(E) Paget disease: increased osteoclastic activity followed by increased osteoblastic activity

118. The characteristics of drug tolerance and physical dependence include all of the following EXCEPT

(A) cross-tolerance among drugs acting on the same pharmacologic receptors
(B) a stereotypic withdrawal syndrome when the drug is abruptly discontinued
(C) magnitude proportional to dose and duration of administration
(D) shifts of the dose–response curve to the right
(E) primarily caused by induction of drug metabolism, resulting in increased drug clearance

119. All of the following muscles can internally rotate the arm at the shoulder EXCEPT

(A) pectoralis major
(B) deltoid
(C) teres major
(D) latissimus dorsi
(E) infraspinatus

120. Buspirone can be accurately described by all of the following phrases EXCEPT

(A) is a partial agonist at 5-hydroxytryptamine$_{1A}$ (5-HT$_{1A}$) receptors
(B) exerts anxiolytic effect after days or weeks of treatment
(C) may cause life-threatening seizures if abruptly discontinued
(D) does not cause muscle relaxation
(E) is safe for use in drug-dependent patients

121. A 25-year-old white woman has been raped. Which statement is LEAST likely to be true about this event?

(A) A weapon was used
(B) The rapist was white
(C) The rapist drank alcohol before the attack
(D) The rapist was 35 years of age
(E) The rapist was 25 years of age

122. Partial seizures that do not respond to phenytoin or carbamazepine therapy may be treated with any of the following drugs EXCEPT

(A) felbamate
(B) ethosuximide
(C) gabapentin
(D) lamotrigine
(E) valproate

123. Branches of the facial nerve include all of the following EXCEPT

(A) chorda tympani
(B) greater petrosal nerve
(C) lesser petrosal nerve
(D) nerve to the stapedius
(E) posterior auricular nerve

124. A 35-year-old woman has major depression. This patient is likely to show all of the following EXCEPT

(A) increased rapid eye movement (REM) sleep
(B) reduced slow-wave sleep
(C) long REM latency
(D) premature morning awakenings
(E) normal sleep onset

125. Adult derivatives of the prosencephalon include all of the following EXCEPT

(A) basal ganglia
(B) thalamus
(C) hypothalamus
(D) midbrain
(E) corpus callosum

126. Before the first episode of schizophrenia, which symptom is LEAST likely to occur in an 18-year-old male patient?

(A) Peculiar behavior
(B) Abnormal affect
(C) Strange perceptual experiences
(D) Gregarious, outgoing behavior
(E) Physical complaints

127. Neural crest cells develop into all of the following EXCEPT

(A) nerve cell bodies found in the dorsal root ganglion of thoracic spinal nerves
(B) nerve cell bodies found in the myenteric plexus of the small intestine
(C) nerve cell bodies found in the intermediolateral horn of the gray matter of the thoracic spinal cord
(D) nerve cell bodies found in the celiac ganglion
(E) nerve cell bodies found in the ciliary ganglion

128. Arteries that contribute to the cerebral arterial circle (of Willis) include all of the following EXCEPT

(A) posterior cerebral artery
(B) middle cerebral artery
(C) anterior cerebral artery
(D) posterior communicating artery
(E) anterior communicating artery

129. Which is LEAST likely to characterize anxiety?

(A) Syncope
(B) Palpitations
(C) Gastrointestinal disturbances
(D) Urinary urgency
(E) Flight of ideas

130. All of the following muscles participate in full abduction of the arm EXCEPT

(A) supraspinatus
(B) deltoid
(C) teres major
(D) trapezius
(E) serratus anterior

131. The differential diagnoses of schizophrenia include all of the following EXCEPT

(A) organic delirium
(B) bipolar disorder
(C) brief psychotic disorder
(D) generalized anxiety disorder
(E) substance abuse

132. Characteristics of smooth and cardiac muscle include all of the following EXCEPT

(A) gap junctions
(B) central nuclei
(C) branching fibers
(D) perinuclear organelles
(E) autonomic and hormonal regulation

133. All of the following statements about marijuana use are true EXCEPT

(A) it is the most widely used illegal drug in the United States
(B) its effects include decreased appetite
(C) its effects include impaired memory
(D) its effects include the "amotivational syndrome"
(E) it is a product of the hemp plant

134. The schematic shows the fever patterns of three different species of malaria.

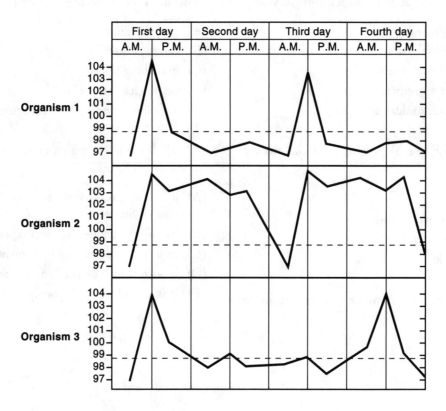

Which statement is NOT correct?

(A) Organism 1 is the most common type of malaria
(B) Organism 3 is associated with membranous glomerulonephritis
(C) Organism 1 commonly relapses
(D) Organism 1 produces the hemoglobinuria associated with "blackwater fever"
(E) Organism 2 has a reduced incidence in patients with sickle cell disease and glucose-6-phosphate dehydrogenase (G6PD) deficiency

135. A 19-year-old man suffers a spinal cord injury in a motorcycle accident. All of the following descriptions about this patient's sexual functioning are true EXCEPT that it

(A) is better if the lesion is of the upper rather than the lower motor neurons
(B) is better if his lesion is incomplete rather than complete
(C) involves erectile problems
(D) results in reduced testosterone levels
(E) results in reduced fertility

136. Tolerance and physical dependence may occur after chronic use of all of the following agents EXCEPT

(A) meperidine
(B) phenobarbital
(C) diazepam
(D) clomipramine
(E) ethanol

137. Which of the following diseases is caused by an organism that differs in morphology from the pathogens causing the other diseases listed?

(A) Trench mouth
(B) Primary syphilis
(C) Relapsing fever
(D) Rat bite fever
(E) Lyme disease

138. Which one of the following associations is NOT correct?

(A) Rapid supination and pronation of the hands—cerebellar function
(B) Stereognosis—sensory cortex
(C) Grasp, snout/suck, and palmomental reflexes—primitive reflexes
(D) Clasp knife reflex—upper motor neuron disease
(E) Romberg's test—lower motor neuron disease

139. Avascular necrosis of bone (osteonecrosis) is LEAST likely to be associated with

(A) Osgood-Schlatter disease
(B) Legg-Perthe disease
(C) long-term use of corticosteroids
(D) sickle-cell disease
(E) fracture of the scaphoid (navicular) bone

DIRECTIONS:

Each set of matching questions in this section consists of a list of four to twenty-six lettered options (some of which may be in figures) followed by several numbered items. For each numbered item, select the ONE lettered option that is most closely associated with it. To avoid spending too much time on matching sets with a large number of options, it is generally advisable to begin each set by reading the list of options. Then for each item in the set, try to generate the correct answer and locate it in the option list, rather than evaluating each option individually. Each lettered option may be selected once, more than once, or not at all.

Questions 140-144

Select the drug that would be the best treatment for the disorders.

(A) Carbamazepine
(B) Felbamate
(C) Valproate
(D) Ethosuximide
(E) Diazepam

140. A child is brought to the clinic after her teacher has observed repeated episodes in which she quit speaking in midsentence, dropped her pencil, and stared into space for a few moments.

141. A 49-year-old dentist complains of occasional, and increasingly frequent, episodes of severe, unilateral facial pain that arises near the mouth, shoots toward the nostril and eye, and seems to be triggered by eating or talking.

142. A 25-year-old woman is brought to the emergency room after loss of consciousness followed by urinary incontinence, tongue biting, muscle rigidity, and jerking movements of her arms and legs. The episode lasted 3 minutes, and she had not yet regained consciousness when she had another similar episode that lasted 5 minutes.

143. A patient is admitted for observation after reports by family members of temporary loss of consciousness during which he exhibited a few involuntary contractions of his legs, without muscle rigidity, tongue-biting, or incontinence.

144. A child is referred to a pediatric neurologist for further evaluation of his mental retardation and mixed seizure disorder, including partial seizures and atonic seizures, which have been refractory to standard therapy.

Questions 145-149

For each site of action, identify the central nervous system drug.

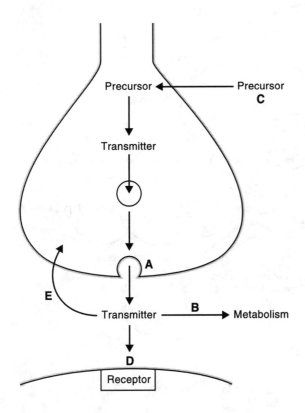

145. Selegiline

146. Paroxetine

147. Clozapine

148. Levodopa

149. Alprazolam

Questions 150-154

Select the pharmacologic agents that match the descriptions of receptor activity.

(A) Phencyclidine
(B) Baclofen
(C) Picrotoxin
(D) Strychnine
(E) Diazepam
(F) Lysergic acid diethylamide
(G) Caffeine

150. γ-aminobutyric acid (GABA) agonist

151. Glycine antagonist

152. N-methyl-D-aspartate (NMDA, excitatory amino acid) receptor antagonist

153. Potentiates GABA receptor activation

154. Antagonist at 5-hydroxytryptamine (5-HT, serotonin) receptors

Questions 155-157

The diagram illustrates the visual pathway of the right side of the brain. Match the visual field defect that would result from lesions located at the numbered sites on the diagram.

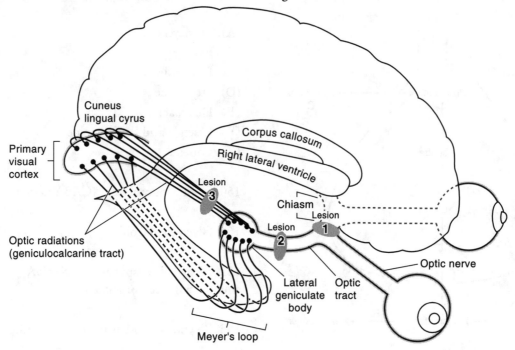

155. Leison 1

156. Leison 2

157. Leison 3

Questions 158-163

For each numbered description of central nervous system (CNS) drug toxicity, select the agent that is most likely to cause the adverse effects.

(A) Levodopa
(B) Trazodone
(C) Haloperidol
(D) Lithium
(E) Phenytoin
(F) Amitriptyline

158. After several years of inpatient and outpatient drug therapy, a patient exhibits involuntary facial grimacing, lip smacking, and tongue protrusion that have become progressively severe.

159. After continuous drug treatment for a nervous system disorder, a 49-year-old woman presents with thickening and bleeding of her gums, broadening of the lips and nose, and mild hirsutism.

160. After 4 years of drug treatment, a patient begins to experience hour-to-hour fluctuations in his ability walk, accompanied by involuntary movements of the face and jerking movements of the hands and feet.

161. A patient presents to the clinic complaining of marked sedation and a sustained and painful penile erection.

162. A patient returning to the clinic for review of his medications shows significant weight gain and hand tremor, and complains of polyuria.

163. A patient is brought to the emergency room after an overdose of unknown medication. She is lethargic and hypotensive (72/48 mm Hg) with dilated pupils (7 mm). The electrocardiogram (ECG) shows a wide QRS complex arrhythmia.

Questions 164-171

The following questions refer to the graph of membrane potentials (MPs), in which line F represents the resting membrane potential of the cell with a typical pump (3 Na$^+$: 2 K$^+$). Match each description with the associated membrane potential.

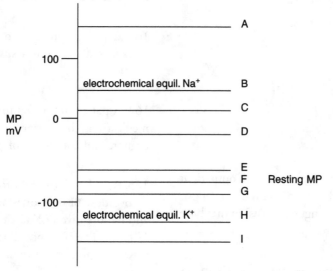

164. Membrane potential line best represents the potential at a skeletal muscle endplate at the peak of its excitation by a motor neuron

165. Membrane potential line that is closest to the electrochemical equilibrium for calcium ions across the axon terminal of a motor neuron

166. Membrane potential line that best represents the potential on the sarcolemma of a skeletal muscle cell at the peak of an action potential

167. Membrane potential line that best represents the potential when the membrane permeability to sodium equals the membrane permeability to potassium

168. If chloride is in electrochemical equilibrium at the resting membrane potential (line F), the potential line that best represents the membrane potential when the permeability to chloride is increased

169. If line F represents a motor neuron at rest, the membrane potential line that best represents the potential on the soma of that motor neuron during an inhibitory postsynaptic potential (IPSP)

170. If line F represents a healthy cardiac muscle cell, the membrane potential line that best represents the potential of that cell when coronary artery disease produces ischemia which slows, but does not stop, the sodium–potassium pump

171. If line F represents the value of the resting membrane potential in a sinoatrial node cell of the heart, the membrane potential line that best represents the value of the resting membrane potential of that cell following increased stimulation by the vagus nerve

Questions 172-175

Select the drug that would antagonize the effects of the numbered pharmacologic agents.

(A) Benztropine
(B) Naltrexone
(C) Methylphenidate
(D) Haloperidol
(E) Flumazanil

172. Propoxyphene

173. Chlordiazepoxide

174. Bromocriptine

175. Tacrine

Questions 176-180

For each site of action, identify the anti-Parkinsonian drugs.

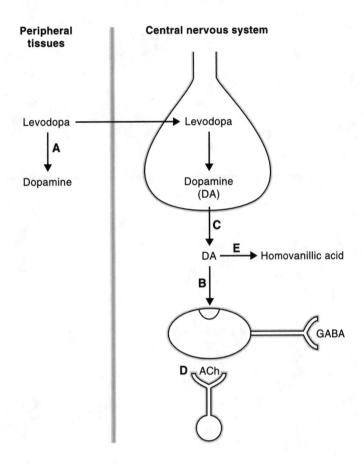

176. Amantadine

177. Benztropine

178. Carbidopa

179. Bromocryptine

180. Selegiline

ANSWER KEY

1. C	31. A	61. B	91. A	121. D	151. D
2. A	32. B	62. E	92. A	122. B	152. A
3. C	33. D	63. D	93. D	123. C	153. E
4. D	34. A	64. C	94. E	124. C	154. F
5. A	35. C	65. D	95. A	125. D	155. A
6. E	36. A	66. B	96. A	126. D	156. C
7. C	37. D	67. B	97. B	127. C	157. G
8. D	38. E	68. B	98. C	128. B	158. C
9. A	39. C	69. D	99. D	129. E	159. E
10. B	40. A	70. B	100. A	130. C	160. A
11. E	41. D	71. B	101. D	131. D	161. B
12. D	42. B	72. D	102. B	132. C	162. D
13. A	43. E	73. E	103. C	133. B	163. F
14. B	44. C	74. D	104. E	134. D	164. D
15. A	45. E	75. E	105. E	135. A	165. A
16. D	46. E	76. D	106. C	136. D	166. C
17. D	47. B	77. B	107. B	137. A	167. D
18. C	48. E	78. B	108. D	138. E	168. F
19. A	49. E	79. B	109. B	139. A	169. G
20. C	50. E	80. C	110. D	140. D	170. E
21. A	51. A	81. A	111. D	141. A	171. G
22. D	52. A	82. C	112. A	142. E	172. B
23. E	53. B	83. D	113. E	143. C	173. E
24. E	54. D	84. B	114. C	144. B	174. D
25. B	55. B	85. C	115. A	145. B	175. A
26. A	56. C	86. C	116. A	146. E	176. C
27. C	57. E	87. D	117. A	147. D	177. D
28. E	58. C	88. B	118. E	148. C	178. A
29. A	59. D	89. C	119. E	149. D	179. B
30. D	60. E	90. C	120. C	150. B	180. E

ANSWERS AND EXPLANATIONS

1. The answer is C. *(Anatomy)*
Postganglionic neurons are derived from neural crest cells. The other cell types are derived from the neural tube or are endodermal in origin.

2. The answer is A. *(Pathology)*
This patient has a classic triad of symptoms for multiple sclerosis (MS), the most common demyelinating disease in the United States. The sudden loss of vision in the left eye, which is painful on movement of the eyes, a poor pupillary light reflex, a swollen optic disc, and flame hemorrhages around the disc margin represent optic neuritis, which is a common complication associated with MS. Optic atrophy is a potential sequela after repeated attacks. MS is two times more common in women than in men. It is more commonly found in temperate climates. MS poses an increased risk in siblings of MS patients. There is an increased concordance rate in monozygotic twins.

MS is an autoimmune disease that is triggered by a viral infection in genetically susceptible individuals with the HLA DR2 haplotype. Grossly, the demyelinating plaques are primarily located in the white matter and have a gray, soft, gelatinous appearance. Favored locations are the angles of the ventricles and the floor of the fourth ventricle. Microscopically, the plaques exhibit gliosis (a proliferation of astrocytes) and a lymphoid (T cell)/plasma cell infiltrate. Approximately 70% of patients present with an episodic course punctuated by acute relapses and remissions with the following constellation of findings: (1) the classic triad of scanning speech, intention tremor, and nystagmus (mnemonic: SIN), (2) paresthesias (numbness and tingling), (3) sensory loss, (4) visual abnormalities (optic neuritis, diplopia), (5) cerebellar ataxia, (6) weakness, (7) urinary incontinence, and (8) preservation of higher intellectual function. The cerebrospinal fluid findings in MS and other demyelinating diseases include: (1) a slight increase (< 20 cells/μl) in the number of lymphocytes (T lymphocytes), (2) slightly increased gamma globulins (mainly IgG, 80%), (3) the presence of oligoclonal immunoglobulin bands (individual monoclonal spikes) on agarose gel electrophoresis (75%–90%), (4) myelin breakdown products (myelin basic protein), and (5) normal glucose levels. Other studies that are useful include evoked response testing and magnetic resonance imaging, which is extremely useful in locating plaques in more than 90% of patients. Aqueous adrenocorticotrophic hormone injections, methylprednisolone, and recently, interferon-β have been used in treatment.

The triad of scanning speed, intention tremor, and nystagmus is not seen in atherosclerotic carotid artery disease, embolization, a hypercoagulable state, or an increase in intracranial pressure from other causes.

3. The answer is C. *(Microbiology)*
The patient is 9 months old and develops high fever, febrile convulsions, and a maculopapular rash immediately after the fever breaks. This scenario is a classic one for roseola, alias exanthem subitum, alias roseola exanthem. Roseola is caused by herpesvirus type 6, which is a double-stranded DNA virus. Roseola occurs in children 6 months to 2 years of age, usually during spring and fall. It has an incubation period of 10 to 15 days. The characteristic presentation is one of a sudden onset of a high fever with an absence of physical findings. The high fevers frequently precipitate febrile convulsions. The fever falls by crisis on the 3rd to 4th day. Within 48 hours after the child's temperature returns to normal, a macular or maculopapular rash starts on the trunk and spreads centrifugally to include the face and extremities. Lymphadenopathy and splenomegaly may occur, since the virus infects lymphocytes. This virus has also been associated with the chronic fatigue syndrome, which is characterized by extreme fatigue, fever, myalgias, depression, and a lymphoproliferative disorder. The other diseases listed have a rash with fever, rather than a rash developing after dissipation of the fever. Varicella, or chickenpox, has macular, then vesicular, and finally pustular lesions.

The measles virus (rubeola) is an RNA virus that belongs to the Paramyxovirus family. It has an incubation period of approximately 7 to 14 days. It is infective 2 days before the initial catarrhal stage through the 5th day of the rash. Rubeola begins with fever (up to 40°C), conjunctivitis (photophobia is the first sign), coryza (excessive mucous production), and cough. This is followed by the pathognomonic Koplik's spots, which are bright red lesions with a white center that develop on the buccal mucosa. In a few days, the patient develops a generalized, blanching, erythematous maculopapular rash (viral induced immune vasculitis), which begins at the hairline and extends down over the body. It gradually resolves with some desquamation over 1 or 2 weeks. Unlike German measles, rubeola is not associated with fetal congenital anomalies. Possible complications include (1) secondary bacterial otitis media, the most common complication, (2) pneumonia, which is responsible for most deaths due to the disease, and (3) subacute sclerosing panencephalitis (SSPE), representing a fatal demyelinating disease that may develop months to years later. Warthin Finkeldey giant cells, which often contain 100 plus nuclei, are a characteristic finding in rubeola. They are found in the lung in pneumonia and in lymphoid tissue throughout the body. Measles is part of the MMR (measles, mumps, rubella) vaccine, which is a live attenuated vaccine.

The rubella virus is an RNA virus in the Togavirus family. It is the cause of German measles. The virus enters through the upper respiratory tract mucosa, replicates in the nasopharyngeal lymphoid tissue, and then spreads via the lymphatics to the posterior auricular and suboccipital lymph nodes. It then enters the blood to produce a viremia. It has an incubation period of 2 to 3 weeks. Painful lymphadenopathy, fever, and malaise occur 5 to 10 days before the onset of the rash. The rash is maculopapular and, like rubeola, represents an immune complex–induced vasculitis. It begins on the face and progresses downwards to involve the extremities. The rash disappears in 3 days, thus the term "3 day measles." The immune complexes may produce a polyarthritis, particularly in adults. Rubella contracted during pregnancy produces teratogenic effects in the developing fetus, the most common of which is nerve deafness.

Parvoviruses are the smallest of the DNA viruses. They produce erythema infectiosum, or fifth's disease, as well as a number of other disorders. Erythema infectiosum is characterized by a confluent rash usually beginning on the cheeks (slapped face appearance), which extends centripetally to involve the trunk. Associated symptoms include fever, malaise, respiratory problems, arthralgias, and joint swelling. Parvoviruses are also associated with (1) aplastic anemia in patients with chronic hemolytic anemias (e.g., sickle cell disease, congenital spherocytosis), (2) repeated abortions, (3) pure red blood cell aplasia (infects the red blood cell precursor stem cell), (4) persistent infection in immunocompromised patients, and (5) arthritis.

The varicella/zoster virus is a DNA virus in the Herpesvirus family (varicella, Herpes, cytomegalovirus, Epstein Barr, herpesvirus 6). Varicella, or chickenpox, is primarily a childhood disease (70%), whereas Herpes zoster, the cause of shingles, is due to reactivation of a latent varicella/zoster infection in the sensory ganglia. The incubation period of chickenpox is 14 to 16 days. The disease is highly contagious 2 days before the vesicles appear until the last lesion dries up. Varicella presents with generalized skin lesions, which begin as macules and progress into a vesicular and pustular stage. The rash spreads centrifugally to the face and out to the extremities. Unlike smallpox (variola) vesicles, which have the same appearance, varicella vesicles appear in varying stages of development as successive crops of lesions appear. Infected squamous cells have intranuclear inclusions similar to those seen in Herpes infections. Pneumonia is more likely to occur in adults and is the most common cause of death in the disease. It is frequently a fatal disease in immunocompromised patients. There is an association with Reye's syndrome. Encephalitis is another potential complication and most commonly involves the cerebellum. It usually resolves without any neurological deficits. Congenital abnormalities are seen in 9% of pregnancies, particularly if it is acquired early in the pregnancy. A new vaccine is presently available.

4. The answer is D. *(Pathology)*
The Weber test is performed by placing the base of a lightly vibrating 512-Hz tuning fork on the midforehead and asking the patient on which side the sound is heard better or if both sides are equal. Normally, the sound should not lateralize to one ear, but be equal in both ears. If a conduction defect is present in the middle ear, it lateralizes to the affected ear, whereas in a sensorineural loss (nerve deafness), it lateralizes to the normal ear. The Rinne test uses the same 512-Hz tuning fork. The vibrating base of the tuning fork is placed on the mastoid bone until the patient can no longer hear it, and then it is quickly positioned close to the ear canal until it is no longer heard. Normally, the sound of air conduction is longer

than the sound of bone conduction. However, in conduction defects, bone conduction is longer than air conduction, because the vibrating bone bypasses the middle ear ossicles and directly stimulates the nerve. In sensorineural loss, the affected ear still retains the normal air conduction greater than bone conduction pattern. The patient in our question has lateralization of the Weber test to the left ear and bone conduction greater than air conduction in that same ear, so it is

a conduction deficit, most likely secondary to otosclerosis. Otosclerosis refers to sclerosis and fixation of the middle ear ossicles. It may be bilateral and has a strong autosomal dominant inheritance pattern. It is the most common cause of conductive hearing loss in adults. Presbycusis is the most common cause of sensorineural hearing loss in the elderly. The findings that would be expected for each of the other choices are as follows:

Clinical Finding	Weber Test	Rinne Test
Presbycusis right ear	Lateralizes to left ear (normal ear)	Air conduction > bone conduction in both ears; therefore, the right ear is affected
Presbycusis left ear	Lateralizes to right ear (normal ear)	Air conduction > bone conduction in both ears; therefore, the left ear is affected
Otosclerosis right ear	Lateralizes to right ear (affected ear)	Bone conduction > air conduction on right (affected ear); bone conduction on left (normal ear)
Normal ears	No lateralization	Air conduction > bone conduction in both ears

5. The answer is A. *(Anatomy)*
The Wernicke area lies in the posterior part of the superior temporal gyrus on the convexity of the brain and extends onto the upper surface of the temporal lobe.

The parietal lobe is the location of sensory association areas. Lesions in this part of the cerebrum generally result in sensory agnosias; that is, the patient either disregards or misinterprets sensory stimuli.

The frontal lobes are associated with the function of human personality, short- and long-range planning, and human initiatives. Complex and intellectual ideas seem to arise in this part of the brain. Aberrant human behavior and dementias are related to lesions in this part of the brain.

The occipital lobe is related to visual function.

The limbic lobe functions in basic human emotions and is also integral to memory and learning processes.

6. The answer is E. *(Pathology)*
The barber has carpal tunnel syndrome with entrapment of the median nerve in the transverse carpal ligament. This condition is commonly seen in people who use their hands a lot, such as jack hammer operators, typists, and tailors. Other causes include rheumatoid arthritis, amyloidosis, and pregnancy. Splinting

of the wrist, physical therapy, and surgical release are the modalities of therapy.

7. The answer is C. *(Microbiology)*
Because the patient is a pig farmer and has generalized aches and pains associated with an exaggerated increase in eosinophils in the peripheral blood, he most likely has trichinosis, which is caused by the nematode *Trichinella spiralis*. The disease is contracted in man by eating raw or poorly cooked pork containing the encysted larvae. The larvae are released after digestion of the cyst wall in the stomach juices. They develop into adult forms that mate in the small intestine. The female worms release additional larvae (not eggs) that penetrate the bowel mucosa and spread hematogenously throughout the body, particularly to the skeletal muscle where they become encysted deep in the muscle. As a rule, the larvae deposited in other organs die. Clinically, patients have fever, muscle pain, periorbital edema (larva penetration), myocarditis, and encephalitis in rare cases. There is a pronounced peripheral blood eosinophilia, since the worms penetrate tissue. The laboratory diagnosis is confirmed by biopsy of muscle to find the cysts, or by serologic tests. Corticosteroids and mebendazole are the treatment of choice.

Regarding the other choices in the question, the nematodes *Strongyloides stercoralis*, *Ascaris lumbricoides*, *Trichuris trichiura*, and *Ancylostoma duodenale* do not have larval forms that encyst in muscle.

8. The answer is D.   *(Pathology)*
Cataracts refer to an opacification in the lens. Those that are secondary to an increase in sorbitol production in the lens are caused by the conversion of glucose into sorbitol by aldolase reductase. Sorbitol is osmotically active and draws water into the lens, leading to the formation of opacifications that interfere with vision. This is a complication commonly seen in diabetes mellitus. The diagnosis is best made by slit lamp examination of the lens. The vast majority of cataracts are associated with the normal aging process. Other associations include intrauterine viral infections (rubella most commonly), trauma, genetic diseases (myoclonic dystrophy), metabolic conditions (galactosemia), drugs (steroid eye drops), hypoparathyroidism (calcium is deposited in the lens), and physical agents (microwaves).

9. The answer is A.   *(Anatomy)*
The dorsal columns of the spinal cord carry sensory information of conscious proprioception from the body. A Romberg sign can be elicited in lesions of this tract by removing another major position sense, namely vision. This patient, when asked to close his eyes, was unable to maintain his position in space.

The lateral spinothalamic tract, now part of the anterolateral system, carries sensory information related to pain and temperature.

Anterior horn cells are the final common pathway to stimulate extrafusal skeletal muscle. The lateral corticospinal tract innervates neurons in the anterior horn of the spinal cord and is the link between the cerebral cortex and spinal cord motor centers. This pathway represents voluntary control of spinal motor mechanism.

The anterior white commissure is the site where second neurons cross in the pain and temperature pathway.

10. The answer is B.   *(Pathology)*
An afebrile patient who complains of itchy eyes, nasal congestion, and increased lacrimation has allergic con-

junctivitis and rhinitis. The discoloration under the eyes is secondary to venous stasis from the nasal congestion. This allergy most commonly has a seasonal association, occurring when different types of pollens are in the atmosphere. It is an IgE mediated, type I hypersensitivity reaction with the release of histamine from mast cells on exposure to specific allergens the patient is sensitized against. A conjunctival or nasal smear for eosinophils helps confirm the diagnosis.

Infection is unlikely in this patient, since he is afebrile and the physical findings are classic for allergy.

There is usually a family history for atopic diseases, such as hay fever and asthma, rather than autoimmune disease.

The findings in this patient are not characteristic of a cluster headache (migraine variant), which presents with sudden development of conjunctival and nasal stuffiness followed by a pounding headache.

11. The answer is E.   *(Microbiology)*
The test for beta lactamase is most useful in determining whether penicillin or cephalosporins are effective in killing *Staphylococcus aureus*, *Haemophilus influenzae*, or *Neisseria gonorrhoeae*. Beta lactam drugs, such as penicillin and the cephalosporins, require an intact lactam ring to exert their antibacterial activity. Beta lactamase is an extracellular enzyme that hydrolyzes the beta lactam ring of penicillin and the cephalosporins, thus rendering them inactive. Some organisms continually synthesize the enzyme (constitutive), whereas others only synthesize the enzyme in the presence of the antibiotic (inducible). The enzyme activity may be blocked by modifying the lactam ring or by adding clavulanic acid and sulbactam, which bind to the lactamase, thus protecting the drug. Rapid assays are available to detect the enzyme.

The Schlichter test, or serum bactericidal test, determines the antibacterial activity of the patient's antibiotic in the serum against the actual organism that is being treated. The Quellung test is used to identify certain organisms, such as *Streptococcus pneumoniae*, *Haemophilus influenzae* type b, and *Neisseria meningitidis*, by using specific antiserum against their capsular polysaccharide. This causes capsular swelling in the presence of homologous antiserum. The Gram stain identifies bacteria and is useful in (1) identifying pathogenic organisms, (2) evaluating the adequacy of a specimen for culture, and (3) providing preliminary data on the choice of treatment. The difference in staining between gram-positive and gram-negative organisms is primarily due to their differences in cell wall lipid content. Gram-negative organisms have a higher lipid content in their cell walls (endotoxin) than gram-positive organisms.

The Kirby-Bauer test is a disk agar diffusion method in which various disks are impregnated with antibiotics of specific concentrations. The disks are placed on Mueller Hinton agar, which has been inoculated with the organisms. After incubation, the zones of growth inhibition around the disks are measured to decide whether the organisms are susceptible (S), have intermediate (I) susceptibility, or are resistant (R) to the antibiotic. The letter S means that the organism is susceptible to the standard oral dose of the antibiotic or the minimal dose of a parenterally administered drug. The letter I means that oral medications are not effective, but the maximal dose of the parenteral agent is effective. The letter R indicates that the antibiotic will not kill the bacteria. *Haemophilus influenzae, Neisseria gonorrhoeae,* and *Streptococcus viridans* are not amenable to the Kirby-Bauer technique.

12. The answer is D. *(Pathology)*
Diabetes mellitus is the most common cause of blindness in the United States. In diabetic retinopathy, the following changes are observed: (1) the formation of microaneurysms due to osmotic damage to the pericytes surrounding the retinal vessels, (2) hemorrhage, (3) exudates, and (4) proliferative retinopathy, which refers to neovascularization (blood vessel formation) with subsequent scarring. Proliferative retinopathy is more likely to be associated with diabetic retinopathy than with hypertensive retinopathy. In hypertensive retinopathy, the following occur: (1) focal spasm of the arterioles, (2) progressive sclerosis (copper wiring, silver wiring) with arteriovenous nicking as thick arterioles cross over venules, (3) flame hemorrhages from rupture of microaneurysms in the retinal vessels, (4) the formation of exudates, and (5) papilledema (swelling of the optic disc). Regarding the exudates, cotton wool exudates (soft exudates with fuzzy margins) are caused by microinfarctions, whereas exudates that have

clear margins (hard exudates) are caused by leakage of protein from increased vessel permeability.

13. The answer is A. *(Anatomy)*
The ventrobasal complex consists of the ventroposterior (VP) and ventrolateral (VL) nuclei. These nuclei contain the third-order neurons in the pathway of somatosensory stimuli to levels of consciousness. Ventroposterolateral (VPL) nuclei serve sensory modalities from the neck down, and the ventroposteromedial (VPM) nuclei serve sensory modalities from the head. Convergence and integration of all sensory modalities arising from the body occur at the ventrobasal complex.

Anterior nuclei participate in neural circuits of the limbic system.

The geniculate nuclei are specifically related to the sensory systems of vision and audition.

The ventroanterior (VA) and ventrolateral (VL) nuclei participate in integration of cerebellum and basal ganglion input to the cerebral cortex.

The hypothalamic nuclei participate in the neuroendocrine and autonomic systems.

14. The answer is B. *(Pathology)*
Any patient with a history of mitral stenosis, dilatation of the left atrium, and an irregularly irregular pulse (atrial fibrillation), who then has the sudden onset of a stroke in the distribution of the left middle cerebral artery (right facial weakness/anesthesia, right hemiplegia/anesthesia of the upper extremities, expressive aphasia involving Broca's area, and receptive aphasia involving Wernicke's speech area) has embolized from the left heart to the left cerebral cortex. Because the patient is afebrile and vegetations are not visible on an electrocardiogram, the embolus most likely originates from a clot in the left atrium that has been dislodged by the vibratory effect of atrial fibrillation, the most common arrhythmia associated with atrial dilatation. The results of a computerized tomography scan are usually negative in early hemorrhagic types of stroke, as in this patient.

Hemorrhagic infarctions of the brain are most commonly secondary to embolism from the left heart to the middle cerebral artery. Less common causes include compression of a cerebral vessel in a herniation (e.g., posterior cerebral artery in uncal herniations), atherosclerotic infarcts, and thrombosis of cerebral veins or the superior longitudinal sinus (child with dehydration). As a rule, hemorrhagic infarctions associated with embolism produce hemorrhage primarily within the gray matter at the periphery of the brain although both the gray and white matter are infarcted (liquefactive necrosis). The restoration of blood flow after dissolution of the embolus is more likely to rupture the weaker gray matter vessels rather than the stronger white matter vessels, thus the predilection for hemorrhage at the periphery. The rate of mortality from embolic infarctions is approximately 30%.

The history of mitral stenosis, left atrial dilatation, and sudden onset of a stroke does not correspond to a subarachnoid hemorrhage, which is most commonly secondary to a ruptured congenital berry aneurysm. It also does not indicate embolism to the right middle cerebral artery, because of the neurologic abnormalities in the dominant left hemisphere. An intracerebral bleed involving the internal capsule is most commonly due to hypertension. An atherosclerotic stroke is more common in the elderly population.

15. The answer is A. *(Microbiology)*
Rheumatic fever is an immunologic disease in which there is a cross-reactivity of antibodies developed against certain strains of group A Streptococcus with certain tissues in the body, including the heart (endocarditis, myocarditis, pericarditis), synovium (arthritis), skin, and basal ganglia. It is an immunologic disease rather than a toxin-induced disease.

Scarlet fever usually begins as a Streptococcal pharyngitis/tonsillitis that is followed by an erythematous rash beginning on the trunk and limbs. The rash is due to elaboration of erythrogenic toxin by the Streptococcus. The face is usually spared, but, if involved, there is a characteristic circumoral pallor. The tongue becomes bright red, thus the term "strawberry tongue." Poststreptococcal immune complex glomerulonephritis is a possible sequela of scarlet fever.

Toxic shock syndrome (TSS) is caused by a toxin-producing strain of *Staphylococcus aureus* that is associated with the use of hyperabsorbent tampons in menstruating women, dressings over operative wound sites, or localized infections with the toxin-producing strains in other sites. TSST-1 is the marker toxin associated with most cases. It presents with a rapid onset of high fever, myalgias, abdominal pain, vomiting, and diarrhea followed in 24 hours by a sunburn-like rash

that occurs during or soon after menses. Hyperemia in the pharynx and vaginal mucosa is also noted. Recovery generally occurs after 7 to 10 days and is marked by desquamation of the rash, particularly on the palms and soles.

Corynebacteria diphtheriae, the cause of diphtheria, is a gram-positive nonmotile bacillus that has a "Chinese letter" appearance on staining. The toxin in diphtheria is bacteriophage related (virus possesses the tox gene) and acts by (1) inhibiting ribosomal synthesis in host cells, and (2) interfering with the beta oxidation of fatty acids. In humans, elongation factor 2, which is responsible for elongating protein chains, is inhibited by the toxin. Diphtheria confined to the oropharynx and larynx is more common in children, where it produces an inflammatory pseudomembrane induced by exotoxin damage of the epithelium. The membrane may obstruct breathing. Drainage of the inflammatory material to the cervical lymph nodes in the neck produces "bull's neck" lymphadenopathy. The toxin also impairs the beta oxidation of fatty acids, which produces fatty change in the liver and in the heart (tabby cat heart). The cardiac muscle is most sensitive to the exotoxin, and cardiac dysfunction is the leading cause of death. The exotoxin also demyelinates peripheral and cranial nerves, resulting in a loss of motor function.

Cholera is caused by *Vibrio cholerae*. Vibrios are gram-negative motile bacteria that love salt and tolerate an alkaline pH environment. *Vibrio cholerae* produces a powerful enterotoxin that stimulates adenylate cyclase in the small bowel, thus producing an isotonic, secretory (noninvasive), high-volume diarrhea with severe fluid losses often described as "ricewater" stools. The disease is contracted by drinking contaminated water or by eating contaminated seafood, especially crustacea (Gulf coast). The El Tor type is more infective than the classic type of Vibrio. Dehydration, normal gap metabolic acidosis (loss of bicarbonate), and hypokalemia develop rapidly.

16. The answer is D. *(Pathology)*
The patient most likely drank methyl alcohol, which was metabolically converted into formic acid. Formic acid produced an increased anion gap metabolic acidosis and optic neuritis, which eventually resulted in atrophy of the optic nerve.

Optic neuritis is an inflammation of the optic nerve that may be secondary to infection (e.g., tuberculosis, syphilis, measles, varicella zoster), multiple sclerosis, systemic lupus erythematosus, or glaucoma. Optic atrophy may result from optic neuritis of any cause (e.g., glaucoma), trauma, ischemia, a long-standing increase in intracranial pressure, or methyl alcohol poisoning, as in this case. Retinal examination reveals a pale disk with absence of the tiny vessels around the nerve.

A demyelinating disease and an increase in intraocular pressure are associated with optic atrophy, but they do not take into account the history of drinking something that affected the patient's vision. Ethyl alcohol and vitamin deficiencies are not commonly associated with optic neuritis or atrophy.

17. The answer is D.   *(Anatomy)*
The longitudinal fissure separates the left and right cerebral hemispheres. The falx cerebri is insinuated into this fissure, further separating the hemispheres. The lower extremity is on the superior aspect of the precentral and postcentral gyri and extends over the midline at the longitudinal fissure.

The collateral fissure is located on the ventral surface of the temporal lobe.

The calcarine fissure is located on the midline of the occipital cortex.

The lateral fissure separates the frontal and parietal lobes from the temporal lobe.

The primary fissure is located on the surface of the cerebellum.

18. The answer is C. *(Pathology)*
This patient has a complete internuclear ophthalmoplegia (INO), which is most commonly due to demyelination of the medial longitudinal fasciculus (MLF) in the dorsal pontine tegmentum. INO is a pathognomonic finding in multiple sclerosis. The figure depicts the MLF, the lateral and medial rectus muscles, and the pons lateral gaze center. Note that the abducens nerve (cranial nerve VI) innervating the lateral rectus muscle, which abducts the eye, does not cross over. However, note the crossover of the oculomotor nerve (cranial nerve III) in the MLF, which innervates the medial rectus muscle. Therefore, when the patient looks to the left, the left lateral rectus abducts the eye to the left, whereas the right medial rectus muscle adducts the eye in the same direction. When the patient looks to the right, the right lateral rectus abducts the eye to the right, whereas the left

medial rectus muscle adducts in the eye in the same direction. Therefore, a demyelinating lesion involving both sides of the MLF at point C, which is what the patient has, disrupts both right and left horizontal gaze, since the medial rectus on both sides is not functioning. A lesion at point A, in the right MLF, affects the ability of the right medial rectus muscle to adduct when the patient gazes to the left, but there is no problem when looking to the right. A problem at point B involving the left side of the MLF affects the left medial rectus muscle, so it cannot adduct when the patient looks to the right.

Hypertension, ischemic cerebral disease, a cerebellar tumor, and a brain stem glioma are not associated with an intermittent history of dizziness and unsteady gait plus a complete INO. Ischemia may be responsible for isolated lesions in the MLF, but complete INO is unusual.

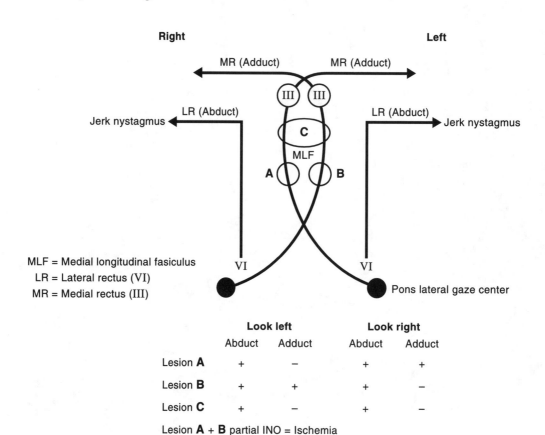

	Look left		Look right	
	Abduct	Adduct	Abduct	Adduct
Lesion **A**	+	−	+	+
Lesion **B**	+	+	+	−
Lesion **C**	+	−	+	−

Lesion **A** + **B** partial INO = Ischemia

Lesion **C** complete INO = Multiple sclerosis

19. The answer is A. *(Microbiology)*
The patient has a characteristic presentation for rubella, or German measles. The rubella virus is an RNA virus that belongs to the Togavirus family. It produces "3-day measles." The incubation time for the virus is 14 to 21 days. Photophobia is conspicuously absent, and painful adenopathy in the locations noted are features not seen in rubeola. The rash, which is an immune complex vasculitis, begins on the face and rapidly spreads to the trunk and extremities within 24 hours. Over the ensuing 2 to 3 days, it becomes more pinpoint in appearance and exhibits mild desquamation. In young women, there is a tendency for arthritis to develop due to antigen–antibody complexes. Splenomegaly is present in 50% of patients. Rubella contracted during pregnancy produces teratogenic effects in the developing fetus. The virus produces a placental and fetal vasculitis, which compromises fetal oxygenation and also causes chromosomal anomalies. The risk of damage is greater the earlier the infection is acquired. Approximately 20% of fetuses infected by the virus develop severe defects including (1) congenital heart lesions (patent ductus arteriosus most commonly), (2) nerve deafness (most common overall defect), and (3) congenital cataracts. Infants may continue to shed the virus for up to 1 year, thus posing a risk for spread of the virus to other susceptible individuals. An attenuated, live vaccine is available, but should not be given while the woman is pregnant but after she delivers. The vaccine is part of the MMR series, which stands for measles, mumps, and rubella. The immunization is usually given at 15 months of age. Patients who are immunocompromised should still get the vaccination, because the dire effects of measles (rubeola) in an immunocompromised host are worse than the risk for receiving the immunization.

Juvenile rheumatoid arthritis does not usually occur in adults. Painful adenopathy in the locations noted for rubella are not a feature of the disease.

Rubeola has a shorter incubation and lacks the painful adenopathy described for rubella. Koplik's spots in the mouth and photophobia are features of rubeola.

Infectious mononucleosis is not usually associated with a rash or arthritis. The adenopathy is usually located in the anterior and posterior cervical areas.

Lyme disease is associated with erythema chronicum migrans, and not a maculopapular rash with the distribution described.

20. The answer is C. *(Pathology)*
The patient most likely has a retinoblastoma. A retinoblastoma, although rare, is the most common intraocular malignancy in children. Retinoblastomas usually occur in a sporadic fashion, but they may also be inherited as an autosomal dominant disease. In either situation, the abnormality is on chromosome 13, which carries an Rb suppressor gene that normally prevents the retinal cells from entering the cell cycle. In the sporadic disease, a spontaneous mutation must inactivate the Rb suppressor genes on both of the chromosomes. However, in the familial form of the disease, one of the suppressor genes is already inactivated at birth, and only one more inactivation is necessary to initiate the tumor. Inactivation of the Rb suppressor gene in familial retinoblastoma is also associated with an increased incidence of osteogenic sarcoma. Other cancers associated with inactivation of the suppressor gene include small cell carcinoma of the lung, breast cancer, and bladder cancer. Retinoblastomas are grossly pigmented tumors that are composed of small cells, which form rosettes (Flexner-Wintersteiner rosettes). Leukocoria, or a white eye reflex, gets most of its notoriety as a diagnostic sign of a retinoblastoma, but it is most commonly the result of a congenital cataract.

21. The answer is A. *(Neuroanatomy)*
The anterior spinal artery supplies the ventral white commissure and bilaterally the anterior horns of the gray matter. Loss of blood supply to the ventral white commissure produces the sensory deficit bilaterally, and loss of blood supply to the anterior motor neurons produces the motor loss.

The posterior spinal arteries supply the dorsal aspects of the spinal cord and generally have a unilateral area of distribution.

The vertebral arteries, although giving rise to the anterior spinal arteries in the posterior cranial fossa, have a much larger area of distribution and many more neurologic deficits would result in their occlusion. Further, the anterior spinal artery depends on the segmental radicular arterial augmentation for complete spinal cord arterial blood supply.

The internal carotid arteries supply the anterior circulation to the cerebral cortex and rostral brain stem.

22. The answer is D. *(Pathology)*
The Weber test is performed by placing the base of a lightly vibrating 512-Hz tuning fork on the mid-forehead and asking the patient on which side the sound is heard better or if both sides are equal. Normally, the sound does not lateralize to one ear, but is equal in both ears. If a conduction defect is present in the middle ear, it lateralizes to the affected ear, whereas in a sensorineural loss (nerve deafness), it lateralizes to the normal ear. The Rinne test uses the same 512-Hz tuning fork. The vibrating base of the tuning fork is placed on the mastoid bone until the patient can no longer hear it, and then it is quickly positioned close to the ear canal until it is no longer heard. Normally, the sound of air conduction is longer than the sound of bone conduction. However, in conduction defects, bone conduction is longer than air conduction, since the vibrating bone bypasses the middle ear ossicles and directly stimulates the nerve. In sensorineural loss, the affected ear retains the normal air conduction greater than bone conduction pattern. This patient has a Weber test that lateralizes to his right ear, and the Rinne test exhibits bone conduction greater than air conduction on the right and air conduction longer than bone conduction on the left. Therefore, the patient has a conduction defect in his right ear most likely secondary to repeated ear infections in the past. Otitis media is the most common cause of conduction defects in children.

Trauma to the head could result in a conduction deficit, but it is not as common as otitis media. Rubella during the mother's first trimester or exposure to cat feces (toxoplasmosis) are unlikely causes, since they produce a sensorineural hearing loss. Gestational diabetes during the pregnancy is not associated with hearing defects in the child.

23. The answer is E. *(Microbiology)*
Onychomycosis is a fungal infection of the nail. It is commonly caused by *Candida albicans*. Maduromycosis, chromoblastomycosis, and sporotrichosis are all subcutaneous mycoses that are usually acquired by puncture wounds of the skin. From this site, they may also involve the underlying bones.

Chromoblastomycosis, or verrucous (wartlike) dermatitis, is a chronic skin lesion associated with several pigmented fungi (Fonsecaea, Phialophora, Cladosporium). These fungi are most frequently introduced into the skin by a splinter. In the subcutaneous tissue, they produce a granulomatous reaction in which the organisms are easily identified by their pigmented, thick-walled bodies. Surgery and oral flucytosine alone or in combination with ketoconazole are treatment options.

Mycetomas (maduromycosis) are localized, tumorous nodules that occur in response to chronic progressive destruction of skin, subcutaneous tissue, fascia, muscle, and bone. In the United States, they are most frequently caused by *Pseudallescheria boydii*, but in other countries Actinomyces, Nocardia, Phialophora, and Aspergillus may be involved. The draining sinuses frequently contain granules containing the infecting agent(s). Those that are nonactinomyces in origin are difficult to eradicate and often require amputation, whereas those associated with Actinomyces are treated with surgery and itraconazole.

Sporotrichosis is caused by the dimorphic fungus *Sporothix schenckii*. A dimorphic fungus is one where the yeast form is present in tissue and the hyphal form in culture. The infection results from traumatic implantation of the fungus that normally grows in the soil. A common source is a prick from a thorn on a rose bush, thus name "rose gardener's disease." It most commonly produces a lymphocutaneous disease characterized by an enlarging, painless nodule at the site of inoculation. Over the course of a the next few weeks, a chain of subcutaneous nodules develop along the lymphatics that frequently suppurate and drain to the skin surface. Cigar-shaped yeast forms are seen in the suppurative nodules, and asteroid bodies (Splendore-Hoeppli phenomenon) are noted within granulomatous microabscesses. Joints may be involved, which accounts for 80% of the extracutaneous disease. The diagnosis is usually made by culture of biopsy material. An oral saturated solution of potassium iodide is used in therapy.

An herpetic whitlow is due to traumatic implantation of herpes simplex type I into the subcutaneous tissue at the tip of the finger. It is a painful, recurrent, vesicular disease with axillary lymphadenopathy, most commonly occurring in dentists.

24. The answer is E. *(Pathology)*
The findings in this patient are most compatible with Meniere disease, which is a type of labyrinthitis involving the cochlea. In Meniere disease, there is an accumulation of fluid (endolymph) in the labyrinth. In a

sensorineural loss (nerve deafness), the Weber test lateralizes to the normal ear, in this case, the left ear. The Rinne test exhibits preservation of air greater than bone conduction in the affected ear, which, in this case, is the right ear.

A demyelinating disease, such as multiple sclerosis, could be associated with vertigo, but the localization of a sensorineural hearing loss in the right ear is against that diagnosis.

A glomus jugulare tumor is a paraganglioma arising from the jugular bulb and tympanic plexus. It is a highly vascular tumor and is associated with a conductive hearing loss, a pulsatile tinnitus, and pulsation of the tympanic membrane that may be inhibited by positive pressure applied to the membrane with a pneumatic otoscope.

A brain stem glioma or a cerebellar tumor are unlikely diagnoses, because the former would have other neurologic signs and the latter would be associated with incoordination and ataxia, rather than vertigo.

25. The answer is B. (Anatomy)
The left cerebral cortex is the location of motor control of speech (Broca area) and motor control of skeletal muscles on the right side of the body. This patient presents with loss of motor speech (motor nonfluent aphasia) and right-sided weakness of extremities that is most significant in the upper limb. The middle cerebral artery supplies the area of cerebral cortex on the lateral side in the area of the lateral sulcus. This region of distribution includes Broca area and the region of precentral and postcentral gyri related topographically to the orofacial and upper limbs.

The anterior cerebral artery distributes blood to the medial surface of the cerebral cortex and to the area of primary motor and sensory cortex related to the lower limb.

The anterior choroidal artery supplies blood to the medial aspects of the temporal lobe including the hippocampal formation.

The posterior cerebral artery supplies the occipital cortex, and loss of blood supply would most likely present first as visual deficits.

26. The answer is A. (Pathology)
The patient most likely has retinitis pigmentosum, which is a degenerative disorder usually beginning in the peripheral part of the retina and progressing centrally (tunnel vision) until even macular vision is destroyed. Retinitis pigmentosum leads to blindness. It may be associated with Friedrich ataxia or abetalipoproteinemia (absent beta apolipoproteins). Friedrich ataxia is associated with neuronal degeneration in the (1) spinocerebellar tracts, posterior columns, pyramidal tracts, and peripheral nerves; (2) retinitis pigmentosum; (3) spinal abnormalities; (4) diabetes mellitus; and (5) cardiac disease. It most commonly has an autosomal recessive inheritance pattern.

Werdnig-Hoffmann disease (upper/lower motor neuron disease in children), multiple sclerosis, tabes dorsalis (neurosyphilis), and retrolental fibroplasia (oxygen-free radical damage to the retina) are not associated with tunnel vision.

27. The answer is C. (Microbiology)
Tenosynovitis in a veterinarian would most likely be due to Pasteurella multocida, which is most commonly contracted by cat (60%–80%) or dog bites. The organism is a gram-negative rod with bipolar staining. If infection occurs within the first 24 hours of a bite, this organism is the most likely offender. It may disseminate to produce a tendinitis, septic arthritis, and osteomyelitis. Penicillin is usually given for infections due to cat bites, whereas ampicillin is used for other bites.

Only Afipia felis (cat-scratch disease) and Pseudomonas mallei (glanders) have a predilection for veterinarians. Pseudomonas aeruginosa and Staphylococcus aureus may be associated with a tenosynovitis, but no more commonly than the general population. Human bites differ from cat/dog bites in that they (1) are more prone to infection than animal bites; (2) frequently contain anaerobes, such as Bacteroides and Fusobacterium species, and aerobes, such as Staphylococcus aureus, Eikenella corrodens, and non–beta-hemolytic streptococci; and (3) often require admission to the hospital, if it is a clench-fist injury over 24 hours old. Treatment must include aerobic and anaerobic coverage. Clindamycin, amoxicillin, and clavulanic acid in combination or cefoxitin or cefotetan alone are used in therapy. Human bites have not been documented to transmit HIV.

Cat-scratch disease is a self-limited disease caused by a gram-negative cell-wall–defective rod, which has been identified as Afipia felis. The disease is most common in young people. Three to 10 days after a cat scratch or contact with a cat, a primary skin papule or pustule develops at the inoculation site. Painful, reactive lymphadenopathy then occurs in the epitrochlear, axillary, or cervical lymph nodes. Granulomatous microabscesses are present. The organisms are best identified with the Warthin-Starry silver stain rather than a Gram stain. The diagnosis is based on the presence of three of the four following criteria: (1) a history of contact with a cat and the presence of a scratch or a dermal lesion, (2) exclusion of other pathogens by tissue culture or serologic tests, (3) a positive skin test reaction for cat-scratch disease, and (4) histopathologic findings in a lymph node of granulomatous microabscesses with silver-stain–positive organisms. Cephalosporins are useful in therapy.

Pseudomonas mallei is the pathogen responsible for producing glanders, a disease associated with horses, mules, and donkeys. In the United States, glanders is usually contracted by inoculation of the organism into an abrasion via contact with an infected horse or by inhalation. The disease is characterized by multiple, noncaseating granulomatous abscesses of the skin, lymphadenopathy, and involvement of the lungs. Chronic disease is called farcy. If left untreated, there is a high mortality rate. Streptomycin and tetracycline are used for therapy.

28. The answer is E.   *(Pathology)*
Tuberous sclerosis is associated with mental retardation, but neurofibromatosis is not. Both conditions have an autosomal dominant inheritance pattern. Tuberous sclerosis is characterized by hamartomatous collections of atypical astrocytes in the brain (i.e., tubers) and calcifications in the brain, as well as angiomyolipomas, hamartomas most commonly located in the kidneys. Neurofibromatosis is associated with an increased incidence of meningiomas, optic gliomas, and acoustic neuromas. Neurofibromatosis is characterized by Lisch nodules, which are hamartomas located in the iris. Neurofibromas may be associated with nodular or pedunculated cutaneous lesions that are frequently pigmented. Tuberous sclerosis also includes cutaneous lesions on the face, called adenoma sebaceum, and subungual fibromas.

29. The answer is A.   *(Anatomy)*
The precentral gyrus of the frontal lobe is the primary motor cortex giving rise to the descending corticospinal tract. The homuncular organization localizes lower limb innervation to the medial aspect of the precentral gyrus. The descending corticospinal tract has its cells of origin in the contralateral cerebral cortex.

Spasticity is one of the cardinal findings in an upper motor neuron syndrome. If the anterior horn cells are involved, the presentation has features of a lower motor neuron syndrome, specifically, a flaccid paralysis.

The fasciculus gracilis is an ascending sensory pathway. A lesion of this pathway may produce ataxia but not paralysis.

30. The answer is D.   *(Pathology)*
Cognitive abnormalities, cerebellar atrophy, and distal sensorimotor peripheral neuropathy all may be associated with alcoholism. Cognitive abnormalities include impairment in recent and remote memory (i.e., Korsakoff's psychosis), confusion, and dementia. Cerebellar atrophy with associated ataxia and mild nystagmus is also a complication associated with alcoholism. The atrophy can be identified by using computed tomography or magnetic resonance imaging. It is related to nutritional deficiency as well as direct toxicity of alcohol on the Purkinje cells. Distal sensorimotor peripheral neuropathy results from a combination of demyelination, which causes sensory disturbances, and axonal degeneration, which causes muscle atrophy. Motor weakness and sensations of burning feet and numbness are common, possibly caused by a direct toxic effect of alcohol or thiamine deficiency.

31. The answer is A.   *(Microbiology)*
Yersinia enterocolitica would most likely be associated with an HLA-B27–positive reactive arthritis. Yersinia are gram-negative coccobacilli that exhibit bipolar staining (safety pin appearance). Transmission of the organism is by the ingestion of contaminated foods, especially pork, milk, and water. It primarily occurs in children, who present with a watery, bloody diarrhea, low-grade fever, and abdominal pain. Aminoglycosides are useful in therapy, although the disease is generally self-limited. Postinfectious complications include the potential for a reactive arthritis and erythema nodosum (localized inflammation of adipose),

particularly in adults. The arthritis develops in individuals who are positive for the HLA-B27 haplotype. The relationship with HLA-B27–positive reactive arthritis is not a feature of the other pathogens listed in the question. Other organisms that have been associated with reactive arthritis include *Yersinia pseudotuberculosis*, Shigella species (mainly *Shigella flexneri*), *Campylobacter jejuni*, and *Chlamydia trachomatis*.

32. The answer is B. *(Pathology)*

Chronic hepatitis associated with degeneration of the lenticular nucleus best characterizes Wilson's disease, an autosomal recessive disease involving a defect in the excretion of copper into bile. Copper accumulation in the hepatocytes produces acute hepatitis, followed by chronic hepatitis. Chronic liver disease results in decreased synthesis of ceruloplasmin, the binding protein for copper. Because total copper is the copper bound to ceruloplasmin plus free copper, the level of total copper in Wilson's disease is decreased, but the level of free copper is increased. The excess free copper is deposited in Descemet's membrane of the eye, producing the Kayser-Fleischer ring, and in the lenticular nuclei, where it produces toxic damage to the neurons, particularly those in the putamen. The definitive diagnosis of Wilson's disease requires biopsy of the liver and quantitation of copper in liver tissue. Penicillamine is used in treatment.

33. The answer is D. *(Neuroanatomy)*

The α-motor neurons represent the "final common pathway" by which the central nervous system influences muscle activity. With the loss of this cell type, there is no reflex response to deep tendon stretch stimulation.

Although descending systems may sprout to innervate other motor neurons in the spinal cord, the specific peripheral distribution of α-motor neurons is not reestablished.

The sensory innervation and γ-system may be retained, but the loss of the α-motor neurons breaks the reflex loop by the loss of extrafusal skeletal muscle stimulation, leading to contraction of the muscle.

This pathway is essential to understanding the findings of individuals with a lower motor neuron syndrome.

34. The answer is A. *(Pathology)*

The photograph of synovial fluid shows a needle-shaped crystal, which appears yellow in color when oriented parallel to the slow axis of the compensator; therefore, it is a monosodium urate (MSU) crystal, and the patient has acute gouty arthritis. The most common mechanism for gout is decreased excretion of uric acid from the kidneys rather than increased synthesis of uric acid crystals. Increased production of uric acid may be caused by an increase in 5-phosphoribosyl-1-pyrophosphate (PPRP) or a decrease in hypoxanthine-guanine phosphoribosyltransferase (HGPRT, activity. A deficiency of HGPRT results in increased PRPP levels, causing increased de novo purine synthesis. Uric acid is the end-product of purine metabolism, so a defect in the urea cycle would not produce these findings. Alcohol does not inhibit HGPRT or have a direct toxic effect on synovial tissue.

The differentiation of MSU crystals associated with gout versus calcium pyrophosphate crystals (CPPD) representing pseudogout is important. Different types of crystals may be identified by synovial fluid (SF) analysis, the two most important being MSU and CPPD. SF analysis via arthrocentesis is performed with strict aseptic technique, and the following tests are usually ordered: (1) volume and gross appearance, (2) a wet prep under polarized light for crystals, and (3) a white blood cell count and differential to distinguish an inflammatory from a noninflammatory joint disease. The SF is first examined under polarized light to see if any crystals are present. If they are, an examination with a first-order red filter in place follows. MSU crystals are usually elongated and needle shaped (monoclinic), whereas the crystals of pseudogout may be either chunky (triclinic) or needle shaped like MSU. Gout is never associated with chunky crystals. Under routine polarized light, the crystals of both gout and pseudogout polarize and they are found either phagocytized by neutrophils or free within the SF fluid. When viewing the SF through a red filter and aligning the crystals parallel to the slow axis of the compensator at the base of the microscope, the crystals of MSU are yellow, whereas the crystals of pseudogout are blue. The polarizing characteristics of MSU define negative birefringence, whereas the findings for CPPD define weakly positive birefringence.

35. The answer is C.   *(Microbiology)*
Erysipeloid, or fish handler's disease, is not a likely hazard in a veterinarian who specializes in large animals. *Erysipelothrix rhusiopathiae* is a gram-positive nonmotile rod that produces alpha hemolysis on blood agar. It is the only gram-positive organism that produces hydrogen sulfide (H_2S). The disease is primarily contracted by butchers or those who work with fish. It is characterized by a localized, nonsuppurative, painful, purple-colored skin rash at the site of inoculation (usually the fingers). Erysipeloid should not be confused with erysipelas, which is caused by a group A streptococcus. Erysipelas is characterized by a raised, erythematous confluent cellulitis that is associated with systemic signs and symptoms. Ampicillin is the treatment of choice.

Brucella species infect the following animals: (1) *Brucella melitensis* infects goats and sheep, (2) *Brucella abortus* is associated with cattle, (3) *Brucella suis* infects pigs, and (4) *Brucella canis* is associated with dogs. Brucella species are gram-negative rods. Most infections in the United States are seen in veterinarians, farmers, and meat packers due to direct contact with infected animal hides, usually cattle (*B. abortus*, most common) and pigs. Infected animals usually develop mastitis, so the disease may also be contracted from unpasteurized milk. Brucellosis in man is usually mild. Severe forms present with disseminated disease, which is spread from the lymphatics throughout the body. Noncaseating granulomatous abscesses are noted in the liver, spleen, and bone marrow. Undulant fever is most commonly due to *B. melitensis*, which is the most severe form of the disease. Serologic tests are the mainstay for diagnosis. Tetracycline plus streptomycin are used in therapy.

Leptospira are tightly wound spirochetes with a crook at the end that resembles a shepherd's staff. They are best visualized by darkfield microscopy. *Leptospira interrogans* is the main pathogen found in the United States. The most important reservoirs for the disease are rodents and domesticated animals, which shed the organisms in the urine into the soil and water where they may live for hours or weeks. The dog is presently the major source of human leptospirosis in the United States. Veterinarians and farmers and those swimming in infected ponds are at increased risk. Indirect contact with infected urine through abraded skin, conjunctival surfaces, and mucosal surfaces allows the organisms to invade the host. Leptospirosis is a biphasic disease and is subdivided into the septicemic phase and the immune phase. Disease severity ranges from a mild (90% of cases) flu-like syndrome with anicteric hepatitis to severe disease (Weil disease), which is associated with jaundice, an extensive hemorrhagic diathesis, and renal failure. In the septicemic phase, the organisms damage the endothelial lining of capillaries (hemorrhagic rash) and spread diffusely throughout the body, most notably the conjunctiva (conjunctivitis and photophobia), the liver (liver cell necrosis), the kidneys (interstitial nephritis), and the central nervous system (meningitis). This phase is terminated by the appearance of antibodies (immune phase) and the presence of numerous organisms in the urine. Urine is an excellent body fluid to examine by dark field microscopy to confirm the disease. The diagnosis is otherwise made by (1) identifying the organisms in the blood or spinal fluid, (2) using serologic tests, or (3) culture of body fluids. High-dose penicillin is used in therapy. Death may occur in 5% to 30% of untreated cases, with renal and/or liver failure.

Q fever is the only rickettsia that may be transmitted without a vector. It is primarily transmitted by inhalation and occasionally by tick bites. Q fever is most frequently contracted by people who have an association with (1) the birthing process of infected sheep, cattle, or goats; (2) the handling of milk in these animals; or (3) exposure to pregnant cats. It characteristically produces (1) an interstitial pneumonia with flu-like symptoms; (2) granulomatous hepatitis (30%); (3) granulomas in the bone marrow, with the characteristic ring granuloma; and, rarely, (4) infective endocarditis. A complement fixation test is the mainstay for the diagnosis. Doxycycline or chloramphenicol may be used in the treatment.

Listeria are gram-positive bacilli that reside intracellularly in monocytes and/or macrophages. Regarding their culture characteristics, they (1) produce beta hemolysis (complete hemolysis) on blood agar in cold temperature, (2) are motile, and (3) are catalase positive. In adults, listeriosis is usually contracted by eating contaminated, ready-to-eat foods, such as soft cheeses and cooked chicken, or by drinking unpasteurized milk. Less frequent modes of transmission include direct contact (butchers, veterinarians) and transplacental transmission to the fetus. In veterinarians, it produces a localized skin infection. When transmitted transplacentally it is associated with stillbirths, neonatal meningitis (10%), and sepsis (high mortality rate). Granulomatous abscesses are noted in disseminated disease, thus the name granulomatis infantisepticum. Listeriosis is a leading cause of meningitis in cancer and renal transplant patients who are immunocompromised. There is an oculoglandular form that is diagnosed with the Anton test. In this test conjunctival inoculation of a guinea pig or rabbit produces a keratoconjunctivitis. Culture techniques are available. Serologic techniques are unreliable. Ampicillin plus gentamicin are used in therapy.

36. The answer is A. *(Pathology)*
Anti–smooth muscle antibody and antimitochondrial antibody are associated with liver disease. Anti–smooth muscle antibody is most commonly seen in autoimmune (lupoid) hepatitis. Antimitochrondrial antibodies are characteristic of primary biliary cirrhosis. Regarding the other choices in the question:

- Antimicrosomal antibodies are seen in Hashimoto thyroiditis and Graves disease.
- Antineutrophil cytoplasmic antibodies are of two types based on immunofluorescent studies—the perinuclear type (p-ANCA) and the cytoplasmic type (c-ANCA). p-ANCA is most commonly associated with polyarteritis nodosa (mnemonic: **P** = **p**olyarteritis), while the c-ANCA is primarily seen in Wegener granulomatosis.
- The anticentromere antibody is seen in a variant of progressive systemic sclerosis, which is called the CREST syndrome (**C** = **c**alcinosis, **R** = **R**aynaud phenomenon, **E** = **e**sophageal motility problems, **S** = **s**clerodactyly, and **T** = **t**elangiectasia).
- Antigliadin antibodies are associated with celiac disease. Gliadin is the alcohol extract of gluten in wheat.
- Anti–parietal cell antibodies are characteristic of pernicious anemia.
- Antihistone antibodies are specific to drug-induced lupus.
- Antiepithelial antibodies are noted in pemphigus vulgaris and bullous pemphigoid.
- Anti–islet cell antibodies are found in type I diabetes mellitus.

37. The answer is D. *(Anatomy)*
Cranial nerves III (oculomotor), VI (abducens), and XII (hypoglossal) exit the ventral surface of the brain stem. The descending corticospinal tract is located ventrally and on the midline of the brain stem until it decussates and courses laterally at the low medulla and spinal cord junction. Therefore, these structures are closely related anatomically and share the same blood supply. Vascular lesions produce concomitant signs of motor dysfunction and cranial nerve involvement. This combination of neurologic complaints helps to localize the level of the brain stem being affected.

Cranial nerve IV exits dorsally, whereas cranial nerves V, VII, VIII, IX, X exit laterally and dorsolaterally from the brain stem.

38. The answer is E. *(Pathology)*
A 23-year-old man with a recent history of chlamydial urethritis followed within a few weeks by bilateral conjunctivitis, painful swelling of his right knee and ankle, and painless ulcers on his penis has Reiter syndrome, which has an HLA-B27 positive haplotype in 90% of cases. Reiter syndrome is defined as a seronegative (rheumatoid factor negative) spondyloarthropathy that most commonly involves young males and is frequently associated with an initial infection caused by chlamydia or intestinal infections secondary to Shigella, Salmonella, Campylobacter, or Yersinia. The arthritis typically begins a few weeks after the infectious episode, and most commonly involves the knees, ankles, and fingers and toes that characteristically appear diffusely sausage shaped; synovial taps reveal Reiter cells, which are monocytes that have phagocytized neutrophils. Low back pain is often associated with sacroiliitis. Indomethacin is the treatment of choice for the arthritis. The conjunctivitis (40%) is noninfectious. Cutaneous lesions include (1) balanitis circinata, which refers to the presence of painless ulcers on the glans penis and urethral meatus, and (2) keratoderma blennorrhagia, which is a hyperkeratotic skin lesion.

39. The answer is C. *(Microbiology)*
Streptococcus bovis, a group D, non-enterococcus, for unexplained reasons, is associated with septicemia and/or endocarditis in patients with colon cancer. When this organism is isolated in the blood in any patient, endoscopic screening or radiographic screening for an occult colorectal cancer is recommended.

Streptococci are gram-positive cocci (in chains or as diplococci) that are catalase negative. They are classified on the basis of the type of hemolysis they exhibit when cultured on blood agar. α-Hemolysis refers to incomplete hemolysis and is associated with a green color from biliverdin pigment. β-Hemolysis is complete hemolysis with a clear zone around the colonies. γ-Hemolysis is the absence of hemolysis in blood agar. The Lancefield antigen groups from A to U are also used to serologically separate out different Streptococci on the basis of the differences in carbohydrate in their cell walls. *Streptococcus viridans* and *Streptococcus pneumoniae* are not classified with the Lancefield system. Group A streptococci (*Streptococcus pyogenes*) are (1) β-hemolytic, (2) possess the M protein, which is a virulence factor that is anti-phagocytic, and, unlike other streptococci, (3) have no growth around a bacitracin disk, indicating susceptibility to bacitracin. Group B streptococci (*Streptococcus agalactiae*) are (1) β-hemolytic, (2) resistant to a bacitracin disk, (3) exhibit sodium hippurate hydrolysis, and (4) react synergistically with *Staphylococcus aureus* hemolysin (CAMP test). Group D streptococci are subdivided into enterococci (*Streptococcus fecalis*, now called Enterococcus) or non-enterococci (*Streptococcus bovis*). They (1) have a variable hemolysis pattern, (2) are resistant to bacitracin, (3) grow in 6.5% salt solution (only enterococci, not non-enterococci, like *S. bovis*), and (4) grow in bile-esculin agar to produce a black discoloration of the agar. *Streptococcus viridans* is (1) α-hemolytic, (2) not inhibited by Optochin (quinine derivative), and (3) is not bile-esculin soluble. *Streptococcus pneumoniae* exhibits (1) α-hemolysis, (2) is inhibited by Optochin, (3) is bile-esculin soluble, and (4) contains a carbohydrate in its cell wall that is precipitated by C-reactive protein in the plasma.

Diseases that are most commonly associated with *Streptococcus pyogenes* include (1) exudative pharyngitis/tonsillitis due to a bacteria (35% of cases, most are viral), (2) rheumatic fever (immunologic disease), (3) retropharyngeal abscess (usually in children less than 4 years of age) or a retrotonsillar (peritonsillar) abscess in older children/adults, (4) scarlet fever, (5) poststreptococcal immune complex glomerulonephritis, (6) impetigo (Staphylococcus to a lesser extent), (7) cellulitis with lymphangiitis ("red streaks"), and (8) erysipelas. Common infections associated with *Streptococcus pyogenes* include (1) pneumonia complicating influenza, (2) meningitis, (3) conjunctivitis, (4) otitis media, (5) orbital cellulitis complicating sinusitis, and (6) puerperal sepsis (postpartum endometritis).

Streptococcus agalactiae (Group B Streptococcus) is (1) the most common cause of neonatal sepsis and meningitis, and (2) a common cause of chorioamnionitis, urinary tract infections, and postpartum endometritis.

Group D *Streptococcus (Enterococcus) faecalis* is commonly associated with infective endocarditis and genitourinary infections.

Streptococcus bovis is a non-enterococcal Group D streptococcus that is associated with septicemia and/or endocarditis in patients with colon cancer.

Streptococcus pneumoniae (*Pneumococcus*) is the most common pathogen associated with (1) community-acquired bronchopneumonia and lobar pneumonia, (2) otitis media, (3) meningitis (adult meningitis), (4) septicemia in splenectomized patients, (5) sinusitis, and (6) spontaneous bacterial peritonitis in the nephrotic syndrome.

Streptococcus viridans is the most common cause of subacute bacterial endocarditis. *Streptococcus mutans* is associated with dental caries.

40. The answer is A. *(Pathology)*

The patient has calcium pyrophosphate dihydrate (CPPD) crystal deposition arthropathy in the setting of chondrocalcinosis. The non-polarized slide of synovial fluid (SF) reveals numerous neutrophils, some of which have phagocytized chunky, triclinic crystals consistent with calcium pyrophosphate and pseudogout. The polarized slide shows the polarization characteristics of this crystal—it is blue if the red filter is in place and the crystal is aligned with the slow axis of the compensator. CPPD, or pseudogout, is a type of degenerative joint disease characterized by the deposition of calcium pyrophosphate in joints, most commonly the knee (> 50%). The disease may be hereditary, idiopathic, associated with metabolic disease (e.g., primary hyperparathyroidism, hemochromatosis), or associated with joint trauma (osteoarthritis). The crystals may deposit in cartilage (chondrocalcinosis), the synovial cavity, or in the synovium. Precipitating events for acute arthritis include surgery or an acute medical illness. The majority of patients show a progressive degeneration of the joints involved. The radiograph appearance of punctate and linear densities in articular hyaline or fibrocartilaginous tissue is almost diagnostic for CPPD.

None of the other choices listed in the question are associated with calcium pyrophosphate crystals.

41. The answer is D. *(Physiology)*
When a nerve cell is at rest, the pump is counterbalancing the leak of Na^+ and K^+ across the cell membrane. When the pump is pumping 3 Na^+ out and 2 K^+ in, the leak must be 3 Na^+ in and 2 K^+ out. If the pump changes to 1 Na^+ out and 1 K^+ in, the continuing leak of 3 Na^+ in but only 2 K^+ out adds net positive charge to the inside of the cell, partially depolarizing the membrane potential. The partial depolarization reduces the electrochemical force moving Na^+ in and increases the electrochemical force moving K^+ out. A new resting membrane potential is established. Here the rate of leak of the ions counterbalances the effect of the pump, that is, the leak is 1 Na^+:1 K^+.

42. The answer is B. *(Pathology)*
Rheumatoid arthritis is associated with ankylosis of the joint space caused by the development of pannus, which overgrows and destroys the articular cartilage. Regarding the other choices in the question

- osteoarthritis is a non-inflammatory joint disease distinguishable by erosion of the articular cartilage. Reactive bone formation occurs at the margins of the joint and produces characteristic osteophytes, or spurs, that are visible on a radiograph.
- chronic gout that results in the formation of tophi causes a very destructive joint disease characterized by erosions of the bone with overhanging margins.
- psoriatic arthritis, in < 10% of cases, produces a very destructive arthritis that usually involves the joints of the hands and causes a characteristic "pencil-in-cup" deformity.
- ankylosing spondylitis is a seronegative spondyloarthropathy usually affecting young males. There is a strong HLA-B27 positive haplotype relationship. The disease usually begins in the sacroiliac area to produce a sacroiliitis. Eventually the vertebral column is involved and the vertebra fuse together forming a "bamboo" spine.

43. The answer is E. *(Microbiology)*
Escherichia coli is more likely to be associated with spontaneous bacterial peritonitis in an alcoholic than *Pseudomonas aeruginosa*.

The Enterobacteriaceae family, of which *Escherichia coli* is a member, are gram-negative, non–spore-forming rods that contain endotoxin in their cell walls. The limulus test is used to detect endotoxin in body fluids. The Enterobacteriaceae (1) ferment glucose to acid, (2) reduce nitrates to nitrites, which is useful in identifying urinary tract infections, (3) have K antigen, which is the capsule antigen that is responsible for a positive Quellung reaction, (4) have flagellar (H) antigens (only *E. coli* and *Salmonella* species), and (5) have somatic (O) antigens. Their capsules suppress phagocytosis. The family Enterobacteriaceae has the following major pathogens: (1) *Escherichia* (2) *Shigella*, (3) *Salmonella*, (4) *Klebsiella*, (5) *Enterobacter*, (6) *Proteus*, (7) *Yersinia*, and (8) *Serratia*. Various *Escherichia coli* strains produce a (1) heat-stable toxin (ST) that stimulates guanylate cyclase; (2) heat-labile toxin (LT) that simulates adenylate cyclase; and (3) verotoxin (O157: H7), which damages endothelial cells and produces the hemolytic uremic syndrome. To isolate and identify these organisms differential media are used. MacConkey's and eosin-methylene-blue (EMB) agars differentiate lactose fermenters, such as *Escherichia coli*, *Klebsiella*, and *Enterobacter*, from nonlactose fermenters (transparent colonies), such as *Salmonella, Shigella, Proteus*, and *Pseudomonas*. In MacConkey's agar, lactose fermenters have pink colonies, whereas nonlactose fermenters have transparent colonies. In EMB agar, lactose fermenters have a metallic green appearance, whereas nonlactose fermenters have transparent colonies. Bile salts and antibiotics are used to suppress growth by other organisms. Highly selective media (*Salmonella-Shigella* agar, Hektoen enteric agar) are also available to separate out pathogenic, nonlactose fermenters from nonpathogenic, nonlactose fermenters. Some of the bacteria swarm over culture media, such as Proteus. *Pseudomonas aeruginosa* produces a greenish pigment called pyocyanin that is helpful in identifying colonies.

Escherichia coli is the most common cause of (1) acute cystitis and pyelonephritis, (2) spontaneous bacterial peritonitis in alcoholics, (3) traveler's diarrhea (enterotoxigenic strain), (4) hemolytic uremic syndrome in children (enterohemorrhagic toxin

O157:H7) due to eating undercooked hamburgers, (5) endotoxic shock, and (6) acute cholecystitis. It is a common pathogen in (1) neonatal meningitis (second most common pathogen); (2) pneumonia in hospitalized patients due to colonization of the airways by the organism; (3) gastroenteritis in infants under 2 years of age (enteropathogenic); (4) enteroinvasive gastroenteritis with bloody diarrhea; (5) peritonitis; (6) wound infections, particularly in people with diabetes; and (7) septicemia (shares the lead with *Staphylococcus aureus*).

Pseudomonas aeruginosa is a pigment producer (pyocyanin) and the most common cause of (1) death due to pneumonia in patients with cystic fibrosis, (2) death due to wound infections in patients with third-degree burns, (3) infections associated with nail punctures through rubber footwear, (4) malignant otitis externa, (5) ecthyma gangrenosum, characterized by black ulcers and/or abscesses of the skin, and (6) hot tub folliculitis from improperly chlorinated hot tubs. It is a common pathogen in hospital-acquired (nosocomial) pneumonia (respirator transmitted); external otitis, or swimmer's ear; purulent conjunctivitis; and septic shock (75% mortality). *Pseudomonas cepacia* is a common terminal pathogen in respiratory disease associated with cystic fibrosis.

44. The answer is C.   *(Pathology)*
Osteoarthritis (OA) is the most common rheumatologic disease in the United States and is characterized by progressive loss of articular cartilage associated with reactive changes at the margin of the joints and in the subchondral bone. It has a predilection for weight-bearing joints, such as the hips and knees. OA is an age-dependent disease, which is found generally in people older than 65 years, predominantly in women. Although the exact etiology of OA is unknown, biomechanical, biochemical, inflammatory, and immunologic factors (HLA-A1 and -B8 haplotypes) have been implicated, and genetic factors play a role in development of OA in the distal interphalangeal joints of the hands. Secondary causes include (1) congenital hip dislocation in children; (2) hemochromatosis; (3) previous trauma (including arthroscopy and arthroscopic surgery); and (4) obesity, which particularly affects the knees. Initially, a process called fibrillation occurs, in which the cartilaginous surface of a joint is eroded, and clefts that penetrate into subchondral bone appear at right angles to the surface. Cartilage fibrillation in

OA can cause fragments of cartilage to break loose and result in the creation of "joint mice." The eventual erosion of the cartilaginous layer in OA can result in reactive bone formation and dense sclerotic bone resembling ivory (eburnation), as bone rubs against bone. Osteophytes (bony spurs) develop along the margins of the joints and are responsible for (1) the "lipping" found in the vertebral bodies, (2) Heberden nodes found at the base of the distal interphalangeal (DIP) joint of the hands, and (3) Bouchard nodes in the proximal interphalangeal (PIP) joints of the hand. Radiographs of affected joints can show both subchondral bone cysts that develop beneath the articular surface and the reduction in joint space. Patients with OA, which is usually asymmetric, slowly develop joint pain with stiffness and enlargement accompanied by limitation of motion. Secondary synovitis is common and is manifested by pain on compression of the joint; pain on passive motion of the joint and crepitus (crackling in the joint) are common. OA in the hip leads to the onset of pain and a limp, accompanied by a loss of hip motion on internal rotation or extension. OA in the knee produces pain and muscle atrophy from disuse. In the spine, OA may involve the intervertebral discs, vertebral bodies, or the posterior apophyseal articulations; pain, stiffness, and compression neuropathies commonly occur.

Rheumatoid arthritis (RA) is a chronic, systemic inflammatory collagen disease that eventually results in progressive destruction of the joint, deformity, and the potential for disability in the patient. It is most common in middle-aged women between 30 and 50 years old, but can involve all ages. It is postulated that RA is triggered by an infectious agent (Epstein-Barr, Mycoplasma, etc) in unison with certain genetic factors (HLA-DR4 haplotype is common). It is an inflammatory disease of the synovium, where an exogenous trigger (infectious agent) activates CD4 T cells in the synovial tissue, which in turn activate B cells, which develop into plasma cells. The plasma cells synthesize immunoglobulin, and IgM autoantibodies develop, in 80% of cases, against the crystallizable fragment (Fc) portion of autologous IgG (rheumatoid factor). IgG antibodies frequently self-associate with each other to form immune complexes (type III hypersensitivity). The immune complexes activate the complement system, certain components of which are chemotactic to neutrophils. The phagocytosis of immune complexes (rheumatoid factor aggregates) by neutrophils produces ragocytes, which can be seen in the synovial fluid. The release of lysosomal enzymes by neutrophils, monocytes, and cytokines (interleukin I and tumor necrosis factor) from lymphocytes, endothelial cells, and monocytes sparks a chronic synovitis with the formation of hyperplastic synovial tissue, called pannus. The pannus spreads over the articular cartilage and destroys it. Subsequent chronic inflammation results in erosions of bone and reactive fibrosis leading to fusion (ankylosis) of the joint space and immobility of the joint. As a rule, the disease is insidious and manifests with symmetric involvement of the joints. The joints that are commonly involved include those in the (1) hands, particularly the metacarpo-phalangeal (MCP) and PIP joints; (2) wrists; (3) foot; (4) elbows; (5) shoulders; (6) knee; and (7) neck, with a predilection for the atlantoaxial joint, leading to possible subluxation and vertebrobasilar insufficiency. Morning stiffness lasting more than an hour is a classic feature of the disease. Advanced RA involving the hands and wrists produces ulnar deviation of the fingers due to

laxity of the soft tissue. A "swan neck" deformity can result from contracture of the interosseous and flexor muscles and tendons causing a flexion contracture of the MCP joint, hyperextension of the PIP joint, and flexion of the DIP joint. A boutonniere's deformity is due to a flexion deformity of the PIP joint and extension of the DIP joint. Baker's synovial cysts can occur in the popliteal fossa and are often confused with popliteal artery aneurysms. RA is a systemic disease that affects many organ systems including the heart, lungs, nervous system, and hematologic system. Laboratory findings include (1) a positive rheumatoid factor, which is also present in diseases other than RA (e.g., infectious endocarditis); (2) an increased erythrocyte sedimentation rate; (3) polyclonal gammopathy, due to chronic inflammation; (4) a positive serum antinuclear antibody test; and (5) radiologic findings demonstrating joint erosions, narrowing of the joint space, and ankylosis. Nonsteroidals or salicylates are the primary treatment, followed by methotrexate. The features of RA differ from those of OA as indicated in the table.

	Osteoarthritis	Rheumatoid Arthritis
Type of joint disease	non-inflammatory	inflammatory
Sex relationship	female predominant	female predominant
Joint involvement	articular cartilage	synovial tissue (pannus)
Age	older individuals	all ages
Weight-bearing joints	yes	smaller joints
Symmetry	asymmetrical	symmetrical
Hands	DIP and PIP	PIP and MCP
Type of disease	degenerative	immunologic
HLA relationship	? HLA A1 and B8	HLA Dr4
Systemic features	no	yes
Laboratory	unremarkable	frequently abnormal
Osteophytes (spurs)	yes	no
Morning stiffness	not prominent	prominent
Ankylosis of joint	no	yes

45. The answer is E. (Anatomy)

Axoaxonic synapses produce either presynaptic inhibition or presynaptic facilitation. They do not initiate action potentials to be conducted in either direction; nor do they block the propagation of action potentials. They appear to alter the influx of calcium ions into the axon terminal. The number of synaptic vesicles released from the axon terminal is proportional to the influx of calcium ions. Therefore, in presynaptic inhibition, the axoaxonic synapse reduces the influx of calcium that occurs when an action potential passes over the axon terminal, and thereby reduces the quantity of neurotransmitter released from the axon terminal.

46. The answer is E.   *(Pathology)*
An autoantibody against IgG (usually IgM) describes the rheumatoid factor (RF), which is more likely to be seen in rheumatoid arthritis (RA) than in ankylosing spondylitis (AS). Ankylosing spondylitis (AS) is a sero-negative (RF negative) spondyloarthropathy that is either seen alone or in association with other disorders such as Reiter syndrome, psoriatic spondylitis, intestinal infections, and inflammatory bowel disease. AS most commonly involves young men between 15 and 30 years of age who are HLA-B27 positive (95% of cases). Approximately 20% of patients who are HLA-B27 positive will develop AS or one of the other variants upon exposure to the environmental factors listed above. Characteristic features include an insidious onset of sacroiliitis, persistence for more than 3 months, and morning stiffness in the lower back that is relieved with exercise, as well as a diminished anterior flexion of the spine, which can be identified with the Schoeber test. The vertebral column is eventually involved with subsequent fusion of the vertebral column and production of the "bamboo spine." Complications include (1) restricted chest movement with development of a restrictive type of lung disease; (2) iridocyclitis, with a potential for visual loss; and (3) aortic valve incompetence with regurgitation in a small percentage of cases. Indomethacin is the treatment of choice.

47. The answer is B.   *(Microbiology)*
Babesia microti is a sporozoan that infects erythrocytes and is transmitted by the bite of an Ixodes tick, the same tick that transmits *Borrelia burgdorferi,* the cause of Lyme disease. In some cases, both diseases are present at the same time. Babesiosis is endemic along the Eastern seaboard in Massachusetts, Long Island, and Martha's Vineyard. Clinically, patients present with chills, fever, headache, and a hemolytic anemia. The majority of people recover from the disease. The laboratory diagnosis is made by (1) examining the peripheral blood and looking for intraerythrocytic organisms that are similar to malaria, (2) serologic tests, and (3) hamster inoculation. Clindamycin plus quinine are used for treatment. Regarding the other choices in the question, all of them are associated with transmission by ticks, but not the same tick associated with Lyme disease.

Colorado tick bite fever is due to an arborvirus that is introduced into the patient by a tick bite. Within 3 to 6 days of a bite, patients experience high fevers, shaking chills, generalized myalgias, headache, abdominal pain, and petechial rash (~10%, unlike Rocky Mountain spotted fever). Absolute leukopenia is characteristic and is related to a maturation arrest in the bone marrow of the granulocytic series. It is a self-limited disease. The diagnosis is made with mouse inoculation and fluorescent antibody staining of the patient's red blood cells, which are infected by the organism.

Relapsing fever is caused by the spirochete, *Borrelia recurrentis.* The disease may be tick-borne or louse-borne. The tick-borne disease is characterized by (1) relapses of high fever, due to the emergence of new antigen types; (2) rash; and (3) neurologic abnormalities. The organisms are visualized in peripheral smears during relapses. The laboratory diagnosis is made by observation of the spirochetes in the blood and by serologic tests. Tetracycline is the treatment of choice.

Ehrlichiosis is a tick-borne disease caused by the rickettsia, *Ehrlichia canis.* The disease resembles Rocky Mountain spotted fever except for the presence of the rash. The organisms live in leukocytes. It primarily occurs in the southern United States. Tetracycline is the treatment of choice.

Rickettsia are obligate intracellular parasites that perpetuate themselves in arthropod vectors. Once introduced into the host by a vector, they invade endothelial cells and produce a vasculitis, which, in some types of rickettsial disease, eventuates in a dark, crusted lesion called an eschar at the site of inoculation. Their pathogenicity is related to their ability to activate endogenous phospholipase A, which enhances inflammation and thrombosis via its stimulation of arachidonic acid metabolism. Rickettsia are also able to leave phagolysosomes. Rocky Mountain spotted fever is the most frequently reported rickettsial disease in the United States. The organism is *Rickettsia rickettsiae.* It has its highest incidence in Oklahoma and North Carolina and is transmitted by the bite of the hard tick, Dermacentor andersoni. Doxycycline or chloramphenicol may be used in treatment. Without treatment, 20% of patients will die, whereas treatment lowers the rate to 5%.

48. The answer is E. *(Pathology)*
Patients with syringomyelia, diabetes mellitus, and tabes dorsalis have an increased incidence of neuropathic arthropathy (Charcot joint). Charcot joint refers to the development of joint disease in neurologic diseases characterized by a loss of pain sensation, proprioception, or both. The combination of neurotrauma in a joint that cannot sense pain, as well as a neurovascular component altering blood flow to the joint, causes destruction of the joint. The joints involved depend on the disease: In diabetes, which is the most common cause of Charcot joint, this disorder primarily involves the feet; in syringomyelia the glenohumeral joint, elbow, and wrist are most affected; in tabes dorsalis the hips, knees, and ankles are most often involved. There is no relationship between osteoarthritis, rheumatoid arthritis, ankylosing spondylitis, or Reiter syndrome and Charcot joint.

49. The answer is E. *(Physiology)*
When an ion is in electrochemical equilibrium, the concentration gradient acting to move that ion across the membrane is counterbalanced by the electrical gradient acting to move that ion in the opposite direction. In this case the concentration gradient is forcing Cl⁻ into the cell while the electrical gradient is forcing Cl⁻ out. If a change is to produce net influx, it must either increase the concentration gradient pushing in or decrease the electrical gradient pushing out. Opening additional Cl⁻ channels does not change either gradient, it merely makes it easier for random diffusion to occur while maintaining the electrochemical equilibrium. Decreasing the Cl⁻ concentration outside or increasing the Cl⁻ concentration inside the cell makes the concentration gradient less than the electrical gradient, thereby producing net efflux. Hyperpolarizing the cell increases the electrical gradient that is pushing out; thus net efflux. Depolarization, however, decreases the electrical gradient. Therefore, the greater concentration gradient produces net influx.

50. The answer is E. *(Pathology)*
A 45-year-old woman who is obese, complains of bilateral hip pain when walking, and whose radiographs reveal narrowing of the joint space and spurs (osteophytes) at the margins of the joints has osteoarthritis (OA). You would expect laboratory tests to show no abnormalities because OA is a noninflammatory joint disease. The various joint diseases are classified in the following four major categories:

Group I: Noninflammatory

- osteoarthritis (most common joint disease)
- neuropathic (Charcot joint)

Group II: Inflammatory

- rheumatoid arthritis (most common autoimmune disease)
- gout (hyperuricemia)
- pseudogout (calcium pyrophosphate)
- systemic lupus erythematosus
- ankylosing spondylitis (HLA-B27 haplotype)
- Reiter disease (urethritis, conjunctivitis, HLA-B27 positive arthritis)
- psoriatic arthritis

Group III: Septic

- infectious arthritis due to bacteria, fungi, and viruses

Group IV: Hemorrhagic

- hemophilia A or B
- trauma
- scurvy

Key synovial fluid (SF) findings that help distinguish these groups include:

Normal SF

- Color: pale yellow
- WBC count: < 200 cells/μl
- Neutrophils: < 25% of total count
- Glucose: < 10 mg/dl difference from serum

Group I: Noninflammatory

- Color: yellow
- WBC count: 200–2000 cells/μl (sometimes from mild secondary synovitis)
- Neutrophils: < 25% of total count
- Glucose: < 10 mg/dl difference from serum

Group II: Inflammatory

- Color: yellow-white
- WBC count: 2000–100,000 cells/μl
- Neutrophils: > 50% of total count
- Glucose: > 25 mg/dl difference from serum
- Crystals: present if gout or pseudogout

Group III: Septic

- Color: yellow-green
- WBC count: 100,000–200,000 cells/μl
- Neutrophils: > 75% of total count
- Glucose: 50 mg/dl or greater difference from serum
- Culture: positive (depending on the organism)

Group IV: Hemorrhagic

- Color: red-brown
- WBC count: 5,000–10,000 cells/μl (same as peripheral blood)
- Neutrophils: > 25% of total count (same as peripheral blood)
- Glucose: < 10 mg/dl difference from serum

51. The answer is A.   *(Microbiology)*
Eosinophilia in parasitic diseases is only present in invasive helminthic infections. *Enterobius vermicularis,* a nematode, is the cause of enterobiasis, or pinworms. It is contracted by the ingestion of embryonated (live) eggs. The larvae develop in the lumen of the small intestine, and adults only have a superficial attachment to the cecum and appendix, so eosinophilia does not occur.

Ascaris lumbricoides is a nematode that infests humans after ingestion of the eggs. The eggs develop into larva that penetrate the small intestine and pass through the lungs, often producing cough and hemoptysis. The larva are then swallowed and form adults, which live unattached in the lumen of the small intestine. Because the larval phase is the only invasive part of the disease, eosinophilia only develops during this phase and not the adult phase. Intestinal obstruction may occur in heavy infestation with tangles of worms obstructing the bowel lumen. Less common findings include acute appendicitis and biliary tract inflammation. The laboratory diagnosis is made by identifying the undeveloped eggs in the stool. Mebendazole or pyrantel pamoate may be used in therapy.

Ancylostoma duodenale and *Necator americanus* (most common) are nematodes that produce hookworm disease. They infect humans by penetration of the unprotected skin of the foot by larvae in infected soil. The larvae migrate through the lungs and are then swallowed. Larvae develop into adults in the small intestine, where they attach themselves to the tip of the villi with buccal capsules containing cutting plates.

Blood is lost in the lumen and also feeds the worms, resulting in iron deficiency in a small number of patients (3%). Clinically, patients develop a dermatitis at the site of larval penetration, cough, occasional hemoptysis as larvae migrate through the lungs, diarrhea, and abdominal pain. Eosinophilia is prominent in the peripheral blood. The laboratory diagnosis is made by finding undeveloped eggs in the stool. Mebendazole or pyrantel pamoate are the treatments of choice.

Strongyloides stercoralis is a nematode that infects humans via penetration of unprotected skin by free-living filariform larvae living in the soil. Like hookworm and ascaris larvae, they pass through the lungs, are swallowed and then develop into adults after the larvae penetrate the mucosa of the duodenum. Adult worms in the duodenal mucosa copulate and the females lay eggs that hatch into rhabditiform larvae, which pass out of the mucosa and into the lumen. From this location, they may reinfect the mucosa and pass through the lung, penetrate the perianal skin and pass through the lung again, or pass out of the body and live in the soil as free-living filariform larvae. Clinically, patients present with cough, epigastric pain, diarrhea, and peripheral blood eosinophilia. Disseminated strongyloidiasis is sometimes seen in immunocompromised hosts. The diagnosis is made by finding rhabditiform larvae in the stool, duodenal aspirates, or by the string test (Enterotest). Thiabendazole is the treatment of choice.

Cutaneous larva migrans is caused by dog and cat hookworms (*Ancylostoma braziliense* or *A. canium*). It is usually contracted by children who are playing on sandy beaches or playgrounds. The larvae penetrate the skin and produce serpiginous tunnels, which cause intense pruritus and scratching (creeping eruption). Adult worms do not form in man, but do develop in infected dogs and cats. The diagnosis is made by direct observation of the tunnels in the skin. Peripheral eosinophilia is prominent. Oral or topical thiabendazole is used in treatment. *Toxocara canis* or *T. cati* is the cause of visceral larva migrans, which is more common in children than in adults. When the eggs are ingested, the larvae penetrate the bowel mucosa and spread throughout the body, particularly the liver, lungs, and eyes. Similar to cutaneous larva migrans, adults do not develop in man. Clinically, patients present with hepatosplenomegaly, pneumonitis, skin rashes, a prominent peripheral blood eosinophilia, and hyper-gammaglobulinemia. The laboratory diagnosis is made by clinical history, serology, and skin tests. Thiabenda-zole is the treatment of choice.

52. The answer is A.   (Pathology)
A 58-year-old man with a 10-year history of gout and nodular masses in the periarticular tissue of the proximal and distal interphalangeal joints of his right hand has tophus formation, which is pathognomonic for chronic gout. Tophi are deposits of monosodium urate (MSU) crystals in tissue.

Gouty arthritis is a heterogeneous group of disorders characterized by hyperuricemia, recurrent attacks of acute arthritis, formation of deposits of MSU (tophi), and uric acid urolithiasis. It is the most common inflammatory arthritis in men older than 30 years.

Gout is a multifactorial inheritance caused by a combination of genetic susceptibility and the effect of certain environmental factors (e.g., alcohol, eating red meats). Hyperuricemia is associated, but not synonymous, with gout because some patients with gout have normal uric acid levels. Primary hyperuricemia with gout refers to hyperuricemia that is a consequence of a disorder in uric acid metabolism that results from (1) decreased excretion (most common mechanism), (2) increased production, or (3) a combination of the two. Secondary hyperuricemia associated with gout can be caused by the same mechanisms as primary gout. There are secondary associations with diabetes mellitus, alcoholism, polycythemia rubra vera, leukemia, multiple myeloma, diuretic therapy, and the treatment of disseminated carcinomas. Uric acid is the end-product of purine metabolism, which is depicted below.

PRPP
↓
Inosine
↙
Purines (e.g., adenine)
↘
Hypoxanthine
↓←Xanthine oxidase inhibited by allopurinol
Xanthine
↓←Xanthine oxidase inhibited by allopurinol
Uric acid → excreted in the kidney

In adult men the uric acid range is 3.5–7.0 mg/dl, whereas in women the range is slightly lower (2.5–6.0 mg/dl), owing to the action of estrogen on the excretion of uric acid by the kidney. Hyperuricemia may result from (1) an increase in production, secondary to high levels of phosphoribosyl pyrophosphate (PRPP), which may be due to low activity of hypoxanthine guanine phosphoribosyl transferase (HGPRT); or (2) a decrease in the excretion of uric acid by the kidney. The latter accounts for the majority (90%) of cases. Complete deficiency of HGPRT is the sex-linked recessive disease called the Lesch-Nyhan syndrome, characterized by mental retardation, self-mutilation, and hyperuricemia. Fewer than 20% of patients with hyperuricemia will develop clinically apparent crystal deposition. However, the duration and magnitude of hyperuricemia correlate directly to the likeli-

hood of developing gouty arthritis or uric acid urolithiasis.

Acute gouty arthritis is sudden, explosive, and most often occurs at night. The first attack most commonly involves the metatarsophalangeal joint (big toe); called podagra, the condition is often triggered by stress, alcohol, drugs, surgery, or an acute medical illness. The interaction of MSU crystals with mononuclear phagocytes stimulates the release of interleukin-1, which initiates the inflammatory reaction and produces many of the systemic signs of the disease, such as fever and absolute neutrophilic leukocytosis. MSU crystals also lyse neutrophils, which release lysosomal enzymes, thus exacerbating inflammation. Interval gout is characterized by a lack of symptoms and physical findings; MSU crystals, however, can still be found in the joints, usually within leukocyte vacuoles.

Chronic gout is characterized by the presence of tophi, which usually occur after 10 years, and a granulomatous reaction surrounding the MSU crystals deposited in the tissue. Deforming arthritis results in the erosion of cartilage and subchondral bone caused by crystal deposition. Bone erosions occur near tophi and have characteristic overhanging margins. Treatment of acute gouty arthritis is aimed at reducing inflammation, and indomethacin is the most commonly used nonsteroidal agent; colchicine is also used as an anti-inflammatory. Underexcretors are treated with uricosuric agents, such as probenecid and sulfinpyrazone; high-dose aspirin is also uricosuric. Overproducers are treated with allopurinol, which is an xanthine oxidase inhibitor that decreases uric acid production.

Regarding the other choices not mentioned in the discussion:

- histologically, a tophus, which produces a granulomatous reaction with multinucleated giant cells, is unlike a rheumatoid nodule, which is characterized by fibrinoid necrosis.
- MSU is a negatively birefringent crystal. Pseudogout has a crystal exhibiting weakly positive birefringence.

53. The answer is B.   (Anatomy)
Inhibition of acetylcholinesterase accentuates cholinergic responses, particularly the actions of the parasympathetic nervous system, which include stimulation of secretion from the nasal mucosa, i.e., rhinorrhea. At the eye, the condition would be miosis rather than mydriasis, and contraction of the ciliary muscles. At the airways the parasympathetics promote bronchoconstriction. Because the sweat glands are innervated by cholinergic sympathetic nerves, sweating is increased.

54. The answer is D.   (Pathology)
A 22-year-old man presenting with a 4-month history of morning stiffness in his lower back, which is relieved by exercise, and diminished anterior flexion of the spine most likely has ankylosing spondylitis (AS). AS is a seronegative (RF negative) spondyloarthropathy that most commonly involves young men between 15 and 30 years old who are HLA-B27 positive (95% of cases). Characteristic features include an insidious onset of sacroiliitis, persistence for more than 3 months, and morning stiffness in the lower back that

is relieved by exercise. A radiograph of the patient's lower back will indicate sacroiliitis. The vertebral column is eventually involved with subsequent fusion of the vertebral column and production of "bamboo spine." Tests for serum uric acid, serum antinuclear antibodies, and alkaline phosphatase level would be normal.

55. The answer is B.   (Microbiology)
The triad of sinus bradycardia, absolute neutropenia, and hepatosplenomegaly is most likely associated with typhoid fever, due to *Salmonella typhi*. The first two findings are secondary to toxins emitted by the bacteria. The pathogenic *Salmonella* species includes typhi, choleraesuis, and enteritidis, alias typhimurium, which is the most common bacteria of this species isolated in the United States. They all contain the O, H, and Vi antigens (virulence factor) as well as endotoxins (fever and complement stimulator) and enterotoxins. Animal reservoirs carry the organisms in nature (e.g., poultry, turtles, cattle, pigs, sheep). *Salmonella* are non–lactose-fermenting gram-negative rods that are motile and produce hydrogen sulfide.

Typhoid fever is contracted by ingesting contaminated food or water. Unlike other types of *Salmonella*, *S. typhi* only has human reservoirs of disease (e.g., Mary Mallon, or "typhoid Mary"). Paratyphoid fever (enteric fever) is a less severe form of the disease and is caused by *S. choleraesuis* and *S. enteritidis* (typhimurium). During the first week, *S. typhi* attaches to and invades the small bowel, particularly the terminal ileum over Peyer's patches, where it is phagocytized but not killed by neutrophils and macrophages. From the small intestine, they are disseminated by the lymphatic system to the regional lymph nodes and into the blood stream. There is hematogenous dissemination throughout the body, most commonly to the liver, spleen, bone marrow, gallbladder, and kidneys. "Rose spots" on the trunk are 2 to 3 mm in diameter, fade on pressure, and disappear in 3 to 4 days. Fever, malaise, constipation, and pain constitute the symptoms and signs during the first week. *Salmonella* may be cultured in the blood (not the stool) during the first week in 90% of cases. Peyer's patches exhibit reactive hyperplasia and a proliferation of macrophages with phagocytized organisms and red blood cells. During the second week, there is a more sustained bacteremia, and the production of the characteristic triad is bradycardia, absolute neutropenia, and hepatospleno-megaly. Diarrhea is present, and fecal smears reveal mononuclear cells rather than neutrophils. Longitudi-nally oriented ulcerations develop in the mucosa over-lying the hyperplastic Peyer's patches (tuberculosis produces transverse ulcers). Organisms are cultured from the stool in the third week (75%) and the urine during the third and fourth weeks. During the third week, there is fever, exhaustion, and improvement unless complications occur (e.g., jaundice, renal fail-ure). Culture is better than the serologic tests (Widal test) for securing the diagnosis. Chloramphenicol is the treatment of choice for typhoid fever around the world, but in this country ciprofloxacin or ofloxacin are commonly used. Carriers are patients who continue to excrete the organism in the stool for more than 3 months after recovery. They are the reservoir for the disease. Ampicillin and ciprofloxacin eliminates the carrier state in patients with normal gallbladder func-tion. Carriers with cholelithiasis must have a cholecys-tectomy. Untreated, typhoid fever has a mortality rate of 10% to 30%, whereas treatment reduces the mortal-ity to ~6%. Recurrence occurs in 5% to 10% of pa-tients and is increased to 20% in patients who are treated with antibiotics, presumably due to the lack of an immune response.

Chagas disease, falciparum malaria, AIDS, and ame-biasis do not have the characteristic triad of sinus bradycardia, neutropenia, and hepatosplenomegaly.

56. The answer is C. *(Pathology)*
Restrictive lung disease, pleural effusion, absolute neu-tropenia, and xerostomia would most likely be associ-ated with rheumatoid arthritis(RA). Extra-articular features of RA include (1) subcutaneous nodules (rheu-matoid nodules), which are areas of fibrinoid necrosis commonly located on the extensor surface of the fore-arm; (2) small vessel vasculitis; (3) fibrinous pericardi-tis; (4) pulmonary manifestations with effusions (pseu-dochylous) and a restrictive type of lung disease; (5) neurologic abnormalities, such as peripheral neuropa-thies and carpal tunnel syndrome (median nerve en-trapment); (6) ophthalmologic disorders, such as uveal tract inflammation; and (7) hematologic problems such as the anemia of chronic inflammation, autoim-mune hemolytic anemia, and autoimmune neutro-penia (Felty syndrome). Autoimmune neutropenia is frequently associated with Sjögren syndrome, which

consists of RA, xerostomia (dry mouth), and kerato-conjunctivitis (dry eyes), as well as autoimmune de-struction of the minor salivary glands and the lacrimal glands. Regarding the other choices in the question:

- sarcoidosis and progressive systemic sclerosis may be associated with restrictive lung disease, but not the other findings listed.
- systemic lupus erythematosus comes closest to the findings in this case, but xerostomia is not a feature; it is also associated with Sjögren syndrome, but not as commonly as RA.
- mixed connective tissue disease is the least likely to display these symptoms.

57. The answer is E. *(Anatomy)*
The tentorium cerebelli is a sheet of dura mater that extends from the occipital bone forward to attach to the petrous portion of the temporal bone. In this location, it lies between the occipital lobes of the cerebrum and the posterior cranial fossa (cerebellum and brain stem).

The falx cerebri separates the right and left cerebral hemispheres.

No meninges are present, except the covering dura, arachnoid, and pia in the region of the frontal lobe opercula, cisterna magna, or cerebellopontine angle.

58. The answer is C. *(Pathology)*
A child with a constellation of findings including fever, disabling arthritis, rash, and blindness is most likely suffering from juvenile rheumatoid arthritis (JRA). JRA is characterized by a chronic synovial inflamma-tion of unknown origin; it most commonly affects the knees, but can also manifest in wrists, ankles, and the atlanto-axial joint in the neck. In general, JRA is more common in girls than boys, but this varies with the type of JRA, which can be divided into the following variant subsets: Still disease (20%), polyarticular (40%), and pauciarticular (40%). Still disease most closely resembles an infectious disease, with spiking fever, a centripetal rash, generalized lymphadenopa-thy, hepatosplenomegaly, transient arthralgias and ar-thritis, and effusions (pericardial and pleural). The polyarticular variant is associated with destructive ar-thritis, particularly if the patient tests positive for the rheumatoid factor. The pauciarticular variant features polyarthritis and inflammation of the anterior uveal

tract 10%–50%), which predisposes the patient to visual loss and blindness. In most cases of JRA, with the exception of the polyarticular variant, the rheumatoid factor is negative. Anemia and leukocytosis are noted in acute attacks. Aspirin is the major anti-inflammatory agent that is used for treatment. Regarding the other choices in the question:

- rheumatic fever features polyarthritis, but it is not destructive
- Lyme disease displays many of these findings, but blindness is not a key feature
- Henoch-Schoenlein vasculitis has palpable purpura, non-disabling arthritis, but is not associated with blindness
- dermatomyositis does not usually involve the joints

59. The answer is D.   (Microbiology)

Black individuals are protected from developing malaria due to *Plasmodium vivax* because of the absence of Duffy antigen, which is the receptor site for the parasite. Duffy antigen is absent in 70% of West Africans. Glucose 6-phosphate dehydrogenase deficiency, sickle cell disease, and β-thalassemia appear to confer protection against death from *P. falciparum*. The presence or absence of D antigen has no significance in the pathogenesis of malaria.

60. The answer is E.   (Pathology)

A giant cell tumor of bone is more likely to involve the epiphysis than the vertebral column. Most giant cell tumors of bone locate around the knee in the distal femur, proximal tibia, or proximal fibula. Histologically they are composed of a non-neoplastic element of multinucleated giant cells and a neoplastic mononuclear fibroblast-like cell that determines the biologic behavior of the tumor. The majority of giant cell tumors behave in a benign fashion. Incomplete removal of the tumor often results in recurrence with more anaplastic mononuclear cells.

Regarding the other choices in the question, osteoblastomas are benign bone tumors most commonly located in the vertebral column. Vertebral fractures are the most common presentation of osteoporosis. Although breast cancer often metastasizes to bone, it most commonly favors the vertebral column. Pott disease is tuberculosis of the vertebral column, which often extends into the psoas muscle to form an abscess.

61. The answer is B.   (Pharmacology)

Huntington disease is a hereditary degenerative brain disease that is characterized by a loss of neurons from the cerebral cortex and striatum, the latter causing severe involuntary movements. It is believed that loss of γ-aminobutyric acid (GABA)–mediated inhibition of dopaminergic neurons produces the motor disturbance. The neurochemical imbalance is opposite that in Parkinson disease and patients may benefit from dopaminergic antagonists, whereas levodopa and other dopaminergic drugs make the condition worse.

62. The answer is E.   (Microbiology)

A patient who has a positive blood culture for coagulase-negative *Staphylococcus* drawn from the right arm and a negative culture from blood drawn from the left arm has a contaminated specimen. If the cultures from both arms were positive, then the organism is clinically significant and could have been associated with a prosthetic heart valve or infective endocarditis, particularly in an intravenous drug abuser. Pneumonia and osteomyelitis are not commonly produced by coagulase-negative *Staphylococci*.

63. The answer is D.   (Anatomy)

The optic nerve (and chiasm) is located lateral to the bifurcation of the internal carotid into its two main terminal branches. An enlargement of the vessel may encroach upon the optic nerve and produce visual field deficits.

The trigeminal nerve exiting the lateral aspect of the pons is related to circumferential branches of the basilar artery.

The oculomotor nerve exits the ventral surface of the midbrain, passing between the posterior cerebral artery and the superior cerebellar artery. If this nerve were affected by an aneurysm at this location, eye movement problems could occur.

The trochlear and the olfactory nerves are not immediately associated with arteries that are commonly affected by aneurysm malformations.

64. The answer is C.   (Microbiology)

Mycoplasma pneumoniae is more likely to be a community-acquired pneumonia than the other organisms and diseases listed, which are more likely to be hospital acquired (nosocomial). Mycoplasmas are the tiniest free-living organisms and lack a cell wall, which is why antibiotics that inhibit cell wall synthesis, such as penicillins and cephalosporins, are ineffective in treatment. They are sometimes designated pleuropneumonia-like organisms, or Eaton agents. On culture, they have a "fried egg" appearance. *Mycoplasma pneumoniae* is the most common cause of primary atypical (walking) pneumonia. It accounts for 15% to 20% of all pneumonias in adolescents and 50% of the pneumonias in crowded conditions, such as military recruit stations. The incubation period is 2 to 3 weeks. Clinically, it is associated with (1) a nonproductive cough, which is the most common symptom (99%); (2) fever; (3) upper respiratory tract symptoms of pharyngitis, chills, earache, and coryza; and (4) an interstitial pneumonia with localized rales and rhonchi without any signs of consolidation or effusion. A chest radiograph shows segmental and interstitial infiltrates. Other associations include (1) bullous myringitis (hemorrhagic vesicles on the membranes); (2) erythema multiforme (targetlike lesions) with a potential for the Stevens Johnson syndrome involving the skin and mucous membranes in a disseminated manner; and (3) a transient, severe cold, autoimmune hemolytic anemia due to anti-I antibodies. The laboratory diagnosis is made by using serologic tests (indirect immunofluorescence, complement fixation) and culture. Cold agglutinin titers are positive in only 40% to 70% of cases, so they are not a good screen for the disease. Erythromycin is the treatment of choice.

65. The answer is D.   (*Pharmacology*)

Conjugation with glucuronide, a Phase II drug metabolism reaction, is the only significant metabolic fate of lorazepam and oxazepam. Other benzodiazepines are oxidatively metabolized to active metabolites, including several that form desmethyldiazepam, including diazepam, clorazepate, prazepam, and chlordiazepoxide. Flurazepam, alprazolam, and triazolam form other active metabolites by oxidative pathways. Drug oxidation usually declines more with old age than do glucuronidation and other Phase II reactions. Hence, drugs metabolized by Phase II reactions may be safer in the elderly.

66. The answer is B.   (*Microbiology*)

Bacteroides and *Fusobacterium* are both anaerobes that are commonly present together in lung abscesses associated with aspiration of infected oropharyngeal material. Lung abscesses are particularly common in alcoholics.

Anaerobes include cocci (*Peptococcus, Peptostreptococcus*), bacilli (*Lactobacillus, Bacteroides*), and spirochetes (*Fusospirochetes*). Strict culture requirements and sampling procedures are required if they are to be identified in tissue. Pathogenic anaerobic organisms (1) are usually part of the normal flora, (2) commonly associated with a foul odor when infecting tissue, (3) commonly produce abscess formation and necrosis, (4) frequently produce gas, (5) frequently are mixed with other aerobes, (6) often require other organisms to grow (e.g., *Pseudomonas*), and (7) usually develop infections slowly.

Bacteroides species comprise most of the normal flora of the intestine. They are gram-negative and usually stain very faintly with the Gram stain. *Bacteroides* infections typically have vessel thrombosis due to the elaboration of heparinases by the organisms. *B. fragilis* is the most common anaerobic isolate and classically is involved in infections below the diaphragm, such as peritonitis, subdiaphragmatic abscesses, pelvic inflammatory disease, and septicemia. They may also infect decubitus ulcers. Only *B. fragilis* is able to establish disease in a site without the presence of other synergic species. *B. melanogenicus* produces a black pigment and classically is involved in anaerobic infections above the diaphragm, such as lung abscesses from aspiration pneumonia.

Fusobacterium are tapered gram-negative anaerobes that frequently intermix with *Bacteroides* in oral and pleuropulmonary disease (abscesses). *Fusobacterium* cause trench mouth in patients with poor dental hygiene. It is associated with periodontitis, gingivitis, and ulcerations.

67. The answer is B.   (*Anatomy*)

The middle cerebral artery distribution includes the area of the left frontal lobe operculum, which usually contains the motor speech center.

The anterior cerebral artery distributes blood to the medial and dorsolateral aspects of the frontal lobe.

Lenticulostriate arteries penetrate the deeper aspects of the cerebrum to distribute to deep cortical nuclei and to fiber systems, including the internal capsule.

The posterior cerebral artery distributes to ventral aspects of the temporal lobe and to most of the occipital cortex.

Posterior communicating arteries send penetrating branches into the core of the cerebrum and the rostral brain stem, including areas of the diencephalon.

68. The answer is B.   *(Microbiology)*

Clostridium perfringens may be associated with both myonecrosis (gas gangrene) and food poisoning. *Clostridia* are anaerobic, spore-forming gram-positive bacilli, whose pathogenic species produce powerful exotoxins. On Gram stains, the spores do not stain (clear space) and require special stains to specifically stain the spore inside the organism.

C. perfringens is nonmotile and produces alpha toxin (hemolytic anemia, myonecrosis) and phospholipase C. In a milk media it is associated with "stormy fermentation," and on blood agar exhibits target hemolysis, which refers to a double zone of beta hemolysis. *C. perfringens* is a cause of (1) skin and soft tissue infections (particularly in people with diabetes), (2) a diffuse spreading cellulitis and fasciitis (synergistic necrotizing cellulitis), (3) septicemia, (4) intra-abdominal infections (peritonitis, gangrenous cholecystitis), (5) pelvic inflammatory disease, (6) "back room abortion" septic endometritis, and (7) a type of food poisoning. Soft-tissue infections are characterized by the formation of gas bubbles and a diffuse, foul-smelling exudate. "Gas gangrene" is predominantly a myonecrosis and is frequently associated with shock, disseminated intravascular coagulation, renal failure, and a hemolytic anemia. High-dose penicillin G is used in therapy, but it frequently does not penetrate the necrotic, avascular tissue. Hyperbaric oxygen therapy is extremely useful, since the organism lacks superoxide dismutase and cannot destroy oxygen-free radicals. Clostridial food poisoning (20% of all cases of food poisoning) has a different pathogenesis than that associated with *C. botulinum, Staphylococcus aureus,* and *Bacillus cereus,* in which there is an ingestion of a preformed enterotoxin. The spores of *C. perfringens* that contaminate meat or poultry are able to germinate if the food is lightly cooked. The ingested organisms proliferate in the small bowel and elaborate an enterotoxin, which produces severe diarrhea and cramping.

C. tetani has a tennis racket appearance due to a spore at its terminal end, and it swarms blood agar plates because of its motility. The spores of *C. tetani* are in the soil and gain entrance into the body via closed wounds and "skin popping" among intravenous drug abusers. Bacterial proliferation in the wound causes the release of a powerful neurotoxin called tetanospasmin, which inhibits spinal afferent fibers by blocking the release of the inhibitory neurotransmitter called glycine, thus resulting in sustained motor stimulation of all voluntary muscles.

C. botulinum is motile, has a subterminal spore, produces heat-resistant spores, and has a heat labile exotoxin. Proliferation of the organisms in contaminated food (usually canned or preserved food, or raw or commercially processed seafood) forms the powerful preformed neurotoxin responsible for food poisoning. The intact toxin attaches to the synaptic vesicles of cholinergic nerves, where it blocks the release of acetylcholine, thus resulting in a descending form of paralysis from the cranial nerves down to the extremities.

C. difficile is associated with pseudomembranous colitis. Administration of antibiotics [e.g., ampicillin (#1 culprit)] to a patient may result in the overgrowth of toxin-producing *C. difficile* in the colon. Patients develop a watery diarrhea, fever, pain, and an absolute leukocytosis while on the antibiotic or at a later date. The pseudomembrane covering the colon is enterotoxin induced and not an example of an invasive enterocolitis. The diagnosis is best made with a toxin assay of stool and not by culture or Gram stain of the stool. Metronidazole (Flagyl) is the treatment of choice, because it is less expensive than oral vancomycin.

69. The answer is D.   *(Anatomy)*

Laminae I, II (substantia gelatinosa) and the spinal nucleus of the trigeminal nerve are somatosensory areas that function in the reception and processing of nociceptive (pain) and temperature afferents. Laminae I, II are related to the body, whereas the spinal nucleus of the trigeminal nerve is related to the region of the face. The modalities served by both nuclei are the same, that is, the response to stimuli is perceived as painful or related to temperature.

Unconscious proprioception is associated with the dorsal nucleus of Clarke in the spinal cord and either the accessory cuneate or mesencephalic nuclei of the trigeminal system.

Visceral sensory neurons involved in reflex stretch mechanisms are located in the intermediate gray of the spinal cord and in the nucleus solitarius of the brain stem.

Deep-tendon reflex afferents are primarily associated with neurons in laminae VI (VII) in the spinal cord and the mesencephalic nucleus of the trigeminal system.

Discriminative touch (two-point; vibration) is associated with the nuclei gracilis and cuneatus from the body regions and the chief (primary, main) sensory nucleus of the trigeminal system in the pons.

70. The answer is B. *(Microbiology)*
Tuberculosis, which is caused by *Mycobacterium tuberculosis*, is the single most important infectious cause of death in the world. Approximately 3 million people worldwide die per year, primarily as the result of overcrowding, AIDS, and multidrug resistance. High-risk groups include (1) patients who are positive for HIV; (2) intravenous drug abusers; (3) immunosuppressed patients; (4) residents in long-term facilities, such as nursing homes; (5) low-income populations; (6) foreign-born persons from high prevalence areas, such as Africa, Central and South America, and the Far East; (7) alcoholics; (8) Hispanics, African Americans, Native Americans, and Eskimos; and (9) patients with chronic diseases, such as diabetes mellitus, end-stage renal disease, and cancer.

71. The answer is B. *(Anatomy)*
Herniation of the tonsils of the cerebellum into the foramen magnum impedes flow of cerebrospinal fluid (CSF) from the foramina of Magendie and Luschka, thereby producing enlargement of all ventricular spaces. This type of herniation is associated with spina bifida and may present immediately or later in life. The tonsils are medial protrusions of the cerebellar hemispheres and are reminiscent of the tonsils protruding into the region of the fauces of the oropharynx. In addition, part of the vermis is called the uvula. These anatomic areas have no known functional significance except that this part of the cerebellum is involved in tonsillar herniation.

Occlusion of the cerebral aqueduct is most likely to cause enlargement in only the lateral and third ventricles.

Arteriovenous malformations of cerebral vessels may cause focal ventricular enlargement in only the lateral ventricles.

Aneurysms of the vertebrobasilar artery occur in the subarachnoid space. They are not likely to cause ventricular enlargement.

Uncal herniation of the medial aspect of the temporal lobe may compress the midbrain and the subjacent cerebral aqueduct, with resultant lateral and third ventricle enlargement. The most devastating aspect of this herniation is compression of the reticular activating system, specifically, the locus ceruleus, resulting in coma. In addition, the posterior cerebral artery and the oculomotor nerve are compressed.

72. The answer is D. *(Anatomy)*
The facial and vestibulocochlear nerves exit the brain stem at the cerebellopontile angle and are the most frequently affected nerves in patients with an acoustic neuroma. Paralysis of facial muscles and complaints about auditory and vestibular (vertigo) system function are frequent in this disease.

The trochlear nerve arises from the dorsal midbrain distant from the site of this tumor.

The oculomotor and abducens nerves arise from the ventral surface of the brain stem at the midbrain and pons, respectively. They are unlikely to be involved with this type of cerebellopontine angle tumor.

The trigeminal nerve arises from the ventrolateral surface of the pons. If an acoustic neuroma is large or takes a deviant path of enlargement, this nerve may be involved.

73. The answer is E. *(Behavioral science)*
An individual with an intelligence quotient (IQ) of 95 is classified as average because the range for average or normal IQ is 90 to 109. The IQ ranges for individuals who are severely mentally retarded, moderately mentally retarded, mildly mentally retarded, and borderline are about 20 to 40, 35 to 50, 50 to 70, and 70 to 79, respectively.

74. The answer is D. *(Behavioral science)*
Anorexia nervosa is most commonly seen in women, in teenagers, and in young adults and is more common

in high than in low socioeconomic groups. Anorexia nervosa is a life-threatening psychiatric illness that has as its main feature an unusual preoccupation with food and body weight. Although anorexic individuals are hungry, they refuse to eat because of fear of gaining weight. Whereas treatment is aimed initially at restoring the nutritional state of the patient, family therapy has been shown to be useful in ongoing treatment of this condition.

75. The answer is E.   *(Anatomy)*
The radial nerve lies in the musculospiral groove of the humerus. While in this groove it is in close contact with the midshaft portion of the humerus. It is separated from the humerus by only a thin portion of the medial head of the triceps muscle. The nerve spirals approximately 270 degrees around the humerus, passing from the medial side of the humerus in the proximal arm to the anterolateral side of the humerus in the distal arm. The nerve is accompanied by the profunda brachii artery.

76. The answer is D.   *(Anatomy)*
The bone of the carpus that most commonly fractures is the scaphoid. The scaphoid is in the floor of the anatomical snuff-box, which is bounded by the tendons of the extensor pollicis longus and the extensor pollicis brevis. Because the blood supply to the scaphoid enters the distal head of the scaphoid and passes through the narrow waist to reach the proximal head, fracture of the scaphoid through the waist can deprive the proximal head of its blood supply and result in necrosis of the proximal head.

77. The answer is B.   *(Anatomy)*
The carpal bone that is most frequently dislocated is the lunate. The ventral surface of the lunate is broader than the dorsal surface. Most of the carpal bones have a dorsal surface that is broader than the ventral surface. Therefore, the lunate is wedge shaped in a direction opposite that of the other carpal bones. When the lunate is dislocated, it typically occurs anteriorly, into the carpal tunnel. Therefore, a dislocation of the lunate may cause median nerve compression in the carpal tunnel.

78. The answer is B.   *(Anatomy)*
The shoulder joint capsule is reinforced by the tendons of the rotator cuff muscles. The supraspinatus tendon reinforces the capsule superiorly, the infraspinatus and teres minor tendons reinforce it posteriorly, and the subscapularis tendon reinforces it anteriorly. The inferior portion of the joint capsule has no tendinous reinforcement. In addition, this portion of the capsule is the most slack to allow mobility in the joint. Therefore, the humeral head is most likely to pass through the inferior part of the joint capsule upon dislocation.

79. The answer is B.   *(Behavioral science)*
Alcohol is the most commonly abused substance in the United States. Marijuana is the most commonly used illegal substance in the United States.

80. The answer is C.   *(Anatomy)*
Research shows that the capillary endothelium provides the most significant barrier to substances having free access to the extracellular spaces of the cells within the brain. Ependymal cells provide a lining of the ventricular spaces. Fenestrated capillary endothelium has specific locations within the brain, for example, the hypothalamus and circumventricular organs. At these locations, the blood–brain barrier does not exist, and blood-borne substances can access the extracellular spaces surrounding the neurons in these brain regions.

81. The answer is A.   *(Behavioral science)*
Among family members, the person most likely to sexually abuse a 9-year-old girl is her father. In fact, 50% of incest is committed by the child's father.

82. The answer is C.   *(Anatomy)*
After the notochord induces the formation of the neural plate, the lateral edges of the plate fold dorsally to form the neural groove. The lips of the neural groove grow toward the midline and fuse to form the neural tube. This closure of the neural tube occurs first in the cervical region and progresses cranially and caudally simultaneously. Failure of the neural tube to close results in a variety of congenital abnormalities that include anencephaly and spina bifida with myeloschisis.

83. The answer is D. *(Behavioral science)*
Although they have limited adverse effects, the selective serotonin reuptake inhibitors (SSRIs) have equal efficacy and take as long to work (at least 3 to 4 weeks) as the tricyclics. Lithium is used primarily to treat the mania of bipolar disorder. Although lithium is no more effective than a tricyclic antidepressant in treating depression, it has antidepressant activity and is used in combination with other antidepressants in patients with unipolar disorder.

84. The answer is B. *(Anatomy)*
The common peroneal nerve is the lateral branch of the sciatic nerve. The sciatic nerve typically divides at the upper border of the popliteal fossa. The common peroneal nerve then lies along the edge of the tendon of the biceps femoris. The tendon attaches to the head of the fibula, and the nerve wraps around the lateral surface of the neck of the fibula and divides into the superficial and deep peroneal nerves. In this position, the common peroneal nerve is in a subcutaneous position and is subject to injury.

85. The answer is C. *(Behavioral science)*
Dependent personality disorder is more common in women than in men. Antisocial, schizoid, and obsessive-compulsive personality disorders are more common in men than in women. Narcissistic personality disorder occurs equally in men and women.

86. The answer is C. *(Anatomy)*
The dorsal column–medial lemniscus system carries the sensory modalities of two-point, epicritic touch, vibration, and conscious proprioception. A tuning fork against bone or skin should be perceived as a vibration sensation.

The spinothalamic system would be tested by evaluating the perceptions of temperature and sharp touch.

The posterior spinocerebellar system carries unconscious proprioception and is evaluated by observing coordination of motor activity such as walking.

The tectospinal system can be evaluated by observing the change in position of the neck, shoulders, and upper trunk to visual and auditory stimuli.

The rubrospinal (extrapyramidal) system can be evaluated by observing muscle tone and coordination of proximal appendicular muscle groups.

87. The answer is D. *(Behavioral science)*
Down and fragile X syndromes are the first and second most common genetic causes, respectively, of mental retardation in the population.

88. The answer is B. *(Anatomy)*
The locus ceruleus, located in the rostral part of the brain stem, synthesizes norepinephrine. The axons from the nucleus project to the cerebral cortex and diffusely innervate the cortical neurons.

The raphae nuclei synthesize serotonin and project axons to the cerebral cortex.

The lateral reticular formation projects to the spinal cord.

The nucleus gracilis in the medulla is part of the dorsal column–medial lemniscus system.

The mamillary bodies are in the diencephalon and project to the thalamus.

89. The answer is C. *(Anatomy)*
Damage to the amygdala results in the Külver-Bucy syndrome, which is characterized by docility and hypersexuality. Damage to the basal ganglia results in movement disorders whereas damage to the hippocampus is associated with memory deficits. The parietal lobes are associated with intellectual processing of sensory information. Damage to the frontal lobes results in problems with mood, orientation, and concentration.

90. The answer is C. *(Anatomy)*
The posterior pituitary is the release site of the neurohormones made by the supraoptic and paraventricular nuclei of the hypothalamus. The axons of these neurons transport the hormones to axon terminals that form neuro-hemal contacts where the hormones are released into the systemic circulation.

The median eminence is the release site for neurohormones manufactured by cells in the arcuate nucleus of the hypothalamus. These releasing and inhibiting factors influence the activity in the anterior pituitary.

The anterior pituitary consists of cells of endodermal origin that manufacture and release systemic hormones (thyrotropin, interstitial cells: stimulating hormone [ICSH], luteinizing hormone [LH], and corticotropin) under the control of the hypothalamus.

The lamina terminalis and the pineal gland are circumventricular organs. The pineal gland synthesizes and releases melatonin and is under the modulatory control of the autonomic nervous system.

91. The answer is A. *(Anatomy)*
The sarcolemma or skeletal muscle cell membrane invaginates to form the T system, or transverse tubule system. This system provides for rapid transmission of the surface membrane excitation to terminal sacs. The sarcolemma depolarization causes a rush of Na^+ ions into the cell and is transmitted into the depths of the cell along membranes of the T system.

The sarcoplasmic reticulum surrounds the myofibrils. These membranes release and then accumulate calcium. The sarcoplasmic reticulum bulges into sacs at the A band–I band junction, creating a triad with the T-tubule.

Junctional or subneural folds are present in the muscle cell surface at the neuromuscular junction.

Rough endoplasmic reticulum is perinuclear in arrangement and does not interact with transverse tubules.

The smooth endoplasmic reticulum of skeletal muscle is called sarcoplasmic reticulum.

92. The answer is A. *(Anatomy)*
Ascending sensory systems are described as having three neurons in the system from periphery to cerebral cortex. The first neuron is in the dorsal root ganglia, the second in the spinal cord or brain stem, and the third in the thalamus. In the pain and temperature pathway, the second neuron cell body is located in the spinal cord dorsal horn. The axons from these cells cross to the opposite side within one segment rostrally of their origin. By contrast, in the dorsal column–medial lemniscus system, for example, those second neurons are located within the nuclei gracilis and cuneatus. Their axons cross to the opposite side within a short segment of the caudal medulla.

93. The answer is D. *(Pharmacology)*
This patient has neuroleptic malignant syndrome, a side effect of high-potency antipsychotic medications like haloperidol. Thioridazine is a low-potency antipsychotic. Use of the antipsychotic clozapine, the antimanic agent lithium, or the antidepressant fluoxetine

is not commonly associated with the development of neuroleptic malignant syndrome.

94. The answer is E. *(Anatomy)*
Hirschsprung disease involves an abnormal dilation of a segment of the colon. The region of the colon distal to this segment is constricted, lacks peristaltic activity, and contains no enteric ganglion cells. These enteric ganglion cells are postganglionic parasympathetic cells derived from the neural crest. These neural crest cells normally migrate and invade the gut but they fail to migrate to the gut in this disease. Endoderm cells form the gut tube lining. Splanchnic mesoderm forms the serosa of the gut tube and the smooth muscle and connective tissue of the gut wall. Somatic mesoderm forms the parietal peritoneum. The hypomere cells, which are the ventral cells of the somite, form much of the muscle and connective tissue of the anterolateral body wall.

95. The answer is A. *(Anatomy)*
Intramembranous ossification is the development of bone from mesenchymal condensation. Mesenchyme cells give rise to osteoblasts, which lay down bone matrix and eventually form bone spicules. When the osteoblasts become enclosed, they are called osteocytes. The frontal, parietal, squamous portion of the temporal, and parts of the occipital bone are derived from intramembranous ossification.

Long bones develop from a cartilage model, which is called endochondral ossification. Growth in length occurs by division of cells in the epiphyseal plate.

Cancellous bone is spongy, or trabecular bone, which can result after either intramembranous or endochondral ossification.

The diaphyseal bone begins development from a cartilaginous model and also involves the production of bone from cells originating from the periosteum. Osteoprogenitor cells develop into osteoblasts from the cellular layer of the periosteum. These osteoblasts secrete bone matrix, increasing the width of the bone.

The ends of bones begin bone formation from a cartilage model. A secondary ossification center develops in the cartilage, and bone is laid down on calcified cartilage.

96. The answer is A. *(Anatomy)*
The pituitary gland is derived from two sources. An evagination of the floor of the third ventricle forms the infundibulum of the hypothalamus and the posterior lobe of the pituitary gland. The anterior lobe and the pars intermedia are formed by the Rathke pouch, which is an evagination of the ectoderm that forms the roof of the stomodeum, or primitive oral cavity. The stomodeum is rostral to the stomodeal membrane and is lined with ectoderm. The pharnyx is caudal to the stomodeal membrane and is lined with endoderm. The branchial pouches are lateral evaginations of the pharyngeal endoderm. The first pharyngeal pouch forms the auditory tube, tympanic cavity, and mastoid air cells. The branchial clefts are invaginations of the body wall ectoderm overlying the branchial pouches. The first branchial cleft forms the external auditory canal. The branchial arches are the mesodermal bars between adjacent branchial pouches and branchial clefts. The first branchial arch forms the mandible, the malleus and the incus, the muscles of mastication and several muscles, and other structures.

97. The answer is B. *(Pharmacology)*
Alcohol amnestic disorder (Korsakoff syndrome) is the result of long-term alcohol abuse.

98. The answer is C. *(Anatomy)*
The dorsal nucleus of Clarke, located in the spinal cord gray matter, gives rise to axons that make up an ipsilateral projection to the cerebellum, the posterior spinocerebellar tract.

The posterior (dorsal) horn is a general area of spinal cord gray matter associated with processing sensory information from numerous sources and projecting it to many areas of the central neuraxis.

The dorsal root entry zone (DREZ), frequently identified as the zone of Lissauer, is located along the dorsolateral sulcus of the spinal cord. The dorsal rootlets are observed in gross specimens attaching to the spinal cord at this site. The zone is thought to be significant in nociception (pain) mechanisms as well.

Rexed Laminae VIII and IX represent motor neurons (anterior motor neuron, α motor neurons) that innervate skeletal muscle.

The γ motor neurons innervate the intrafusal muscle cells of the muscle spindles.

99. The answer is D. *(Behavioral science)*
Although methadone, like heroin, causes physical dependence and tolerance, it also has advantages for the heroin addict. Methadone suppresses heroin withdrawal symptoms, has longer duration of action, and causes less euphoria, drowsiness, and depression than heroin.

100. The answer is A. *(Anatomy)*
The oculomotor nerve emerges from the midbrain and passes between the two cerebral peduncles. The nerve then passes between the superior cerebellar artery and the posterior cerebral artery before entering the dura of the lateral wall of the cavernous sinus. Because of the close relationship between the oculomotor nerve and the superior cerebellar, posterior cerebral, and basilar arteries, an aneurysm of any of these three arteries can compress the oculomotor nerve.

101. The answer is D. *(Pathology)*
Hemiballismus is associated with a lesion of the subthalamic nucleus of the motor system. Lesions in this nucleus produce uncontrolled flailing and involuntary movement, especially of the upper extremity.

Amyotrophic lateral sclerosis, a disease of the lower motor neurons, produces weakness in skeletal muscles, which may eventually lead to paralysis and muscle atrophy.

Dysdiadochokinesia is a disorder relater to cerebellar disease. The patient is unable to perform patterns of repetitive motor activity, such as alternating supination and pronation of the hands.

Athetosis refers to slow writhing movements of the limbs. This finding is characteristic of lesions in areas of the basal ganglia that are not subthalamic.

102. The answer is B. *(Anatomy)*
The roots of the brachial plexus are the anterior rami of spinal nerves C_5–T_1. These five roots form the three trunks of the plexus. Each trunk divides into an anterior and a posterior division. The divisions form the three cords of the brachial plexus. The dorsal scapular nerve is a branch of the C_5 root. The suprascapular nerve is a branch of the upper trunk. The upper subscapular nerve and the thoracodorsal (middle

subscapular) nerve are branches of the posterior cord. The lateral pectoral nerve is a branch of the lateral cord.

103. The answer is C.   *(Behavioral science)*
In schizophrenia, the most common type of hallucination is auditory. Other types of hallucinations, such as cenesthetic (altered sensations of body organs), visual, olfactory, and kinesthetic, can also occur.

104. The answer is E.   *(Anatomy)*
From the lateral ventricles, cerebrospinal fluid (CSF) flows through the foramen of Monro into the third ventricle, through the cerebral aqueduct, into the fourth ventricle, through the foramina of Magendie and Luschka, out of the brain and into the subarachnoid space. In the subarachnoid space, the CSF circulates around the spinal cord and brain. Eventually, the CSF is reabsorbed through the arachnoid villi into the superior sagittal sinus (a dural sinus).

The foramen of Magendie is out of sequence in choice A. The fourth ventricle and foramen of Luschka are out of sequence in choice B. CSF does not flow through the septum pellucidum, which is the medial boundary of the lateral ventricle, so choice C cannot be correct. The order in choice D is essentially the reverse of the normal direction of CSF flow.

105. The answer is E.   *(Pharmacology)*
Clozapine is more effective than traditional antipsychotic agents against the negative symptoms of schizophrenia, such as withdrawal. The traditional antipsychotic agents are effective against positive symptoms of schizophrenia, such as hallucinations, delusions, talkativeness, and strange behavior.

106. The answer is C.   *(Anatomy)*
The ansa cervicalis is formed by nerve fibers from the anterior rami C_1–C_3. It gives rise to nerves that innervate the infrahyoid strap muscles: sternohyoid, sternothyroid, and omohyoid. The geniohyoid muscle is innervated by cervical nerve fibers that are carried with the hypoglossal nerve. The mylohyoid is innervated by a branch of the mandibular division of the trigeminal nerve. The cricothyroid and crioarytenoid

muscles are intrinsic muscles of the larynx and are innervated by branches of the vagus nerve.

107. The answer is B.   *(Pharmacology)*
Whereas barbiturates induce hepatic cytochrome P-450 drug-metabolizing enzymes and may thereby increase the metabolism of other drugs, benzodiazepines have little effect on these enzymes. Both barbiturates and benzodiazepines suppress rapid eye movement (REM) sleep, and a rebound in REM sleep is observed when they are discontinued. Although diazepam has been useful as a muscle relaxant in muscle spasm and spasticity, barbiturates lack this effect. Only barbiturates are contraindicated in acute intermittent porphyria because they induce γ-aminolevulinic acid synthetase and they accelerate porphyrin synthesis in these patients. Neither barbiturates nor benzodiazepines have analgesic activity, which is defined as the ability to relieve pain without loss of consciousness. In fact, some studies suggest that barbiturates produce hyperalgesia in certain situations.

108. The answer is D.   *(Anatomy)*
The phrenic nerve lies on the anterior surface of the anterior scalene muscle. The nerve is held tightly against the surface of the muscle by the deep cervical fascia. The roots of the brachial plexus and the subclavian artery pass posterior to the anterior scalene muscle and anterior to the middle scalene muscle.

109. The answer is B.   *(Behavioral science)*
Manic episodes usually have a rapid onset and, when untreated, last approximately 3 months.

110. The answer is D.   *(Anatomy)*
Although the la and lb afferents from skeletal muscle are difficult to distinguish from one another because they are similar in size, they can be distinguished by monitoring their reflex responses. The la sensory neurons carry impulses from the muscle spindles, which are sensitive to an increase in length of the muscle. The lb sensory neurons carry impulses from the Golgi tendon organs, which are sensitive to an increase in tension. During a contraction the muscle increases its tension on the Golgi tendon organs, which produces an increase in the number of action potentials

in the lb neurons. Contraction, however, shortens the muscle, creating slack in the muscle spindle, which decreases the number of action potentials coming from the muscle spindles over the la neurons.

111. The answer is D. *(Physiology)*

The "all-or-none" law for action potentials states that when two or more stimuli of threshold or greater strength are applied to a membrane, they generate equivalent action potentials (when all other conditions are unchanged), and when the stimuli are of subthreshold strength, they generate no action potential. A stimulus that is stronger than another suprathreshold stimulus does not produce a larger action potential (all the sodium channels that can open do open in response to a stimulus that is of threshold strength). In this situation, only the first four stimuli are strong enough to produce action potentials. The refractory period prevents action potentials from summating; mechanical contractions in muscle can summate, action potentials cannot.

112. The answer is A. *(Physiology)*

In a typical nerve cell, the electrochemical equilibrium for Na^+ is approximately $+60$ mV and for K^+ it is approximately -97 mV. If the membrane is equally permeable to both ions, the membrane potential would be roughly midway between $+60$ and -97 mV. When the membrane potential is closer to the K^+ electrochemical equilibrium (as it is in a typical cell), it indicates that the permeability to K^+ is much greater than the permeability to Na^+. When the membrane potential is a steady value as it is in a typical motor neuron at rest, it indicates no net gain or loss of electrical charge due to ion movement. If the pump is transporting 3 Na^+ out and 2 K^+ in, it must be balancing the movement of 3 Na^+ in and 2 K^+ out; therefore, more Na^+ is moving into the cell than K^+ is moving out.

113. The answer is E. *(Microbiology)*

Epidemic typhus, due to *Rickettsia prowazekii*, is transmitted by a louse. Rickettsia are obligate intracellular parasites that perpetuate themselves in arthropod vectors. Once introduced into the host by a vector, they invade endothelial cells and produce a vasculitis, which, in some types of rickettsial disease, eventuates in a dark, crusted lesion called an eschar at the site of inoculation. Their pathogenicity is related to their ability to activate endogenous phospholipase A, which enhances inflammation and thrombosis via its stimulation of arachidonic acid metabolism. Rickettsia are also able to leave phagolysosomes, thus avoiding their destruction. The rickettsial diseases are as follows.

Disease	Arthropod Agent	Eschar	Rash Distribution
Typhus group			
Epidemic typhus	Louse; *Rickettsia prowazekii*	None	Trunk→ extremity
Brill Zinsser	Recurrence of above	None	Trunk→ extremity
Endemic (murine)	Rat flea; *R. typhi*	None	Trunk→ extremity
Scrub typhus	Mite; *R. tsutsugamushi*	Present	Trunk→ extremity
Spotted fever group			
Rocky Mountain spotted fever	Tick; *R. rickettsia*	None	Extremity→ trunk
Rickettsialpox	Mite; *R. akari*	Present	Trunk→ extremity
Other types			
Q fever	Inhalation, tick; *Coxiella burnetii*	None	None

The other organisms in the question are transmitted by ticks. Relapsing fever is caused by *Borrelia recurrentis*, a spirochetal organism, and is transmitted by ticks or lice. Babesiosis is an intraerythrocytic parasite transmitted by the tick Ioxides dammini, the same vector that transmits Lyme disease. Rocky Mountain spotted fever, due to *Rickettsia rickettsia*, is transmitted by ticks.

114. The answer is C. *(Anatomy)*
The axillary nerve passes out of the axilla by passing through the quadrangular space. The lateral border of the space is the surgical neck of the humerus. The medial border of the space is the long head of the triceps. The long head of the triceps keeps the axillary nerve pressed against the surgical neck of the humerus. Fracture of the humerus at this site may lead to a laceration of the axillary nerve.

115. The answer is A. *(Pathology)*
This patient has a distal sensorimotor neuropathy due to osmotic damage of the Schwann cells (demyelination) and axonal degeneration (muscle atrophy). The peripheral neuropathy associated with diabetes is typically distal, symmetric, and has a "stocking glove" distribution. Osmotic damage is caused by conversion of glucose in the Schwann cell into sorbitol by aldolase reductase. The osmotically active sorbitol draws water into the cell and destroys it. Careful control of hyperglycemia is useful in preventing this complication. Amitriptyline, Tegretol, and capsaicin cream to relieve the pain have been tried with varying success.

Vitamin deficiencies, subacute combined degeneration (demyelination) associated with B_{12} deficiency, and nonenzymatic glycosylation (glucose combining with amino acids) are not implicated in the neuropathy associated with diabetes mellitus. However, a similar type of neuropathy in alcoholics is associated with thiamine deficiency.

116. The answer is A. *(Behavioral science)*
Cocaine intoxication is marked by aggression, agitation, hypersexuality, euphoria, irritability, impaired judgment, and combativeness. Stupor is not commonly part of the clinical picture for cocaine intoxication.

117. The answer is A. *(Pathology)*
Osteogenesis imperfecta (too little bone), or brittle bone disease, is the most common hereditary bone condition and, in most cases, is an autosomal dominant disease. Resulting from abnormal collagen synthesis, osteogenesis imperfecta causes abnormalities in the skeleton (frequent pathologic fractures), eyes (blue sclera from too little collagen), ears (hearing deficits),

joints (laxity), and teeth (dentin deficiency causes blue–yellow discoloration).

Achondroplasia is an autosomal dominant disease characterized by impaired formation of cartilage and premature closure of the epiphyseal plates of long bones. People with achondroplasia have a normal-sized head and vertebral column but shortened arms and legs.

Osteopetrosis (too much bone), or marble bone disease, results from an overgrowth and sclerosis of cortical bone caused by a defect in osteoclasts. In osteopetrosis, which can be an autosomal dominant or recessive disease, bone replaces the marrow cavity, requiring extramedullary hematopoiesis, in which other hematopoietic sites produce blood cells, for survival. Complications of the disease include pathologic features and anemia. Because osteoclasts derive from monocytes, marrow transplantation is sometimes performed.

Osteoporosis, a decrease in bone mass, is the most common metabolic abnormality of bone in the United States. In women, it is most commonly caused by estrogen deficiency after menopause, resulting in the excessive release of interleukin-1 by macrophages and monocytes. Interleukin-1 activates the osteoclasts, creating an imbalance between osteoclastic activity (resorption of bone) and osteoblastic activity (formation of bone); the increased osteoclastic activity causes a bone mass deficit for which osteoblasts are unable to compensate. If not contraindicated, estrogen is the gold standard for the prevention of osteoporosis and should be given to all postmenopausal women. And because most of the bone is lost in the first 3 to 6 years after menopause, early estrogen replacement is the key to the prevention of osteoporosis.

Paget disease of bone (osteitis deformans) occurs primarily in elderly males and refers to abnormal bone thickening and architecture that relate to an initial period of excessive bone resorption followed by excessive bone formation. The new bone has a haphazard arrangement, called mosaic bone, and is extremely soft despite its increased thickness. The disease may involve one bone or many bones including, in decreasing order of frequency, the pelvis, skull, and femur. Additional features associated with Paget disease include (1) excessively high serum alkaline phosphatase levels caused by the osteoblastic phase of the disease, (2) the development of arteriovenous fistulas within the soft bone producing high-output cardiac failure, (3) pathologic fractures, (4) enlargement of the head, and (5) an increased risk of developing osteogenic sarcoma owing to excessive osteoblastic activity. The etiology of Paget disease is unknown, although recent speculation has implicated either a slow virus infection or something related to the measles virus.

118. The answer is E. *(Pharmacology)*
Tolerance and physical dependence often accompany chronic use of central nervous system depressants. The mechanism appears to involve cellular adaptations of the affected neuronal circuits, such that larger doses of the drug are required to produce the same magnitude of effect, and the dose–response curve is shifted to the right. Physical dependence occurs simultaneously with tolerance as the neurons adapt to the continued presence of the drug to maintain their functional state. When the drug is abruptly removed, rebound hyperexcitability occurs as the depressant effect of the drug is removed, resulting in a withdrawal syndrome. Although pharmacokinetic tolerance can occur simultaneously, it is neither necessary nor sufficient to cause physical dependence.

119. The answer is E. *(Anatomy)*
The infraspinatus muscle is an external rotator of the shoulder. The deltoid muscle has many functions. The middle part of the muscle is an abductor; the anterior part of the muscle is an internal rotator and a flexor. The posterior part of the muscle is an external rotator and an extensor. The latissimus dorsi is an internal rotator and an extensor. The pectoralis major and teres major muscles are adductors and internal rotators. The internal rotators of the shoulder are more numerous and stronger than the external rotators. A lesion of the upper trunk of the brachial plexus results in loss of almost all the external rotators but spares some of the internal rotators. Therefore, a patient with such a lesion maintains the arm in an internally rotated position.

120. The answer is C. *(Pharmacology)*
Buspirone and other 5-hydroxytryptamine$_{1A}$ (5-HT$_{1A}$) agonists exert a delayed anxiolytic effect. In contrast to benzodiazepines, buspirone does not cause

sedation or muscle relaxation and has no anticonvulsant effect. Tolerance and dependence do not occur with buspirone, and it appears safe for use in patients with a history of drug-dependence problems. The primary side effects are nausea, dizziness, headache, and restlessness.

121. The answer is D. *(Behavioral science)*
Most rapists are less than 25 years of age. Weapons are often used in rape attacks, alcohol is often involved, and rapists tend to rape women of the same race.

122. The answer is B. *(Pharmacology)*
Several new drugs have been introduced for the treatment of refractory partial seizures, including all of those listed except ethosuximide. Felbamate may be particularly useful in patients with pediatric epileptic encephalopathy (Lennox-Gastaut syndrome). Ethosuximide is the drug of choice for generalized absence seizures (petit mal epilepsy) and is not useful in treating partial seizures.

123. The answer is C. *(Anatomy)*
The first branch of the facial nerve is the greater petrosal nerve, which arises from the geniculate ganglion. It carries preganglionic parasympathetic fibers. The chorda tympani arises from the facial nerve just before the facial nerve emerges from the facial canal. It carries preganglionic parasympathetic and taste fibers. The nerve to the stapedius arises from the facial nerve as the nerve passes the stapedius muscle on the posterior wall of the tympanic cavity. The posterior auricular nerve becomes a branch of the facial nerve as it emerges from the facial canal. It innervates the posterior auricular muscles and provides cutaneous sensory innervation to the posterior pinna. The lesser petrosal nerve is a branch of the glossopharyngeal nerve. It contains preganglionic parasympathetic fibers that lead to the otic ganglion.

124. The answer is C. *(Behavioral science)*
Rapid eye movement (REM) latency, that is, the time until initiation of REM after sleep onset, is short in unipolar depression. Normal sleep onset, premature morning awakenings, increased REM, and reduced

slow-wave sleep are characteristic of unipolar depression.

125. The answer is D. *(Anatomy)*
The rostral end of the neural tube develops three brain vesicles: the prosencephalon, the mesencephalon, and the rhombencephalon. The prosencephalon subsequently divides into the telencephalon and the diencephalon. The telencephalon develops into the cerebral hemispheres (including the basal ganglia and the corpus callosum). The diencephalon develops into the thalamus, the hypothalamus, and the epithalamus. The mesencephalon develops into the midbrain. The rhombencephalon divides into the metencephalon and the myelencephalon. The metencephalon develops into the pons and the cerebellum. The myelencephalon develops into the medulla.

126. The answer is D. *(Behavioral science)*
Before the first episode of schizophrenia, the premorbid personality of the patient is often quiet, obedient, and passive. This individual does not form friendships; often is introverted, daydreams, and avoids social activities. Physical complaints such as back pain and headache as well as anxiety may coincide with onset of the symptoms of schizophrenia. In addition, abnormal mood changes and strange perceptions often occur.

127. The answer is C. *(Anatomy)*
Neural crest cells develop into the sensory cells of the peripheral nervous system, including the cells of the dorsal root ganglia and the cells of the sensory ganglia of the cranial nerves, for example, the trigeminal ganglion, the geniculate ganglion, the spiral ganglion, the vestibular ganglion, and the ganglia of the ninth and tenth cranial nerves. The neural crest also develops into the postganglionic nerve cells of the autonomic nervous system, including those in the sympathetic paravertebral ganglia (sympathetic chain), the sympathetic prevertebral ganglia (e.g., the celiac ganglion), the parasympathetic ganglia of the head (e.g., the ciliary ganglion), and the parasympathetic ganglion cells in the walls of the viscera (e.g., myenteric plexus). Preganglionic autonomic cells (e.g., preganglionic sympathetic cells in the intermediolateral cell column) are derived from neural ectoderm cells.

128. The answer is B. *(Anatomy)*
The cerebral arterial circle is a group of communicating arteries that provides collateral channels between arteries on the right side and the left side and between branches of the vertebral arteries and the internal carotid arteries. The two vertebral arteries join to form the basilar artery at the pons–medulla junction. The basilar artery divides into the two posterior cerebral arteries at the pons–midbrain junction. Each posterior cerebral artery communicates with the internal carotid artery of the same side through the posterior communicating artery. The anterior cerebral artery is a direct branch of the internal carotid artery. The two anterior cerebral arteries communicate through the anterior communicating artery. The middle cerebral artery is a direct branch of the internal carotid artery (as are the anterior cerebral, posterior communicating, and ophthalmic arteries) and does not contribute to the cerebral arterial circle.

129. The answer is E. *(Behavioral science)*
Anxiety is characterized by restlessness, dizziness, palpitations, syncope, tingling in the extremities, tachycardia, tremor, gastrointestinal disturbances, as well as urinary urgency and frequency. Flight of ideas (thoughts following each other in quick succession) is characteristic of mania.

130. The answer is C. *(Anatomy)*
Full abduction of the arm requires both abduction of the humerus at the glenohumeral joint and upward rotation of the scapula. The trapezius and serratus anterior muscles rotate the scapula upward. The deltoid and supraspinatus muscles abduct the humerus at the glenohumeral joint. The teres major muscle adducts and medially rotates the humerus. If a patient has a paralyzed trapezius (accessory nerve lesion) or serratus anterior (long thoracic nerve lesion), only about 90 to 120 degrees of abduction are possible.

131. The answer is D. *(Behavioral science)*
Psychotic symptoms such as hallucinations and delusions are not seen in generalized anxiety disorder but are seen in schizophrenia and may be seen in all of the other choices. Although psychotic symptoms can

be present in organic delirium often due to substance abuse, unlike schizophrenia, the hallucinations are less well organized and more likely to be visual rather than auditory in nature. In bipolar disorder, serious mood symptoms are seen along with psychosis. In brief psychotic disorder, a severe stressor often precedes the psychotic symptoms, which last from 1 day to 1 month.

132. The answer is C. *(Anatomy)*
Cardiac muscle consists of long, branching fibers whereas smooth muscle cells or fibers are unbranched. Cardiac muscle is striated and resembles skeletal muscle in its arrangement of contractile elements. Cardiac fibers that are specialized to conduct impulses are called Purkinje fibers.

Central nuclei, one per cell, are common to smooth and cardiac muscle. Skeletal muscle has multiple nuclei per cell.

Gap junctions are a component of the cardiac muscle intercalated disk, in addition to desmosomes and a fascia adherens (zonula adherens). Gap junctions join smooth muscle cells, allowing for a wavelike spread of contraction.

Both smooth and cardiac muscles are innervated by sympathetic and parasympathetic nerves and are hormonally regulated. Smooth muscle responds to oxytocin, and both respond to hormones (biogenic amines) secreted by the adrenal medulla.

Typical organelles such as mitochondria, a Golgi complex, lipofuscin pigment, and glycogen are found near the nucleus in both.

133. The answer is B. *(Behavioral science)*
Increased rather than decreased appetite is an effect of marijuana use. Marijuana is the most widely used illegal drug in the United States, with effects including impaired memory and the "amotivational syndrome," that is, lack of desire to work and increased apathy.

134. The answer is D. *(Microbiology)*
Malaria is caused by sporozoans of which four Plasmodium species are pathogenic to man, namely, *Plasmodium vivax, falciparum, malariae,* and *ovale.* Organism 1 represents *P. vivax;* 2, *P. falciparum;* and 3, *P. malariae.* The chart is helpful in summarizing their frequency, distribution, and effect on red blood cell (RBC) size (normal or macrocytic). The chart also shows the presence or absence of relapse caused by reinfection of the liver.

Organism	Frequency	Tropics	Subtropics	Temperate	Red Blood Cell (RBC)	Relapses
P. vivax	55%	X	X	X	↑	Yes
P. falciparum	40%	X	X	—	↔	No
P. malariae	5%	—	X	X	↔	No
P. ovale	Rare	Africa	S. America	—	↑	Yes

The female Anopheles mosquito is the vector for malaria. The sexual cycle (schizogony) develops in the mosquito, whereas the asexual cycle (sporogony) develops in man. Reinfection of hepatocytes by merozoites, which occurs in *Plasmodium vivax* (organism 1) and *ovale* (not represented), is the reason for relapses of the disease and repetition of the cycle. Patients with sickle cell disease or glucose-6-phosphate dehydrogenase (G6PD) deficiency are resistant to *P. falciparum* infections (organism 2). Patients who are Duffy blood-group negative (black population) are resistant to *P. vivax* infections, because the organisms need the Duffy blood group to parasitize the RBC.

The pathogenesis of anemia in malaria involves both intravascular and extravascular hemolysis of RBCs, the latter by macrophage removal of infected cells.

The clinical presentation for the "benign" forms of malaria is characterized by periodic paroxysms of shaking chills, owing to rupture of the RBCs, followed by high fever and pronounced diaphoresis as the temperature falls. *P. vivax* (organism 1; most common type of malaria) has a tertian pattern, which is a fever spike every 48 hours. *P. malariae* (organism 3) has a quotidian fever pattern, which is a fever spike every 72 hours. *P. falciparum* (organism 2) has a quotidian, or intermittent fever pattern. Splenomegaly is a consistent feature in malaria. The spleen is frequently dark black because of the hematin pigment from extravascular hemolysis. *P. falciparum* is the most severe form of the disease. Parasitemia is greatest for *P. falciparum* and least for *P. malariae.* In falciparum malaria (malignant pernicious malaria), the RBCs aggutinate and stick to the blood vessels, resulting in central nervous system hemorrhage (classic "ring hemorrhages" in the brain) and disseminated intravascular coagulation. In addition, falciparum malaria in the brain produces small areas of reactive gliosis known as Durck glial nodules. Massive intravascular hemolysis results in hemoglobinuria, which, in the presence of an acid pH, converts the hemoglobin to a black pigment, thus the term "blackwater fever." Another feature of falciparum malaria is focal liver cell necrosis, leading to jaundice and liver failure. *P. malariae* (organism 3) is associated with an immune complex glomerulonephritis (membranous type) presenting as the nephrotic syndrome.

The laboratory diagnosis of malaria is secured by noting the parasites in the peripheral blood (thin and thick smears). *P. falciparum* differs from the other types in that only ring forms and gametocytes (banana-shaped organisms) are present. The other types have all stages represented in the blood (ring forms, schizonts, merozoites, and gametocytes).

Chloroquine is used to prevent all types of malaria. It kills blood schizonts and is gametocidal to all malaria species, except *P. falciparum.* Mefloquine is the drug of choice for resistant strains. Primaquine primarily eradicates *P. vivax* and *ovale*, because it has schizonticidal properties for organisms located in the liver. It is gametocidal to *P. falciparum.* One problem is the danger of precipitating hemolysis in patients who have a deficiency of G6PD (Heinz body anemia).

135. The answer is A. *(Behavioral science)*
The prognosis for sexual functioning of this 19-year-old man who has suffered a spinal cord injury in a motorcycle accident is better with lower rather than upper motor neuron lesions and with an incomplete rather than a complete lesion. Problems with erection are common after spinal cord injury. Testosterone levels and fertility are often reduced after spinal cord injury.

136. The answer is D. *(Pharmacology)*
Tolerance and physical dependence can occur after chronic administration of most central nervous system depressants, including ethanol, barbiturates, benzodiazepines (diazepam), and opiates (meperidine). Tolerance and physical dependence are not associated with most antiepileptics, antidepressants, neuroleptics, and lithium.

137. The answer is A. *(Microbiology)*
Fusobacterium are tapered gram-negative anaerobes that frequently intermix with Bacteroides in oral and pleuropulmonary disease (abscesses). Fusobacterium cause trench mouth, or Vincent's disease, which consists of periodontitis, gingivitis, and ulcerations in the mouth of patients who have poor dental hygiene. Pencillin G or V is useful in therapy. Fusobacterium are also pathogens in human bites, particularly those associated with fights and wounds over clenched fists.

The other diseases listed in the question are spirochetal diseases. Primary syphilis is caused by *Treponema pallidum*, which is most commonly transmitted by sexual intercourse. Relapsing fever is due to *Borrelia recurrentis*, which is transmitted by a tick or a louse. Rat bite fever is caused by *Streptobacillus moniliformis* or *Spirillum minus* (rarely). It is contracted in rat infested slum areas. The disease begins approximately 10 days after a rat bite. Fever, chills, headache, vomiting, and migratory arthralgias and myalgias are noted. *Streptobacillus moniliformis* is also the cause of Haverhill fever, which is transmitted by drinking contaminated raw or unpasteurized milk. Lyme disease is due to *Borrelia burgdorferi*, which is transmitted by the bite of a tick called *Ioxides dammini*. It initially produces erythema chronicum migrans, a red, concentrically enlarging rash that develops in the area of the tick bite. Chronic arthritis develops in later stages of the disease.

138. The answer is E. *(Anatomy)*
Romberg's test primarily evaluates joint position, which is a function of the dorsal columns. The patient

is asked to stand with the feet together and eyes closed. Loss of balance with the eyes closed that is corrected by opening the eyes indicates dorsal column disease (e.g., tabes dorsalis). Loss of balance with the eyes open or closed indicates a cerebellar problem, but that is not the primary purpose of the test.

Rapid supination and pronation of the hands evaluates the fine motor coordination of the cerebellum. Slow or irregular supination and pronation is called dysdiadochokinesia, which is commonly seen in Parkinson's disease. Stereognosis refers to the ability to recognize objects placed in the hand or numbers written on the palm by the examiner. It evaluates the sensory cortex. The grasp, snout/suck, and palmomental reflexes are primitive reflexes that are characteristic of newborns. However, when they are present in adults, they are abnormal. During the grasp reflex, the patient holds onto the examiner's index finger when the examiner is stroking the palm. This reflex indicates a premotor lesion. In the snout/suck reflex, percussion of the upper lip causes a puckering of the mouth or sucking movement. It indicates frontal lobe disease. In the palmomental reflex, or Radovici's sign, scratching or pricking of the thenar eminence produces twitching of the chin. This is associated with pyramidal tract disease or tetany. The clasp-knife reflex is seen in spasticity associated with upper motor neuron disease. When the patient's arm is forcibly drawn toward the examiner's chest, the arm suddenly gives, like opening the blade of a pocket knife.

139. The answer is A. (Pathology)
Avascular necrosis is an infarction of bone that is associated with (1) long-term corticosteroid use, such as in patients with systemic lupus erythematosus (most common cause), (2) sickle-cell disease, (3) trauma, (4) Legg-Perthe disease, or (5) Keinböck disease involving the scaphoid (navicular) bone. Osgood-Schlatter disease is a localized inflammation that produces pain in the tibial tuberosity at the point of attachment of the patellar tendon, which results in prominence of the tibial tuberosity that persists throughout life. It usually occurs during the pubertal growth spurt and is not an example of avascular necrosis.

The most common complaint in avascular necrosis of bone is pain either directly over the bone or referred to a different site. A radiograph of the bone reveals increased density due to reactive bone formation.

Legg-Perthe disease is an avascular necrosis involving the femoral head, which is more common in boys than girls, and normally develops between 3 to 12 years of age. It begins as a slowly evolving limp, with pain referred into the groin area. If it heals, the leg is usually shorter on the affected side. The scaphoid bone is the most common fracture site of all of the carpal bones, and it is very susceptible to avascular necrosis and nonunion. With the hand clenched into a fist, the fingers point to this bone.

140-144. The answers are: 140-D, 141-A, 142-E, 143-C, 144-B. (Pharmacology)
Phenytoin and carbamazepine are often used for the chronic prophylaxis of generalized tonic–clonic seizures, whereas status epilepticus is usually treated with intravenous diazepam followed by intravenous phenytoin. Carbamazepine is also the drug of choice for trigeminal neuralgia, with phenytoin as an alternate. Ethosuximide is the drug of choice for generalized absence seizures except when other types of seizures are also present. Valproate is effective in most forms of generalized seizures, including myoclonic seizures and mixed seizure disorders, but is usually considered to be an alternative drug except for myoclonic seizures, in which it is usually the drug of choice. Felbamate is the first drug to be shown effective in epileptic encephalopathy (Lennox-Gastaut syndrome) in randomized clinical trials.

145-149. The answers are: 145-B, 146-E, 147-D, 148-C, 149-D. (Pharmacology)
Most central nervous system drugs affect neurotransmitter synthesis, storage, release, degradation, or receptor activation. Selegiline blocks monoamine oxidase-B, which inactivates dopamine, and thereby augments dopamine concentrations in the brain. Paroxetine is a selective inhibitor of neuronal serotonin reuptake and is used in treating depression. Clozapine acts in part by blocking dopamine D_4 receptors and is therefore useful in treating schizophrenia, particularly resistant schizophrenia.

Levodopa is the precursor to the neurotransmitter dopamine. When administered systemically, it crosses the blood–brain barrier and is converted to dopamine by central neurons. As with selegiline, it is useful in treating Parkinson disease. Alprazolam, a benzodiazepine, activates receptors coupled with the γ-aminobutyric acid (GABA)–chloride ionophore and thereby augments GABA receptor-mediated neuronal membrane hyperpolarization.

150-154. The answers are: 150-B, 151-D, 152-A, 153-E, 154-F. *(Pharmacology)*

A number of drugs appear to act on γ-aminobutyric acid (GABA) receptors or metabolism, including the GABA agonist, baclofen, GABA antagonists such as picrotoxin, and potentiators of GABA-receptor activation, the benzodiazepines. Several antiepileptic drugs including gabapentin may also act via GABA receptors or inhibit GABA metabolism (vigabatrin). The benzodiazepines such as diazepam potentiate the effect of GABA-receptor activation. Strychnine produces its convulsive effects by blocking glycine receptors. Excitatory amino acid (glutamate, aspartate) receptors include the subclass activated by *N*-methyl-D-aspartate (NMDA). The NMDA receptors are antagonized by the anesthetic and psychotomimetic agents ketamine and phencyclidine (PCP). Lysergic acid diethylamide, a potent hallucinogen, is an ergot alkaloid derivative with antagonist effects at central 5-hydroxytryptamine (5-HT, serotonin) receptors.

155-157. The answers are: 155-A, 156-C, 157-G. *(Anatomy)*

The illustration diagrams the right side of the visual pathway from the chiasm to the right primary visual cortex. Lesion number one is located within the optic chiasm and would compromise axons from the nasal halves of the retinas (cross fibers). The temporal visual fields project to these retinas, so the resulting defect is a bitemporal hemianopia, a condition also known as tunnel vision. Lesion number two is in the right optic tract, so the left visual field information projecting from the right retinal halves of both eyes is blocked, resulting in a left homonymous hemianopia. Remember, any lesion posterior the the optic chiasm results in a defect that is the same for both eyes and is termed homonymous. Lesion number three disrupts the upper portion of the optic radiations, which carry information from the lower left visual fields for both eyes. The resultant deficit would be a left inferior homonymous quadrantanopia. When a portion of the

optic radiations of a side is affected, the resultant defect is quadrantal; the entire optic radiations of a side would have to be involved for the defect to be a hemianopia.

Selection B would not be a choice because the lesion would have to be bilateral, involving the lateral aspects of the chiasm to result in a binasal hemianopia. Selections D, F, and H are incorrect because most of the defects in the diagram are on the right side, causing left visual field defects. The left side visual pathway would have to contain the lesions to result in right side visual field defects. Selection E is also incorrect because a left superior homonymous quadrantanopia would require the lesion to be in the Meyer loop (lower optic radiations).

The right visual field projects to the left halves of the retinas (temporal half on the left and nasal half on the right) and conversely the left visual field projects to the right halves of the the retinas (temporal half on the right and nasal half on the left). Information processed in the right retinal halves is projected to the right optic tract and conversely, the information processed in the left retinal halves is projected to the left optic tract. The optic tracts terminate within the lateral geniculate bodies of the thalamus of the appropriate side. Also, information from the nasal halves of the retinas cross in the chiasm and project to the contralateral side. The temporal halves of the retinas do not cross, but project to the same side (ipsilateral) optic tract. Axons from neurons within the lateral geniculate bodies comprise the optic radiations (geniculocalcarine tract) that project to the primary visual cortex above and below the calcarine fissure. This portion of the cerebral cortex is located in the occipital lobe. The upper halves of the visual fields project to the lower retinal halves and the lower visual fields project to the upper retinal halves. Information is then projected to the appropriate side geniculate body. The upper fibers of the optic radiations project input from the lower visual field of the appropriate side and the converse is true for the lower fibers of the optic radiations. Remember, the lower optic radiation fibers project downward through the temporal lobe (the Meyer loop) of the cerebrum before continuing to the primary visual cortex (lingual gyrus). Another easy way to remember this is the **rule of L's:** **L**ower retina projects to the **L**ateral portion of the lateral geniculate body, which projects through the Meyer Loop, which projects to the **Lingual** gyrus. The upper optic radiation fibers project straight back through the parietal lobe of the cerebrum to the primary visual cortex (cuneus).

For a schematic illustration of the processes involved, please refer to the visual pathways diagram. **(Note: all lesion sites are indicated with the capital letters that are choices in the question.)**

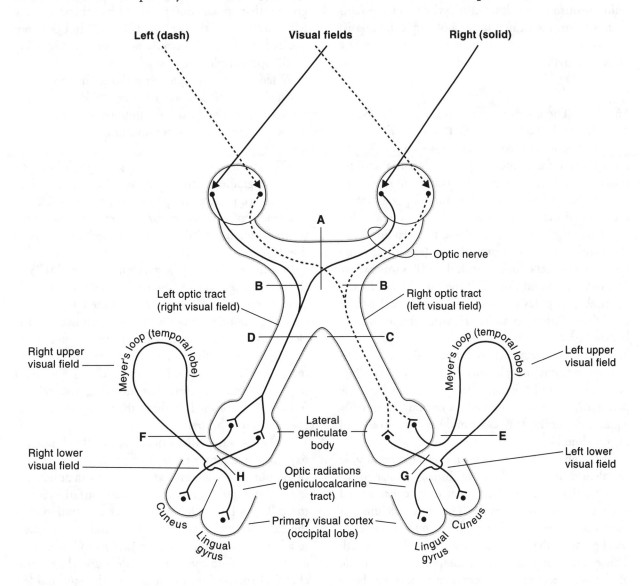

158-163. The answers are: 158-C, 159-E, 160-A, 161-B, 162-D, 163-F. *(Pharmacology)*
Chronic levodopa therapy frequently leads to dyskinesias and variations in response, known as the "on–off" phenomenon, which probably result from deterioration of dopaminergic neurons and decreased activation of levodopa to dopamine. Trazodone may cause painful priapism through a central nervous system mecha-

nism in some patients and frequently causes sedation. Haloperidol and other high-potency neuroleptic drugs may cause tardive dyskinesia in some patients, usually after months or years of treatment. This condition is believed to result from upregulation of dopamine receptors. Lithium frequently causes a benign tremor, weight gain, polyuria, polydipsia, or both during chronic administration, whereas nausea and vomiting are usually signs of acute overdosage. Among the adverse effects of chronic phenytoin administration are changes in connective tissue leading to gingival hyperplasia and facial coarsening (lips and nose) as well as mild hirsutism. Overdoses of tricyclic antidepressants such as amitriptyline may cause cholinergic (mydriasis) and adrenergic blockade (hypotension) as well as severe cardiac arrhythmias, coma, and seizures.

164-171. The answers are: 164-D, 165-A, 166-C, 167-D, 168-F, 169-G, 170-E, 171-G. *(Physiology)* The electrochemical equilibrium for sodium (line B) is the value of the membrane potential (MP) if sodium is the only ion that can cross the cell membrane. Line H, the electrochemical equilibrium for potassium, is the value of the MP if potassium is the only ion that can cross the membrane. When both sodium and potassium can cross the membrane (and there is no appreciable effect of other ions), the MP is somewhere between line B and line H. If the membrane is more permeable to potassium (as it is in a normal resting cell), the MP is closer to line H; when the membrane is more permeable to sodium, it is closer to line B. Stimulation of the muscle endplate by the motor neuron opens numerous cholinergic channels that allow both sodium and potassium to cross. At its peak the permeability to sodium and potassium is roughly equal, making the MP about midway between B and H, i.e., line D.

Although a nerve membrane is much less permeable to calcium than to sodium, calcium is similar to sodium in that it is a cation that is more concentrated outside the cell than inside. Therefore calcium has both a large concentration gradient and a strong electrical gradient that tend to move the ion into the cell. This electrochemical gradient disappears if the inside of the cell becomes more electrically positive. How positive it must become depends on the difference in the ion concentration outside compared to inside. For sodium ions the concentration outside is about 10 times greater than the concentration inside and electrochemical equilibrium is about +60 mV (line B). For calcium ions the concentration outside is more than 1000 times greater than the concentration inside. Therefore, electrochemical equilibrium must be at a value that is even more positive than the value for sodium, i.e., line A.

At rest the sarcolemma, i.e., the skeletal muscle membrane, is more permeable to potassium than to sodium, and the resting MP is at line F. During an action potential, sodium permeability becomes much greater than potassium permeability; therefore, the MP moves above the midpoint (line D) but does not rise as high as line B because potassium permeability is still appreciable.

When the permeability to sodium and potassium is equal, the MP is approximately midway between the sodium electrochemical equilibrium and the potassium electrochemical equilibrium. Best answer is line D.

When an ion is in electrochemical equilibrium, the electrical gradient across the membrane exactly balances the concentration gradient for that ion. No net movement of that ion occurs, no matter how much the permeability to that ion increases. MP stays at line F.

During an inhibitory postsynaptic potential (IPSP), the postsynaptic membrane on the neuron cell body (soma) responds to the neurotransmitter with an increase in chloride permeability. For most neurons the electrochemical equilibrium for chloride is not at the resting MP but rather at a more negative MP. Therefore, the MP goes toward the more negative value; it hyperpolarizes. However, the continuing permeability of sodium keeps the MP above the potassium electrochemical equilibrium.

When ischemia (inadequate blood flow) reduces oxygen delivery to a portion of the heart, the membrane pumps at that area are unable to maintain the low sodium and high potassium concentration inside the cells. As intracellular sodium concentration rises the electrochemical equilibrium for sodium decreases to a less positive value (perhaps near line C). As intracellular potassium concentration decreases the electrochemical equilibrium for potassium changes to a less negative value (perhaps line F). If the ratio of the membrane permeability for sodium compared to potassium remains unchanged, the new MP is less negative than the original MP, but not completely depolarized. Best answer is line E.

A major effect of vagal stimulation at the sinoatrial node is to increase the membrane permeability to potassium. This response moves the resting MP closer to the potassium electrochemical equilibrium. However, the continuing permeability to sodium keeps the resting value above the electrochemical equilibrium for potassium.

172-175. The answers are: 172-B, 173-E, 174-D, 175-A. *(Pharmacology)*
An overdose of any natural or synthetic opiate, such as propoxyphene, can be countered with an opiate receptor antagonist such as naloxone or naltrexone. The effects of benzodiazepines such as chlordiazepoxide can be blocked with the specific benzodiazepine receptor antagonist flumazenil. The central nervous system effects of bromocriptine, an ergot alkaloid that specifically activates dopamine receptors, can be antagonized with a dopamine receptor antagonist such as haloperidol. Tacrine is a centrally acting cholinesterase inhibitor. Its effect would be partly blocked by a muscarinic receptor antagonist such as benztropine or atropine.

176-180. The answers are: 176-C, 177-D, 178-A, 179-B, 180-E. *(Pharmacology)*

Levodopa, the precursor to dopamine, can be administered to patients with Parkinson disease because, unlike dopamine, levodopa crosses the blood–brain barrier. However, before levodopa enters the brain, a considerable amount is metabolized peripherally. Carbidopa, which does not cross the blood-brain barrier, acts to prevent the peripheral metabolism of levodopa so that most of it enters the brain where it can be converted to dopamine in nigrostriatal neurons.

Bromocriptine is a dopamine receptor agonist that can substitute for dopamine in patients with Parkinson disease who have a deficiency of this neurotransmitter.

Amantadine, an antiviral compound, also acts to release dopamine from central neurons and can be used adjunctively in Parkinson disease.

Benztropine and trihexyphenidyl are muscarinic receptor antagonists that block the excessive cholinergic activity resulting from dopamine deficiency in patients with Parkinson disease

Selegiline inhibits monoamine oxidase type B and thereby reduces the degradation of dopamine. It may be used alone or in combination with levodopa or a dopamine agonist.

Test 2

QUESTIONS

DIRECTIONS:
Each of the numbered items or incomplete statements in this section is followed by answers or by completions of the statement. Select the ONE lettered answer or completion that is BEST in each case.

1. A 28-year-old woman says that she has always been "a nervous person." She feels tense all the time, shows sympathetic and parasympathetic symptoms, and has insomnia. This woman's condition is most likely to be

(A) post-traumatic stress disorder
(B) generalized anxiety disorder
(C) obsessive-compulsive disorder
(D) agoraphobia
(E) panic disorder

2. Which of the following is associated with ependymal cells rather than microglial cells?

(A) Blepharoplasts
(B) Rod cells
(C) Gitter cells
(D) Reservoir for HIV
(E) Neuronophagia

3. A 25-year-old man has a negative Dick test and a positive Schick test. These results indicate that he has

(A) neutralizing antibodies against diphtheria
(B) neutralizing antibodies against scarlet fever
(C) a defect in cellular immunity
(D) had the full complement of diphtheria-pertussis-tetanus (DPT) shots as a child
(E) had poststreptococcal glomerulonephritis as a child

4. Xenodiagnosis is used in the diagnosis of a disease that is transmitted by the bite of a

(A) body louse
(B) deer tick
(C) reduviid bug
(D) mosquito
(E) rat flea

5. Which of the following vaccines can be administered to a patient with known anaphylactic reactions to eggs?

(A) *Haemophilus influenzae* type B vaccine
(B) Influenza vaccine
(C) Measles vaccine
(D) Mumps vaccine
(E) Yellow fever vaccine

6. The pediatric disease that most closely resembles amyotrophic lateral sclerosis (ALS) is

(A) Schilder disease (adrenoleukodystrophy)
(B) tabes dorsalis
(C) Werdnig-Hoffmann disease
(D) Gaucher disease
(E) Niemann-Pick disease

7. A 5-year-old boy presents with a 2-month history of progressive dysarthria, difficulty initiating swallowing, and right-sided weakness. Examination demonstrates diminished right conscious proprioception and 2-point discrimination, atrophy of the left side of the tongue and spastic right hemiparesis mostly affecting use of the right lower extremity. This most likely represents

(A) right pontine glioma
(B) left pontine glioma
(C) left lateral medullary infarct
(D) left medial medullary glioma
(E) right medial medullary glioma

8. Compared with serum, cerebrospinal fluid (CSF) has

(A) a higher chloride concentration
(B) a higher protein concentration
(C) the same glucose concentration
(D) more lymphocytes per microliter
(E) a greater concentration of gamma globulins

9. A 12-year-old boy has *Neisseria meningitidis* meningitis. His mother and sister are found to be asymptomatic carriers of the organism. They should be treated with

(A) oral vancomycin
(B) rifampin
(C) penicillin
(D) amoxicillin
(E) doxycycline

10. Which of the following diseases is a lysosomal storage disease that is associated with the synthesis of abnormal myelin?

(A) Tay-Sachs disease
(B) Niemann-Pick disease
(C) Metachromatic leukodystrophy
(D) Hurler disease
(E) Hunter disease

11. Across the cell membrane of a skeletal muscle cell in the resting state with a nonelectrogenic pump ($1 Na^+ : 1K^+$)

(A) both sodium and potassium are in electrochemical equilibrium
(B) the rate of sodium influx is equal to the rate of potassium efflux
(C) the rate of sodium influx is much less than the rate of potassium efflux
(D) the rate of sodium influx is much greater than the rate of potassium efflux
(E) sodium leaks into the cell but there is no potassium efflux

12. A 35-year-old woman has oligoclonal bands in a high-resolution electrophoresis of her spinal fluid. This laboratory test was most likely prompted by a chief complaint of

(A) loss of recent memory
(B) seizure activity
(C) dizziness and paresthesias
(D) severe occipital headaches
(E) tunnel vision

13. Respiratory precautions are unnecessary in patients who have

(A) untreated tuberculosis
(B) untreated coccidioidomycosis
(C) pertussis
(D) diphtheria
(E) influenza

14. Small cystic lesions in the lenticular nucleus, thalamus, and internal capsule are most closely associated with

(A) hypertension
(B) embolism
(C) a demyelinating disease
(D) a genetic disease
(E) a neoplastic process

15. Alternating hemiplegia is best described as

(A) a neurological deficit involving pairs of cranial nerves
(B) a neurological deficit involving limbs on one side and cranial nerves on the other side
(C) a neurological deficit involving four limbs (quadriplegia)
(D) neurological deficits involving cranial nerves and limbs on the same side
(E) neurological deficits that move from side to side with each visit

16. Pale infarctions in the central nervous system (CNS) best characterize the lesions associated with

(A) embolic stroke
(B) hypertensive bleed
(C) atherosclerotic (ischemic) stroke
(D) ruptured berry aneurysm
(E) ruptured arteriovenous malformation

17. Which of the following is more likely associated with *Klebsiella pneumoniae* than *Escherichia coli*?

(A) A hospitalized patient who has pneumonia
(B) Endotoxic shock
(C) Hemolytic uremic syndrome in children
(D) An alcoholic who has lobar pneumonia
(E) Acute pyelonephritis

18. A 35-year-old woman presents with a 7-day history of a severe occipital headache, which she describes as "the worst headache I have ever had in my life." Xanthochromia is noted in her cerebrospinal fluid (CSF). Her headache is most closely associated with

(A) a subarachnoid hemorrhage
(B) a brain tumor
(C) multiple sclerosis
(D) an intracerebral hemorrhage
(E) viral meningitis

19. Both fenfluramine and phentermine

(A) produce central nervous system stimulation
(B) act to suppress appetite
(C) are effective in treating narcolepsy
(D) have been used in children with attention deficit disorders
(E) affect noradrenergic neurotransmission

20. Laminar necrosis and watershed infarcts characterize disease most likely secondary to

(A) hypertension
(B) atherosclerosis
(C) infection
(D) demyelinization
(E) a genetic disease

21. Which of the following groups of organisms are associated with food poisoning secondary to ingesting preformed toxins?

(A) *Staphylococcus aureus, Clostridium botulinum* (infant), *Bacillus cereus*
(B) *Salmonella, C. botulinum* (infant), *C. botulinum* (adult)
(C) *S. aureus, B. cereus, C. botulinum* (adult)
(D) *S. aureus, Salmonella, Clostridium perfringens, C. botulinum* (adult)
(E) *S. aureus, C. botulinum* (infant), *B. cereus, C. botulinum* (adult)

22. Which of the following most likely causes a communicating (nonobstructive) hydrocephalus?

(A) Tuberculous meningitis
(B) Stenosis of the duct of Sylvius
(C) Ependymoma of the fourth ventricle
(D) Blockage of the arachnoid granulations
(E) Colloid cyst of the third ventricle

23. As a result of a unilateral lower motor neuron lesion of the hypoglossal nerve

(A) the tongue would deviate toward the same side as the lesion when protruded
(B) the patient would not be able to protrude the tongue
(C) taste would be lost on one side of the tongue
(D) the tongue would deviate toward the opposite side of the lesion when protruded
(E) there is marked spasticity in the affected side of the tongue

24. In the central nervous system (CNS), oligodendrocytes share a similar function with

(A) gemistocytes
(B) astrocytes
(C) Schwann cells
(D) microglial cells
(E) ependymal cells

25. Which of the following helminths primarily produces gastrointestinal symptoms, without lung involvement, during the course of its infection?

(A) *Dirofilaria immitis*
(B) *Strongyloides stercoralis*
(C) *Trichuris trichiura*
(D) *Ascaris lumbricoides*
(E) *Necator americanus*

26. A 70-year-old man has a history of transient episodes of vertigo, dysarthria, and dysphagia. He also has numbness of the ipsilateral face and contralateral limbs that lasts for 10 to 15 minutes and then resolves without any deficits. The mechanism for this patient's disease is most closely associated with

(A) a demyelinating disease
(B) deficiency of dopamine
(C) ischemia involving the vertebral artery
(D) a cerebellar tumor
(E) a neoplasm of the brain stem

27. The repolarization phase of an action potential is due to

(A) increasing sodium permeability and increasing potassium permeability
(B) increasing sodium permeability and decreasing potassium permeability
(C) decreasing sodium permeability and an immediate increasing potassium permeability
(D) decreasing sodium permeability and a delayed increase potassium permeability
(E) increasing activity of the sodium potassium pump

28. A 42-year-old man complains of a frontal headache when he wakes up in the morning. It lasts into the afternoon and then subsides. The headache has been present for a few months. A computerized tomography (CT) scan shows a frontal lobe mass with focal areas of calcification. You strongly suspect the patient has

(A) an astrocytoma
(B) a pinealoma
(C) a meningioma
(D) an oligodendroglioma
(E) a glioblastoma multiforme

29. Bowel obstruction is most likely associated with

(A) typhoid fever
(B) shigellosis
(C) intestinal tuberculosis
(D) schistosomiasis
(E) taeniasis

30. A 32-year-old patient has decreased pain and temperature sensation in the upper extremities, atrophy of the intrinsic muscles of his hand, and brisk deep tendon reflexes in the upper extremity. The clinical findings strongly suggest

(A) amyotrophic lateral sclerosis
(B) multiple sclerosis
(C) syringomyelia
(D) subacute combined degeneration
(E) Guillain-Barré syndrome

31. The nucleus that gives rise to motor fibers that innervate muscles of larynx, pharynx, and palate is the

(A) hypoglossal nucleus
(B) nucleus ambiguus
(C) nucleus solitarius
(D) dorsal motor nucleus of the vagus
(E) Edinger-Westphal nucleus

32. Which one of the following is a manifestation of apoptosis?

(A) Red neurons
(B) Lafora bodies
(C) Lewy bodies
(D) Pick's bodies
(E) Globoid cells

33. A patient with diarrhea has a fecal smear that is negative for leukocytes. The patient's diarrhea is most likely caused by

(A) *Campylobacter* enteritis
(B) shigellosis
(C) typhoid fever
(D) enterotoxigenic *Escherichia coli*
(E) amebiasis

34. Which range of blood alcohol concentration defines legal intoxication?

(A) 0.01%–0.05%
(B) 0.06%–0.08%
(C) 0.08%–0.15%
(D) 0.40%–0.50%
(E) 0.60%–0.90%

35. Which one of the following would be true if only the left optic nerve was severed?

(A) Shining a light in the left eye would elicit the pupillary reflex in both eyes
(B) Shining a light in the left eye would elicit the pupillary reflex in the opposite eye only
(C) Shining a light in the right eye would elicit the pupillary reflex in both eyes
(D) Shining a light in the right eye would elicit the pupillary reflex in the opposite eye only
(E) The left pupil would be permanently dilated

36. A 40-year-old neuropathologist developed a rapidly progressive dementia and died. At autopsy, the cerebral cortex revealed a "bubbles and holes" spongiform change. The pathogenesis of the central nervous system (CNS) changes relates to

(A) a decrease in acetylcholine (ACh) levels
(B) an increase in aluminum levels
(C) neuronal damage by amyloid
(D) a slow virus disease
(E) deficiency of galactocerebrosidase

37. Calcium initiates a skeletal muscle contraction by

(A) binding to tropomyosin
(B) being released primarily from the sarcolemma during an action potential
(C) binding to troponin
(D) covering actin binding sites
(E) binding to myosin crossbridges

38. The most common central nervous system infection is primarily transmitted by

(A) traumatic implantation
(B) a mosquito
(C) ascending infection along peripheral nerves
(D) local extension from a primary site in the skull
(E) the hematogenous route

39. The antipsychotic effects of phenothiazines such as thioridazine are attributable to blockade of

(A) muscarinic receptors
(B) dopaminergic receptors
(C) adrenergic receptors
(D) serotoninergic receptors
(E) histaminergic receptors

40. Which of the following diseases is associated with multinucleated macrophages and abnormal myelin synthesis?

(A) Subacute sclerosing panencephalitis
(B) Parkinson's disease
(C) Rabies
(D) Herpes encephalitis
(E) Krabbe's disease

41. Inhibitory postsynaptic potentials (IPSPs) commonly occur at which of the following sites?

(A) The anterior gray horn of the cord, dorsal root ganglia, and muscle endplates
(B) The anterior gray horn of the cord and dorsal root ganglia, but not at muscle endplates
(C) The anterior gray horn of the cord, but not at dorsal root ganglia or muscle endplates
(D) The anterior gray horn of the cord and muscle endplates, but not at dorsal root ganglia
(E) Dorsal root ganglia and muscle endplates, but not at the anterior gray horn of the cord

42. An increased spinal fluid protein concentration, obliterative vasculitis, and scarring at the base of the brain are characteristic of

(A) tuberculous meningitis
(B) Guillain-Barré syndrome
(C) neurosyphilis
(D) aseptic meningitis
(E) *Neisseria meningitidis* meningitis.

43. A 37-year-old patient is an intensive care unit nurse whose job requires that she remain very alert. Which of the following antidepressants is best for this patient?

(A) Trimipramine
(B) Desipramine
(C) Amitriptyline
(D) Doxepin
(E) Imipramine

44. Which of the following disorders would most likely be present in an elderly individual with a pathologic fracture due to a lytic lesion in bone?

(A) Fibrous cortical defect (nonossifying fibroma)
(B) Multiple myeloma
(C) Metastatic prostate cancer to bone
(D) Osteochondroma
(E) Osteoporosis

45. Along which of the following is the propagation of inhibitory postsynaptic potentials (IPSPs) the most rapid?

(A) Axons of myelinated alpha motor neurons
(B) Axons of unmyelinated alpha motor neurons
(C) Axons of myelinated Ia sensory neurons
(D) Axons of unmyelinated Ia sensory neurons
(E) IPSPs are not propagated along axons

46. A radiolucent defect in bone that is a cause of a pathologic fracture and nocturnal pain in the legs in children is

(A) a fibrous cortical defect (nonossifying fibroma)
(B) an aneurysmal bone cyst
(C) fibrous dysplasia
(D) an enchondroma
(E) an osteoma

47. Patients receiving clozapine must be monitored frequently for the occurrence of

(A) aplastic anemia
(B) hepatitis
(C) agranulocytosis
(D) hyperprolactinemia
(E) tardive dyskinesia

48. A 65-year-old woman with rheumatoid arthritis complains of an inability to swallow dry crackers. She also states that her eyes "feel like they have sand in them." This woman is most likely to have a/an

(A) autoimmune destruction of the minor salivary and lacrimal glands
(B) positive anti-Smith (Sm) antibody
(C) abnormal esophageal motility study
(D) positive anti-centromere antibody
(E) history of night blindness

49. Which of the following describes the change in dimensions that occur within the sarcomeres of a skeletal muscle as it shortens during a contraction?

(A) The A band gets narrower, the I band gets narrower, and the H zone gets narrower
(B) The A band is unchanged, the I band gets narrower, and the H zone gets narrower
(C) The A band is unchanged, the I band gets narrower, and the H zone is unchanged
(D) The A band gets narrower, the I band is unchanged, and the H zone gets narrower
(E) The A band gets narrower, the I band gets narrower, and the H zone is unchanged

50. Which fiber tract is primarily involved with correlating movement of the eyes with signals from the vestibular nuclei?

(A) Medial lemniscus
(B) Corticobulbar tract
(C) Dorsal longitudinal fasciculus
(D) Medial longitudinal fasciculus
(E) Stria terminalis

51. Prolonged apnea may occur in patients with a genetically determined abnormal variant of cholinesterase following intravenous administration of

(A) succinylcholine
(B) tubocurarine
(C) mivacurium
(D) pancuronium
(E) succinylcholine or mivacurium

52. A young woman with photophobia, morning stiffness in her hands, and an unexplained pericardial effusion would most likely have a positive test for

(A) an HLA-B27 haplotype
(B) serum antinuclear antibodies
(C) antistreptolysin (ASO) antibodies
(D) rheumatoid factor
(E) syphilis serology

53. In the Papez circuit of the limbic system, between which combination is the hypothalamus placed on the basis of function?

(A) Cingulate cortex–hippocampus
(B) Hippocampus–thalamus
(C) Thalamus–hippocampus
(D) Thalamus–cingulate cortex
(E) Parahippocampal gyrus–thalamus

54. In which of the following combinations of autoantibodies are both antibodies used in the diagnosis of the same autoimmune disease?

(A) Anti-SS-A (Ro) and anti-centromere antibodies
(B) Anti-Smith (Sm) and anti–double-stranded DNA antibodies.
(C) Anti-ribonucleoprotein and anti-histone antibodies
(D) Anti-SS-B (La) antibodies and anti–single-stranded DNA antibodies
(E) Anti-mitochondrial and anti-microsomal antibodies

55. Transient muscle fasciculations followed by skeletal muscle relaxation may occur following the intravenous administration of

(A) tubocurarine
(B) vecuronium
(C) atracurium
(D) pancuronium
(E) succinylcholine

56. Which one of the following disease processes is most likely to produce a bitemporal hemianopsia?

(A) Tumor in the orbit
(B) Aneurysm of the posterior cerebral artery
(C) Pituitary tumor
(D) Transverse sinus thrombosis
(E) Uncal herniation

57. Which effect of morphine can be attenuated by atropine?

(A) Analgesia
(B) Respiratory depression
(C) Antitussive effect
(D) Constipation
(E) Miosis

58. A 42-year-old woman with clinical features that suggest combinations of systemic lupus erythematosus, progressive systemic sclerosis, and polymyositis without any evidence of renal disease would most likely have a positive test for

(A) anti–double-stranded DNA antibodies
(B) anti–single-stranded DNA antibodies
(C) anti-Scl-70
(D) anti-Jo-1
(E) anti-ribonucleoprotein antibodies

59. A patient complains about being "high strung." This patient often feels tense, has a rapid heartbeat, sweating, and a dry mouth for no apparent reason. This patient is likely to

(A) be suffering from panic disorder
(B) be a man
(C) have developed this problem between age 35 and 45
(D) have gastrointestinal problems
(E) be helped by treatment with lithium

60. In which of the following conditions are consciousness and attention most impaired?

(A) Stupor
(B) Delirium
(C) Somnolence
(D) Clouding of consciousness

61. Bipolar disorder is best described as

(A) being more common in lower socioeconomic groups
(B) having a strong genetic component
(C) having a better prognosis than major depressive disorder
(D) being more common in African-American patients than in Caucasian patients
(E) being characterized by chronic impairment between episodes

62. An acutely ill 6-year-old child presents with a 2-day history of high fever, chills, and localized pain and tenderness in the upper right thigh. Cutaneous erythema and swelling are noted in this area. There was a history of blunt trauma to this area approximately 1 week ago. A radiograph reveals soft-tissue swelling around the proximal femur but no evidence of a fracture in the femur. A technetium radionuclide scan exhibits uptake in the area of the metaphysis of the proximal femur. A complete blood cell count exhibits an absolute neutrophilic leukocytosis with left shift and toxic granulation in neutrophils. The pathogenesis of this patient's disease is most closely related to

(A) a fracture
(B) avascular necrosis
(C) an infectious process
(D) a neoplastic process
(E) an autoimmune disease

63. Which nerve is most likely to be injured by a fracture of the medial epicondyle of the humerus?

(A) Median nerve
(B) Radial nerve
(C) Ulnar nerve
(D) Medial brachial cutaneous nerve
(E) Musculocutaneous nerve

64. Which of the following skin diseases has a different pathogenesis from the others listed?

(A) Pityriasis rosea
(B) Pemphigus vulgaris
(C) Vitiligo
(D) Bullous pemphigoid
(E) Dermatitis herpetiformis

65. A 54-year-old man has a stroke and then experiences depression. Which area of the brain is most likely to be damaged?

(A) Temporal lobe
(B) Frontal lobe
(C) Parietal lobe
(D) Occipital lobe
(E) Cerebellum

66. Which of the following skin diseases most closely resembles a squamous cell carcinoma of the skin in its gross and microscopic appearance?

(A) Lichen planus
(B) Actinic keratosis
(C) Keratoacanthoma
(D) Ichthyosis vulgaris
(E) Erythema nodosum

67. Which factor has been implicated most strongly in the etiology of Alzheimer disease?

(A) Reduction in brain level of acetylcholinesterase
(B) Reduction in brain level of choline acetyltransferase
(C) Thiamine deficiency
(D) Endocrine disorder
(E) Folic acid deficiency

68. A 42-year-old man has recurrent development of vesicular and bullous lesions in sun-exposed areas. He has had to avoid alcohol because it seems to coincide with these episodes. One would expect this patient to have

(A) a history of abdominal pain
(B) an increase in δ-aminolevulinic acid in his urine
(C) an increase in porphobilinogen in his urine
(D) colorless urine during these attacks
(E) a decrease in red blood cell uroporphyrinogen decarboxylase

69. If a patient has a total lesion of the median nerve within the carpal tunnel, which of the following movements of the thumb is no longer possible?

(A) Abduction
(B) Adduction
(C) Flexion
(D) Extension
(E) Opposition

70. The most common type of hallucination seen in delirium is

(A) auditory
(B) visual
(C) gustatory
(D) kinesthetic
(E) cenesthetic

71. A patient complains of a loss of strength in the thumb, and there is a flattening of the thenar eminence. The nerve that is most likely injured is the

(A) ulnar
(B) median
(C) radial
(D) anterior interosseous
(E) posterior interosseous

72. Which combination of the following classic histologic findings in skin is correctly matched with the skin disorder producing these changes?

(A) Psoriasis—Pautrier's microabscess
(B) Urticaria pigmentosum—eosinophil infiltration of superficial dermis
(C) Mycosis fungoides—Munro's microabscess
(D) Molluscum contagiosum—Civatte bodies
(E) Lepromatous leprosy—Grentz zone

73. The lowest risk factor for divorce is

(A) religious differences
(B) socioeconomic differences
(C) marriage in middle age
(D) premarital pregnancy
(E) a short courtship

74. Atrophy of the epidermis rather than hyperkeratosis is most likely a feature of

(A) systemic lupus erythematosus
(B) chronic eczema
(C) lichen planus
(D) psoriasis
(E) ichthyosis vulgaris

75. Muscles capable of supinating the forearm are innervated by the

(A) median and ulnar nerves
(B) radial and ulnar nerves
(C) median and radial nerves
(D) musculocutaneous and radial nerves
(E) musculocutaneous and median nerves

76. Which term is associated with the most severe state of depression?

(A) Irritability
(B) Euthymia
(C) Dysphoria
(D) Euphoria
(E) Anhedonia

77. On angiography, which vessel follows the contour of the corpus callosum?

(A) Middle cerebral artery
(B) Vertebral artery
(C) Posterior cerebral artery
(D) Superior cerebellar artery
(E) Anterior cerebral artery

78. A 49-year-old woman known to have a cerebral neoplastic mass of considerable size within the deep cortex and white matter of her temporal lobe is being managed with therapeutics and pain medication. A visiting nurse scheduled for a routine visit finds the woman lying on the floor unconscious and is unable to arouse her. The nurse observes that the pupils are nonreactive and generally dilated in appearance. Although respiration and pulse are present, they are weak and she continues to be unresponsive. The nurse immediately calls for transport. What is the most likely reason for the observations on this patient?

(A) The patient overdosed on barbiturates
(B) The mass produced a temporal lobe displacement compressing the brain stem
(C) The vertebrobasilar perfusion of the patient collapsed
(D) The patient slipped and hit her head
(E) An acute episode of Alzheimer disease

79. The record of a 56-year-old man shows that he has various neurologic problems that can be called a "posterior fossa syndrome." The most likely reason is

(A) occlusion of segmental radicular arteries
(B) atherosclerosis of the common carotid artery
(C) aneurysm of the anterior cerebral artery
(D) vertebral–basilar insufficiency
(E) rupture of an aneurysm between the anterior cerebral vessels

80. Which of the following statements about heroin addicts is true? They

(A) are usually in their late 40s
(B) are more likely to be women
(C) are likely to die from complications of withdrawal from the drug
(D) can be treated with methadone because it is not addicting
(E) are more commonly found in large cities

81. A patient presents with inability to abduct and adduct digits II through V and clawing of the digits that is most prominent in digits IV and V. Which nerve is most likely to be injured?

(A) Ulnar nerve
(B) Medial nerve
(C) Radial nerve
(D) Lower trunk of the brachial plexus
(E) Upper trunk of the brachial plexus

82. Which statement about pain relief from chronic pain is true?

(A) Patients are at high risk for drug addition
(B) Pain medication should be given only when the patient is experiencing distress
(C) Behavior modification is the first line of treatment for pain caused by cancer
(D) Most patients in pain are undermedicated in the United States
(E) Drug addiction commonly occurs in terminal patients

83. When a patient flexes the wrist, the hand deviates toward the medial side. Which nerve is most likely to be injured?

(A) Ulnar nerve
(B) Median nerve
(C) Radial nerve
(D) Anterior interosseous nerve
(E) Posterior interosseous nerve

84. Which of the following symptoms is most likely to occur with withdrawal from nicotine?

(A) Delirium tremens
(B) Weight gain
(C) Euphoria
(D) Excitability
(E) Abstinence

85. Calcitonin affects the

(A) calcification of the osteoid
(B) ruffled border of the osteoclast
(C) canalicular processes of the osteocyte
(D) acid phosphatase matrix vesicles of the osteoblast
(E) alignment of hydroxyapatite crystals along collagen fibrils

86. Which of the following Brodmann areas represents the primary motor cortex?

(A) 3,1,2
(B) 4
(C) 6
(D) 17
(E) 41

87. Winging of the scapula usually indicates a lesion of the

(A) spinal accessory nerve
(B) suprascapular nerve
(C) thoracordorsal nerve
(D) long thoracic nerve
(E) lateral pectoral nerve

88. Which of the following statements applies to apoptosis?

(A) It is mediated only by natural killer (NK) cells
(B) DNA fragmentation is a frequent observation
(C) Cells, but not cytokines, induce it
(D) The target cell nucleus remains intact
(E) It results in osmotic disruption of target cells

89. A 30-year-old female with a longstanding history of epileptic seizures has undergone electroencephalogram (EEG) recordings to locate the focus of the epileptic seizure. Results indicate that the focus is within the inferior aspects of the left frontal lobes, just in front of the precentral gyrus. During surgery to remove the diseased brain area, extensive brain mapping is required. Given the site of the diseased tissue, the surgical team would plan to thoroughly test which one of the following cortical functions?

(A) Visual field alterations
(B) Somatosensory discrimination
(C) Motor skills associated with speech
(D) Word association skills
(E) Muscular control in toe and finger movement

90. Uncal herniation will result in an

(A) ipsilateral dilated pupil and contralateral third nerve palsy
(B) ipsilateral third nerve palsy and contralateral sixth nerve palsy
(C) ipsilateral third nerve palsy and sparing of the pupillary light reflex
(D) ipsilateral sixth nerve palsy and sparing of the pupillary light reflex
(E) ipsilateral dilated pupil and ipsilateral third nerve palsy

91. In smooth muscle, myosin light chain kinase (MLCK)

(A) phosporylates the light chains of actin filaments
(B) dephosporylates the light chains of actin filaments
(C) is inactivated by increasing levels of cyclic adenosine monophosphate (cAMP)
(D) is inactivated by increasing inositol triphosphate levels
(E) is activated by calcium (Ca^{++}) binding to troponin

92. Bupropion may exert its antidepressant effect by blocking the neuronal reuptake of

(A) dopamine
(B) serotonin
(C) norepinephrine
(D) serotonin and norepinephrine
(E) glutamate

93. Inside many smooth muscle cells there is a relatively high chloride concentration, and at the resting membrane potential, the ratio of CI^-_o to CI^-_i is less than the value required for electrochemical equilibrium. Increasing the membrane permeability to chloride in these cells will cause

(A) depolarization
(B) hyperpolarization
(C) a decrease in the electrochemical equilibrium for CI^-
(D) more rapid influx and efflux of CI^- but no change in the membrane potential
(E) no change in the influx or efflux of CI^- and no change in the membrane potential

94. Clinical examination of a patient reveals a loss of pain and temperature sensation in the arms and upper chest region with no appreciable loss of touch and vibratory sensation or motor control. There is no loss of sensation or motor control in the regions above or below the arms and upper chest. Which of the following is the most likely cause?

(A) Transection of the cord in the upper cervical region
(B) Hemisection of the anterior half of the spinal cord in the upper cervical region
(C) Hemisection of the dorsal half of the spinal cord in the upper cervical region
(D) Compression of the dorsal roots in the cervicothoracic portion of the cord
(E) Lesions radiating out from the central canal in the cervicothoracic portion of the cord

95. In 1994, an increased number of encephalitis cases developed in and near marshland areas in Southern California. There was an increased amount of rainfall that year. Which of the following vectors was most likely responsible for the outbreak?

(A) Louse
(B) Tick
(C) Bug
(D) Mosquito
(E) Flea

96. A rock collector, who just returned from the Sonoran desert in Arizona, presents with fever, and enlarged, painful draining inguinal lymph nodes. This patient most likely has a disease that was transmitted by the bite of a

(A) louse
(B) tick
(C) bug
(D) mosquito
(E) flea

97. A lack of dystrophic calcification associated with the inflammatory process would most likely be noted in

(A) cysticercosis
(B) trichinosis
(C) congenital toxoplasmosis
(D) herpes encephalitis
(E) congenital cytomegalovirus infection

98. Which of the following is more likely a feature of atypical pneumonia rather than a pneumonia caused by *Streptococcus pneumoniae*?

(A) High fever
(B) Nonproductive cough
(C) Gram-positive sputum stain
(D) Sudden onset
(E) Rust-colored sputum

99. Which of the following is the best marker of disease activity in HIV-positive patients when they develop overt AIDS?

(A) Anti-gp120
(B) p24 antigen
(C) Ratio of CD_4 T-helper cells to CD_8 T-suppressor cells
(D) Mitogen assay for T-cell function
(E) Total lymphocyte count

100. Which of the following organisms is the most common cause of disseminated helminthic infection in patients with impaired cellular immunity?

(A) *Strongyloides stercoralis*
(B) *Ancyclostoma duodenale*
(C) *Enterobius vermicularis*
(D) *Ascaris lumbricoides*
(E) *Trichuris trichiura*

101. Which of the following relationships is correct?

(A) Black widow spider—painful bite with envenomation of a necrotoxin
(B) Brown recluse spider—painful bite with envenomation of a neurotoxin
(C) Scorpion—abdominal pain with a board-like rigidity that is confused with a surgical abdomen
(D) Bees and wasps—most common cause of death due to a venomous bite
(E) Chigger—causative agent of scabies

102. The most common bacterial infection associated with intravenous drug abuse would most likely produce

(A) skin and soft-tissue infections
(B) osteomyelitis
(C) infective endocarditis
(D) embolic strokes that produce cerebral abscesses
(E) pneumonia

103. Which of the following associations is correct?

(A) Carbon monoxide poisoning—necrosis of the globus pallidus and degeneration in the substantia nigra
(B) Wernicke's encephalopathy—absence of the tail of the caudate nucleus
(C) Huntington's chorea—ring hemorrhages in the mamillary bodies and periventricular area
(D) Alzheimer's disease—lenticular degeneration
(E) Wilson's disease—senile plaques

DIRECTIONS:

Each of the numbered items or incomplete statements in this section is negatively phrased, as indicated by a capitalized word such as NOT, LEAST, or EXCEPT. Select the ONE lettered answer or completion that is BEST in each case.

104. Axonal injury results in all of the following EXCEPT

(A) swelling of the perikaryon
(B) dissolution of the Nissl substance
(C) disappearance of the axon nucleolus
(D) decrease in the cytoplasmic basophilia
(E) peripheral displacement of the nucleus

105. Which of the following statements about tetanus immunization is NOT true?

(A) Tetanus toxoid immunization is recommended for individuals before they enter college
(B) Tetanus toxoid is not recommended for nonimmunized patients who have clean minor wounds that have been properly cleaned and débrided
(C) Tetanus toxoid alone is recommended for immunized patients who have dirty wounds and have not had a booster shot in more than 5 years
(D) In patients who have been fully immunized, booster shots protect the patient for 10 years
(E) Tetanus toxoid and immune globulin are recommended for nonimmunized patients who have dirty wounds

106. All of the following are true concerning fast skeletal muscle fibers EXCEPT

(A) some are red; some are white
(B) some have many mitochondria; some have few mitochondria
(C) some have a high concentration of myoglobin; some have a low concentration of myoglobin
(D) some have slow myosin adenosine triphosphatase (ATPase); some have rapid myosin ATPase
(E) some have many capillaries around them; some have few capillaries around them

107. Which of the following musculoskeletal injury relationships is NOT correct?

(A) Greenstick fracture—commonly seen in children
(B) Colle's fracture—associated with a fall on the outstretched hand
(C) Supracondylar fracture—associated with injury to the radial nerve and brachial artery leading to ischemic contracture in the forearm
(D) Clavicular fracture—most common newborn fracture
(E) Rotator cuff injury—pain at the tip of the shoulder and inability to abduct the arm

108. All of the following would result from a lesion of the oculomotor nerve EXCEPT

(A) the eye would be in lateral and inferior (down and out) position
(B) the pupillary light reflex would be disrupted
(C) there would be a ptosis of the eyelid
(D) the pupil would be constricted
(E) all muscles of the eye would show flaccid paralysis except the lateral rectus and superior obliques muscles

109. Which of the following bone disease or x-ray relationships is NOT correct?

(A) Osteogenic sarcoma—sunburst appearance
(B) Ewing's sarcoma—onion skinning
(C) Osteoid osteoma—radiolucent nidus surrounded by dense sclerotic bone
(D) Osteogenic sarcoma—Codman's triangle
(E) Avascular necrosis—lytic area in bone with absence of reactive bone formation

110. All of the following are correct concerning fluoxetine and sertraline EXCEPT

(A) selectively block serotonin reuptake by central nervous system neurons
(B) effectively used in treating mood depression
(C) cause considerable sedation and should be taken at bedtime
(D) may cause a small weight loss
(E) unlikely to cause adverse cholinergic and cardiovascular effects

111. A 65-year-old man has noticed a progressive increase in hat size and pain in the pelvic bones. His serum alkaline phosphatase is markedly elevated. A physical exam including rectal exam is normal. Radiographs of his skull and pelvic bones reveal irregular thickening of the bone. There is a mixture of sclerotic bone with areas of bone lysis. One would LEAST expect which of the following as a further complication of this patient's disease?

(A) Pathologic fractures
(B) Enlargement of the sella turcica
(C) High-output cardiac failure
(D) Replacement of the bone matrix with mosaic bone
(E) An increased incidence of osteogenic sarcoma

112. Which of the following would be LEAST LIKELY to prevent conduction of nerve impulses along a preparation of mammalian nerve fibers in a fluid medium?

(A) extracellular sodium is replaced by potassium
(B) extracellular sodium is replaced by an impermeant cation
(C) the resting membrane potential is decreased to -30 mv
(D) the sodium potassium pump is momentarily stopped
(E) tetrodotoxin, a sodium channel blocker, is present

113. Which of the following skin disorder relationships is NOT correctly matched?

(A) Acute eczema—scaling and lichenification
(B) Acne rosacea—sebaceous gland hyperplasia
(C) Acanthosis nigricans—phenotypic marker for gastric adenocarcinoma
(D) Discoid lupus—liquefactive degeneration of the basal cell layer
(E) Merkel cell carcinoma—neoplasm resembling small cell carcinoma of the lung

114. Examination of a patient reveals a sensory deficit on the skin of the lateral side of the hand. All of the following nerves can be sites of lesions that result in this sensory deficit EXCEPT

(A) lower trunk of the brachial plexus
(B) median nerve
(C) radial nerve
(D) ventral ramus of C_6
(E) lateral root of the median nerve

115. All of the following are correct concerning phenylzine and tranylcypromine EXCEPT

(A) inhibit both monoamine oxidase A and monoamine oxidase B
(B) antidepressant activity occurs within 1 to 2 days after starting treatment
(C) may cause orthostatic hypotension, weight gain, and ejaculatory delay
(D) hyperpyrexia may occur if used concurrently with tricyclic antidepressants
(E) consumption of foods rich in tyramine may cause hypertension in patients receiving these drugs

116. A 17-year-old who is going to have his first schizophrenic episode in 2 months is at present likely to show all of the following EXCEPT

(A) strange perceptions
(B) peculiar behavior
(C) somatic problems
(D) increased level of social activities
(E) interest in the occult

117. All of the following drugs may lower the seizure threshold EXCEPT

(A) ciprofloxacin
(B) amitriptyline
(C) chlorpromazine
(D) lorazepam
(E) loxapine

118. A midshaft fracture of the humerus may result in laceration of the radial nerve. Such an injury can result in all of the following EXCEPT

(A) wristdrop
(B) an inability to supinate the forearm
(C) an inability to extend the thumb
(D) an inability to make a tight fist
(E) a weakness of thumb abduction

119. All of the following statements concerning drug interactions in the central nervous system are correct EXCEPT

(A) carbamazepine induces hepatic drug-metabolizing enzymes
(B) the depressant effects of ethanol are potentiated by tricyclic antidepressants, opiates, and benzodiazepines
(C) valproate can inhibit the metabolism of other drugs, including phenytoin and carbamazepine
(D) acute administration of large quantities of ethanol induces hepatic cytochrome P450 enzymes
(E) ingestion of protein or pyridoxine may reduce the effectiveness of levodopa in Parkinson's disease

120. All of the following symptoms are characteristic of avoidant personality disorder EXCEPT

(A) sensitivity to rejection
(B) timidity
(C) social withdrawal
(D) inferiority complex
(E) peculiar appearance

121. All of the following statements concerning sedative-hypnotic drugs are correct EXCEPT

(A) midazolam causes retrograde amnesia when it is administered intravenously as a preanesthetic medication or for minor surgical and diagnostic procedures
(B) zolpidem is an imidazopyridine derivative that binds to benzodiazepine receptors and is indicated for short-term treatment of insomnia
(C) in the management of ethanol withdrawal, a long-acting benzodiazepine such as chlordiazepoxide is substituted for ethanol and then gradually withdrawn
(D) in treating patients with anxiety who are otherwise healthy, therapeutic doses of benzodiazepines have little effect on respiratory or cardiovascular function
(E) benzodiazepines may be safety prescribed for elderly patients at the same doses used for younger patients without risk of adverse effects

122. A lesion of the upper trunk of the brachial plexus can result in all of the following EXCEPT

(A) an inability to abduct the arm at the shoulder
(B) a weakness in external rotation of the arm at the shoulder
(C) a cutaneous sensory deficit on the lateral side of the distal arm
(D) a weakness in flexion of the arm at the shoulder
(E) an inability to pronate the forearm

123. Central nervous system stimulants such as methylphenidate and the amphetamines are used in treating all of the following conditions EXCEPT

(A) drug-induced respiratory depression
(B) narcolepsy
(C) attention deficit disorder
(D) obesity
(E) hyperkinetic syndrome in children

124. A lesion of the lower trunk of the brachial plexus can result in all of the following EXCEPT

(A) an inability to abduct and adduct digits II through V
(B) a clawing of digits II through V
(C) a sensory deficit on the entire dorsal and ventral surfaces of the hand
(D) an inability to oppose the thumb
(E) an inability to adduct the thumb

125. All of the following drugs have a very strong drug dependence liability EXCEPT

(A) phencyclidine
(B) nicotine
(C) heroin
(D) cocaine
(E) morphine

126. Examination of a patient reveals paralysis of the abductor pollicis brevis muscle. All of the following nerves can be sites of lesions that resulted in this paralysis EXCEPT

(A) medial root of the median nerve
(B) lower trunk of the brachial plexus
(C) anterior interosseous nerve
(D) median nerve
(E) ventral roots of C_8 and T_1

127. Pancuronium has all of the following attributes EXCEPT

(A) acts as a nondepolarizing neuromuscular blocker
(B) has little effect on autonomic ganglia
(C) is administered parenterally
(D) is eliminated by hepatic metabolism
(E) overdose can cause respiratory paralysis

128. Nerve fibers in the posterior cord of the brachial plexus innervate all of the following muscles EXCEPT

(A) latissimus dorsi muscle
(B) subscapularis muscle
(C) teres major muscle
(D) teres minor muscle
(E) infraspinatus muscle

129. Neostigmine can rapidly reverse the muscle paralysis caused by all of the following agents EXCEPT

(A) pancuronium
(B) succinylcholine
(C) vecuronium
(D) tubocurarine
(E) metocurine

130. A complete lesion of the upper trunk of the brachial plexus results in damage to nerve fibers found in all of the following nerves EXCEPT

(A) radial nerve
(B) lateral pectoral nerve
(C) recurrent branch of the median nerve
(D) musculocutaneous nerve
(E) axillary nerve

131. The neuromuscular blockade produced by pancuronium may be potentiated in all of the following situations EXCEPT

(A) administration of furosemide
(B) administration of isoflurane
(C) administration of lidocaine
(D) administration of gentamicin
(E) a patient with myasthenia gravis

132. Nerves that contain nerve fibers from the C_8 and/or T_1 spinal cord segments include all of the following EXCEPT

(A) medial antebrachial cutaneous nerve
(B) lateral pectoral nerve
(C) recurrent branch of the median nerve
(D) deep branch of the ulnar nerve
(E) superficial branch of the ulnar nerve

133. The pharmacologic effects of tubocurarine include all of the following EXCEPT

(A) skeletal muscle relaxation
(B) hypotension
(C) release of histamine
(D) increased intraocular pressure
(E) ganglionic blockade

134. Nerves that contain posterior division nerve fibers include all of the following EXCEPT

(A) the thoracodorsal nerve
(B) the posterior interosseous nerve
(C) the lower subscapular nerve
(D) the axillary nerve
(E) the medial pectoral nerve

135. The pharmacologic effects of halogenated inhalational anesthetics such as halothane include all of the following EXCEPT

(A) decreased respiratory tidal volume and minute volume
(B) dose-dependent arterial hypertension
(C) uterine relaxation
(D) decreased cardiac contractility
(E) analgesia

136. Which anatomic structure is NOT considered a part of the limbic system?

(A) Cingulate gyrus
(B) Hippocampus
(C) Parahippocampal gyrus
(D) Superior temporal gyrus
(E) Hypothalamus

137. Adverse effects of morphine include all of the following EXCEPT

(A) respiratory depression
(B) constipation
(C) diuresis
(D) nausea and vomiting
(E) pruritus and flushing of the skin

138. A 55-year-old patient with bipolar disorder is placed on lithium therapy. Which condition is this patient LEAST likely to experience?

(A) Hypothyroidism
(B) Gastric distress
(C) Tremor
(D) Mild cognitive impairment
(E) Food intolerance

139. Chronic administration of opiate analgesics usually results in tolerance to all of the following effects EXCEPT

(A) sedation
(B) miosis
(C) analgesia
(D) constipation
(E) miosis and constipation

140. Organelles typically present in the axon include all of the following EXCEPT

(A) vesicles
(B) neurotubules
(C) mitochondria
(D) neurofilaments
(E) rough endoplasmic reticulum

141. All of the following are correct concerning lithium EXCEPT

(A) its low therapeutic index necessitates serum level monitoring
(B) it appears to act by inhibiting post-receptor signal transduction
(C) it is primarily used as a mood stabilizer in bipolar affective disorder
(D) diuretics may lower lithium serum levels, necessitating increased lithium doses
(E) chronic use may lead to hypothyroidism

142. All of the following statements about the femoral nerve entering the thigh are true EXCEPT

(A) it passes posterior to the inguinal ligament
(B) it lies lateral to the femoral artery
(C) it lies medial to the femoral vein
(D) it is external to the femoral sheath
(E) it lies anterior to the iliopsoas muscle

143. The following opioid receptors are correctly characterized EXCEPT

(A) mu—mediates supraspinal analgesia, miosis, euphoria, and sedation
(B) delta—primarily associated with smooth muscle relaxation in the gut and biliary tract
(C) kappa—a spinal opioid receptor mediating analgesia and sedation
(D) sigma—activated by pentazocine and other partial/mixed agonists; mediates dysphoria and psychotomimetic effects

144. All of the following are believed to be true concerning the mechanism of contraction of smooth muscle EXCEPT

(A) excitation of contraction can occur without an action potential
(B) calcium influx from the extracellular space helps initiate a contraction
(C) intracellular calcium ions bind to calmodulin
(D) the calcium-calmodulin complex inhibits myosin light chain kinase
(E) the actin-myosin complex utilizes adenosine triphosphate (ATP) for energy

145. If an accident caused a hemisection on the right side of the spinal cord in the midthoracic region, which of the following would be the LEAST likely to be lost or diminished?

(A) Temperature sensation from the right side below the area of injury
(B) Vibratory and 2-point discrimination from the right side below the injury
(C) Unconscious proprioception from the right side below the area of injury
(D) Voluntary movement of the right leg
(E) Pain sensation from the left side below the area of injury

146. Which of the following statements concerning rabies and rabies immunization is NOT correct?

(A) Rabies may be contracted by aerosolization in bat-infested caves
(B) Fluorescent antibody testing of corneal scrapings detects rabies antigen in people suspected of having rabies
(C) Full immunization is unnecessary in domestic dog and cat bites if the animals show no signs of rabies after 10 days of observation
(D) Animal bites from skunks, coyotes, foxes, or raccoons are considered rabid and full immunization is recommended
(E) In bites from wild animals suspected of being rabid, thorough cleansing of the wound site with soap and water and an injection of half of the dose of the human diploid vaccine to the wound site are recommended as prophylactic measures

147. All of the following statements about synovial joints are true EXCEPT

(A) the synovial epithelium secretes the synovial fluid
(B) the fibrous capsule is lined on its inner side by the synovial membrane
(C) the synovial membrane lines the intra-articular portion of the bone
(D) the articular surface of the bone is covered by cartilage
(E) the articular cartilage is covered by the synovial membrane

148. Which of the following statements concerning influenza and influenza vaccination is NOT true?

(A) In the elderly population, vaccination is more useful in preventing illness than reducing deaths caused by influenza
(B) Vaccination is generally recommended for all individuals who are 65 years of age or older
(C) Vaccination is recommended for adults and children with chronic pulmonary and cardiovascular diseases
(D) In young adults, amantadine prophylaxis is 70% to 90% effective in preventing influenza type A
(E) Vaccination should be avoided by patients who are allergic to eggs

149. Within a muscle, the muscle fibers may be grouped as motor units. All of the following statements about motor units are true EXCEPT

(A) all the muscle fibers within a single motor unit are innervated by a single efferent neuron
(B) the force of contraction of a muscle may be gradually increased by gradually increasing the number of motor units that are depolarizing and contracting
(C) during a sustained maximal contraction of a muscle, all the motor units are depolarizing synchronously
(D) each muscle cell within a motor unit always contracts maximally when the motor unit depolarizes
(E) different motor units within the same muscle may cause different movements

150. All of the following have radiodense abnormalities that are usually visible on an x-ray of the skull EXCEPT

(A) an astrocytoma
(B) old age
(C) hypoparathyroidism
(D) cysticercosis
(E) a meningioma

DIRECTIONS:

Each set of matching questions in this section consists of a list of four to twenty-six lettered options (some of which may be in figures) followed by several numbered items. For each numbered item, select the ONE lettered option that is most closely associated with it. To avoid spending too much time on matching sets with a large number of options, it is generally advisable to begin each set by reading the list of options. Then for each item in the set, try to generate the correct answer and locate it in the option list, rather than evaluating each option individually. Each lettered option may be selected once, more than once, or not at all.

Questions 151-155

Select the opiate that best matches the numbered descriptions.

(A) Propoxyphene
(B) Butorphanol
(C) Fentanyl
(D) Dextromethorphan
(E) Methadone

151. A high-potency, short-acting opiate that is often used to provide or supplement anesthesia for cardiac surgery; recently available as a transdermal skin patch formulation for severe pain

152. An orally effective, long-acting opiate that is used to facilitate abstinence in patients who are addicted to intravenous opiates

153. An orally effective but weak opiate used for minor pain in combination with acetaminophen or aspirin

154. A stereoisomer of a potent opiate analgesic that lacks significant analgesic effects but retains antitussive activity

155. A mixed agonist/antagonist opiate that is available in a parenteral and an intranasal formulation for treatment of moderate to severe pain

Questions 156-159

Select the general anesthetic that best matches the numbered descriptions.

(A) Halothane
(B) Nitrous oxide
(C) Ketamine
(D) Diethylether
(E) Thiopental

156. A "complete" anesthetic that produces analgesia, amnesia, unconsciousness, and muscle relaxation, while permitting adequate oxygenation without cardiovascular or respiratory depression

157. An incomplete anesthetic whose minimum alveolar concentration (MAC) is greater than 100% that provides excellent analgesia for minor surgery and causes only minimal cardiovascular depression

158. Sensitizes the heart to catecholamines, thereby predisposing patients to cardiac arrhythmias; it has a low MAC and a relatively low blood-gas partition coefficient

159. A potent analgesic and amnesic agent that produces a cataleptic state in which the patient appears awake but is unresponsive to pain

Questions 160-164

For each of the pathophysiological descriptions, select the schematic of the spinal cord that best illustrates the location of the lesion (dark shaded area).

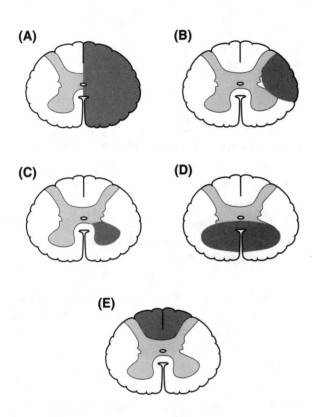

(A)   **(B)**

(C)   **(D)**

(E)

160. Infarction (damaged tissue area) in this part of the spinal cord would produce signs and symptoms associated with an unsteady gait due to ataxia, and loss of voluntary motor skills, especially in distal parts of extremity.

161. Infarction in this part of the spinal cord would result in diminution of sensory localization of sharp stimuli and may produce persistent paresthesias of tingling and numbness; accompanying these sensory findings, weakness of voluntary motor activity would be detected bilaterally.

162. Axon demyelinization in this fiber pathway results in loss of two-point touch discrimination, a Romberg's sign, and decreased conscious proprioception in the right side of the body.

163. Infarction in this part of the spinal cord results only in deficits described as a lower motor syndrome.

164. A traumatic lesion of this nature produces a constellation of neurological findings best described as a Brown-Sequard syndrome.

Questions 165-169

Select the neuroleptic drug that best matches the numbered descriptions.

(A) Clozapine
(B) Risperidone
(C) Haloperidol
(D) Prochlorperazine
(E) Fluphenazine
(F) Promethazine

165. A high-potency butyrophenone that produces little sedation and postural hypotension but has a high incidence of acute extrapyramidal side effects

166. A drug that is particularly useful for the treatment of resistant schizophrenia and in patients with predominantly "negative" schizophrenic symptoms but may cause agranulocytosis

167. A phenothiazine drug that is available as a long-acting injectable preparation for chronic maintenance therapy

168. A new atypical antipsychotic drug that acts on dopamine D2 and 5-HT2 receptors but does not cause agranulocytosis

169. A phenothiazine drug that is often used for the treatment of nausea and vomiting

Questions 170-174

Select the one lettered heading below that matches the symptoms with the location of the responsible pathology. Use each answer only once.

(A) Left pons
(B) Right pons
(C) Cerebellar-pontine angle
(D) Left hemisphere
(E) Right hemisphere

170. Inability to abduct the right eye and left hemiparesis

171. Decreased hearing in the left ear and weakness in muscle of facial expression on the left

172. Weakness of the muscles in lower part of face on the right and right hemiparesis of extremities

173. Inability to abduct the left eye and prominent asymmetry of the face on the left side

174. Weakness in right upper limb and a Broca's aphasia

Questions 175-178

Select the muscle relaxant drug that best matches the numbered descriptions.

(A) Baclofen
(B) Diazepam
(C) Pancuronium
(D) Cyclobenzaprine
(E) Dantrolene

175. Administered intravenously to patients with malignant hyperthermia, where it acts to inhibit the release of calcium from the sarcoplasmic reticulum of skeletal muscle

176. Reduces spasticity in patients with spinal cord injuries without causing significant sedation by activating $GABA_B$ receptors

177. Used in acute muscle spasm due to minor injuries but is not effective in cerebral palsy or spinal cord injury; acts on the brain stem and/or spinal cord to reduce elevated muscle tone and cause significant sedation

178. A competitive nicotinic receptor antagonist that is primarily used to provide adequate skeletal muscle relaxation for surgery

Questions 179-180

Match the following cross-sections and gross specimen of the brain with the clinical description that they most likely represent.

(A) An elderly woman who hit her head on the edge of a desk and has fluctuating levels of consciousness in the emergency room

(B) A major league baseball player who was hit on the side of the head with a baseball bat and has signs of increased intracranial pressure

(C) A 55-year-old black man with essential hypertension presents with a sudden onset of hemiplegia

(D) A 35-year-old woman with polycystic kidney disease who complains of a severe occipital headache

(E) A 56-year-old man with a ventricular aneurysm who presents with a sudden onset of hemiplegia

180.

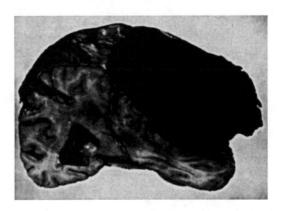

179.

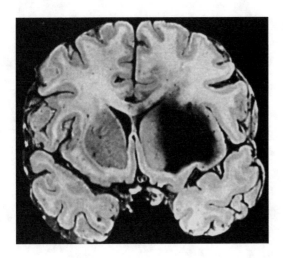

ANSWER KEY

1. B	31. B	61. B	91. C	121. E	151. C
2. A	32. A	62. C	92. A	122. E	152. E
3. B	33. D	63. C	93. A	123. A	153. A
4. C	34. C	64. A	94. E	124. C	154. D
5. A	35. C	65. B	95. D	125. A	155. B
6. C	36. D	66. C	96. E	126. C	156. D
7. D	37. C	67. B	97. D	127. D	157. B
8. A	38. E	68. E	98. B	128. E	158. A
9. B	39. B	69. E	99. B	129. B	159. C
10. C	40. E	70. B	100. A	130. C	160. B
11. B	41. C	71. B	101. D	131. A	161. D
12. C	42. A	72. E	102. A	132. B	162. E
13. B	43. B	73. C	103. A	133. D	163. C
14. A	44. B	74. A	104. C	134. E	164. A
15. C	45. E	75. D	105. B	135. B	165. C
16. C	46. A	76. E	106. D	136. D	166. A
17. D	47. C	77. E	107. C	137. C	167. E
18. A	48. A	78. B	108. D	138. E	168. B
19. B	49. B	79. D	109. E	139. E	169. D
20. B	50. D	80. E	110. C	140. E	170. B
21. C	51. E	81. A	111. B	141. D	171. C
22. D	52. B	82. D	112. D	142. C	172. D
23. A	53. B	83. B	113. A	143. B	173. A
24. C	54. B	84. B	114. A	144. D	174. D
25. C	55. E	85. B	115. B	145. A	175. E
26. C	56. C	86. B	116. D	146. E	176. A
27. B	57. E	87. D	117. D	147. E	177. D
28. D	58. E	88. B	118. B	148. A	178. C
29. C	59. D	89. C	119. D	149. C	179. C
30. C	60. A	90. E	120. E	150. A	180. B

ANSWERS AND EXPLANATIONS

1. The answer is B. *(Behavioral science)*
Generalized anxiety disorder is characterized by persistent anxiety lasting at least 6 months, with tension, sympathetic and parasympathetic symptoms, and insomnia. In this condition, the symptoms of anxiety cannot be related to a specific person or situation; instead, anxiety is "free floating."

2. The answer is A. *(Pathology)*
Ependymal cells line the cerebral ventricles and have blepharoplasts that are visible with special stains. They are useful histologic markers that document the ependymal origin of a brain tumor. Microglial cells are derived from macrophages and are the phagocytic cells of the central nervous system. When activated, microglial cells are called gitter cells and have a foamy appearance. Neuronophagia (e.g., viral encephalitis, poliomyelitis) occurs when microglial cells phagocytize breakdown products of the neuron. Rod-like microglial cells are seen in neurosyphilis. Macrophages are primarily responsible for carrying HIV into the central nervous system and are the reservoir cell for the virus.

3. The answer is B. *(Microbiology)*
The patient has a negative Dick test and a positive Schick test, which indicates that he has neutralizing antibodies against the group A streptococcus that causes scarlet fever. In both tests, the antigen that is injected is the toxin. If neutralizing antibodies are present, they neutralize the toxin and skin reactions do not occur. This indicates that the patient is immune to the specific strain of bacteria producing the disease. For example, the patient's negative Dick test means that he has neutralizing antibodies that will protect him against the strain of streptococcus that produces scarlet fever, but not against strains that may be associated with pharyngitis or other infections. Absence of the antibodies allows the toxin to host an inflammatory reaction, which indicates a lack of immunity. If the patient had a full complement of diphtheria-pertussis-tetanus (DPT) immunizations, neutralizing antibodies against diphtheria should be present. The presence of a reaction for the Schick test is a not a test of cellular immunity, because it is an antigen–antibody reaction.

4. The answer is C. *(Pathology)*
Xenodiagnosis is used in the diagnosis of Chagas disease, which is caused by *Trypanosoma cruzi*, a hemoflagellate. There are four morphologic forms of hemoflagellates. In man, they may be intracellular, in which they are called leishmanial forms; or, they may be located extracellularly in the blood, in which they are called trypanosomes. The insect vectors may have leptomonads (promastigotes) or crithidial (epimastigote) forms. Leishmaniasis (cutaneous, mucocutaneous, and visceral) only has the leishmanial, intracellular forms present in man. In African trypanosomiasis, only the extracellular, or trypanosomal form, is present in man. Chagas disease has both the intracellular (leishmanial) and extracellular (trypanosomal) forms.

Chagas disease is rampant in South America and is the major cause of progressive heart failure and death in that area. *T. cruzi* is a flagellated protozoan that is transmitted to man by the bite of the Reduviid bug, or kissing bug, which usually occurs during the night. Shortly after the bite, the bug defecates on the wound site and the sleeping host rubs the organisms into the wound. Periorbital inflammation develops, which is called Romana's sign. Trypanosomes circulate in the blood and leishmanial forms invade (1) the reticuloendothelial cells, producing hepatosplenomegaly; (2) the heart muscle, causing myocarditis and arrhythmias; (3) the brain, producing a meningoencephalitis; and (4) into the gastrointestinal tract, where the leishmania destroy the ganglion cells in the distal esophagus and rectum to produce acquired achalasia and Hirschsprung disease, respectively. Laboratory diagnosis is made by (1) finding trypanosomes in the blood, (2) finding leishmanial forms in tissue, (3) culture, (4) serology, and (5) xenodiagnosis.

Xenodiagnosis is a method of inoculation in which sterile Reduviid bugs are fed or offered the blood of an infected patient. After a few weeks, the bug's intestinal contents are examined for presence or absence of the organism. Only 5% of patients die in the acute stage of heart failure, whereas in chronic disease, heart failure is a common cause of death. Nifurtimox is the drug of choice.

5. The answer is A. *(Microbiology)*
Haemophilus influenzae type B vaccine is not an egg-based vaccine and is safe to administer to a patient with a history of anaphylactic reactions to eggs. Influenza, measles, mumps, and yellow fever vaccines are egg-based. Vaccines often contain materials other than the active-immunizing antigens, such as preservatives, antibiotics (e.g., neomycin, streptomycin) to prevent bacterial overgrowth, adjuvants to enhance immunogenicity, and stabilizers. Patients who are allergic to neomycin should not receive the measles-mumps-rubella (MMR) and oral polio vaccines. Patients who are allergic to streptomycin should not receive the live or the killed polio vaccine.

6. The answer is C. *(Pathology)*
Werdnig-Hoffmann disease most closely resembles amyotrophic lateral sclerosis (ALS). Both of these diseases involve the degeneration of motor neurons.

ALS appears to be increasing in incidence. In 5% to 10% of cases, there is an autosomal dominant pattern with strong age-dependent penetrance. Proposed etiologies include oxidative stress, viral infection, immunologic disease, or some unknown environmental factor. Currently, the oxidative stress theory is favored because a defect in the zinc-copper binding superoxide dismutase (SOD1) coded on chromosome 21 was discovered. Because SOD1 is an antioxidant that converts the superoxide free radical into peroxide and oxygen, reduced activity causes apoptosis (individual cell necrosis) of spinal motor neurons. Inhibition of glutamate transport potentiates the toxicity associated with the reduced SOD1 levels. ALS most commonly presents with both upper motor neuron signs (e.g., spastic paralysis) and, eventually, lower motor neuron signs (e.g., muscle atrophy, fasciculations). Atrophy of the intrinsic muscles of the hand and forearms with hand weakness and spastic changes in the lower legs are early signs. Antioxidant cocktails have now been developed, which offer some symptomatic improvement.

Werdnig-Hoffmann disease is a progressive muscular atrophy noted in infants. It often presents as the floppy child syndrome.

7. The answer is D. *(Anatomy)*
This is a description of a medial medullary syndrome. Contralateral loss of motor innervation producing upper motor neuron signs and symptoms, contralateral loss of modalities carried by the dorsal column-medial lemniscal tract, and ipsilateral paralysis of the tongue with lower motor neuron characteristics are the cardinal features of this syndrome. Medial medullary syndrome may occur from vascular disease affecting penetrating vessels of the anterior spinal artery or vertebral arteries. The pyramids, medial lemniscus, and hypoglossal nerves are most affected.

In contrast, a lesion in the pons would be more likely produce to peripheral signs and symptoms related to the abducens, facial, or trigeminal nerves.

The third choice is not correct because the hypoglossal nerve and nucleus are located in the medial aspects of the medulla. Also, the pyramidal and medial lemniscal pathways reside on the midline.

Based on the clinical findings, the right medial medulla would not be the affected site. The motor paralysis and the sensory deficits are found on one side, but both of these systems cross at the medulla-spinal cord junction, so lesions above the decussation would produce clinical findings on the opposite side. The cranial nerve lower motor neuron symptoms are on the left and would be produced by an ipsilateral nerve palsy. If the right medulla was lesioned, the tongue findings would be detected on the right.

8. The answer is A. *(Pathology)*
Compared with serum, cerebrospinal fluid (CSF) has a higher chloride concentration. CSF is an ultrafiltrate of plasma. It is produced primarily by the choroid plexus cells in the lateral ventricles. From the lateral ventricles, CSF flows through the foramen of Munro into the third ventricle, through the aqueduct of Sylvius, and into the fourth ventricle. It then exits the fourth ventricle through the foramina of Luschka and Magendie and enters the subarachnoid space located between the arachnoid and pia mater. The CSF in the subarachnoid space cushions the brain and spinal cord. CSF is resorbed through the arachnoid villi, extending into the dural venous sinuses located along the summit of the brain. The venous sinuses empty into the jugular venous system.

CSF has a lower glucose, lower protein (15 to 45 mg/dl), less lymphocytes, and higher chloride (120 to 130 mEq/dl) than serum. These differences help distinguish serum from CSF in trauma cases.

9. The answer is B. *(Microbiology)*
Rifampin achieves high mucosal concentrations and is the drug of choice for chronic carriers of *Neisseria meningitidis, Staphylococcus aureus,* and *Haemophilus influenzae.* In addition, it is an important antituberculous agent. Its mechanism of action is that it binds to DNA-dependent RNA polymerase, thus effectively inhibiting transcription of mRNA from DNA. Similar to alcohol, it may induce the cytochrome P-450 microsomal system in the liver and cause an increase in the synthesis of γ-glutamyl transferase as well as an increase in the metabolism of other drugs metabolized in the liver (e.g., anticonvulsants).

10. The answer is C. *(Pathology)*
Metachromatic leukodystrophy is a lysosomal storage disease associated with the synthesis of abnormal myelin. The term *leukodystrophy* refers to the abnormality in myelin synthesis. Metachromatic leukodystrophy is an autosomal recessive disease characterized by an arylsulfatase A deficiency, leading to the accumulation of sulfatides in lysosomes that stain positively with periodic acid-Schiff stain and various metachromatic stains. The clinical findings include various visceral lesions, mental retardation, peripheral neuropathy, and abnormal myelination in the central nervous system associated with reactive gliosis. It is diagnosed by the absence of arylsulfatase A in the urine.

Tay-Sachs disease is an autosomal recessive GM_2 gangliosidosis characterized by a hexosaminidase (α-subunit) deficiency and an accumulation of GM_2 ganglioside in lysosomes. It is commonly found in Ashkenazi Jews, in which there is a 1 in 30 carrier rate. The patients are normal at birth but develop abnormalities by 6 months of age, including severe mental retardation, blindness (cherry red spot in the macula), and muscle flaccidity. The lipid has a whorled configuration in lysosomes when viewed by electron microscopy. It is a uniformly fatal disease.

Niemann-Pick disease is an autosomal recessive lysosomal storage disease associated with a sphingomyelinase deficiency and the accumulation of sphingomyelin in macrophages and neurons. The type A variant is most common. It is characterized by severe mental retardation, hepatosplenomegaly, deterioration of psychomotor function, and foamy macrophages. Zebra bodies are noted in the lysosomes when viewed by electron microscopy. The disease is fatal in early life.

Hurler disease is an autosomal recessive mucopolysaccharidosis characterized by a α-1-iduronidase deficiency and an accumulation of dermatan and heparan sulfate. It is associated with coarse facial features, severe mental retardation, hepatosplenomegaly, clouding of the cornea, a high incidence of coronary artery disease, joint stiffness, and vacuoles in lymphocytes that contain the mucopolysaccharides in lysosomes.

Hunter disease is a sex-linked recessive mucopolysaccharidosis characterized by a deficiency in L-iduronosulfate and an accumulation of dermatan and heparan sulfate in lysosomes. It is a milder form of Hurler disease.

11. The answer is B. *(Physiology)*
Only if the membrane potential (MP) is at the value of electrochemical equilibrium for sodium (around +60 mv) is there no net movement of sodium across the cell membrane; only at electrochemical equilibrium for potassium (around -100 mv) is there no net movement of potassium. For all MP values between +60 and -100 there is an influx of sodium and an efflux of potassium. When the pump is nonelectrogenic (does not contribute to the MP), the resting MP occurs at that value at which the rate of sodium influx equals the rate of potassium efflux. If the membrane is equally permeable to both sodium and potassium, then the resting MP will be about midway between +60 and -100 mv. Because the rate of flux of an ion is a product of permeability to that ion and the distance from electrochemical equilibrium for that ion, then when potassium is more permeable than sodium, as it is in a typical cell at rest, the point at which the rate of sodium influx equals that of potassium efflux is much closer to the potassium electrochemical equilibrium.

12. The answer is C. *(Pathology)*
A woman who has oligoclonal bands in her spinal fluid most likely has a demyelinating disease, the most common of which is multiple sclerosis. Dizziness and paresthesias are common findings in demyelinating diseases. Memory loss, seizure activity, occipital headaches, and tunnel vision are not associated features of demyelination.

Oligoclonal bands are identified as narrow bands in the gamma globulin region. They are the product of different clones of plasma cells in the central nervous system (CNS) as a secondary response to chronic inflammation. They are present in other demyelinating diseases in the CNS, including subacute sclerosing panencephalitis and Guillain-Barré syndrome.

13. The answer is B.   *(Microbiology)*
Respiratory precautions are unnecessary in patients who have pulmonary involvement caused by any of the systemic fungal infections. In coccidioidomycosis, the disease is contracted by inhaling arthrospores from the soil. Granulomas in the lungs contain spherules, which contain endospores that are not infective.

Respiratory precautions in patients who have untreated tuberculosis are unnecessary 2 to 3 weeks after therapy is initiated. In pertussis (whooping cough), precautions are unnecessary 1 week after therapy is initiated. Diphtheria requires precautions until the cultures are negative. Influenza requires respiratory precautions for the entire duration of the illness. Airborne precautions are recommended for (1) varicella, until all the lesions are crusted (only for those who are not immune), (2) rubeola (measles) for 4 days after the rash starts, (3) mumps for 9 days after onset of parotid swelling, and (4) rubella for 7 days after the rash appears.

14. The answer is A.   *(Pathology)*
Small cystic lesions in the lenticular nucleus, thalamus, and internal capsule are most closely associated with lacunar infarctions, which are most commonly secondary to hypertension. They account for 20% of all strokes. The small arterioles supplying these areas are branches of the middle cerebral artery. They exhibit arteriolar sclerosis, which thrombose and cause microinfarctions (liquefactive necrosis) that leave cystic spaces ranging in size from 1 to 15 mm. Multiple lesions are commonly observed. They account for a number of syndromes including (1) a pure motor hemiparesis if the posterior limb of the internal capsule is infarcted and (2) a pure sensory stroke if the infarct is in the ventrolateral thalamus. In some cases, these infarcts are associated with diabetes mellitus, which also produces small vessel disease.

Embolism usually produces hemorrhagic infarctions in the distribution of the middle cerebral artery. They generally occur at the periphery of the cerebral cortex.

The plaques of a demyelinating disease are softened rather than cystic areas in the brain.

Genetic diseases are an uncommon cause of cystic lesions in the brain.

Cystic astrocytomas may occur in the cerebellum.

15. The answer is C.   *(Anatomy)*
Alternating hemiplegia is a neurological deficit involving limbs on one side and cranial nerves on the opposite side. This is most often related to cranial nerves III, VI, and XII. Although the involvement of the body may be the same, if the lesion is in the midbrain the eye is affected; if it is located in the pons specifically, the lateral rectus muscle is involved; and if the lesion is located in the medulla, the tongue is affected.

16. The answer is C.   *(Pathology)*
Pale infarctions in the central nervous system (CNS) best characterize the lesions associated with an atherosclerotic (ischemic) stroke. The four major causes of a cerebrovascular accident, or stroke, in order of frequency, are ischemia (60% to 90% of cases), intracerebral hemorrhage (e.g., hypertensive bleed), subarachnoid hemorrhage (e.g., ruptured berry aneurysm, arteriovenous malformation), and embolic infarction (e.g., hemorrhagic infarction). As a general rule, ischemic strokes are pale (80% of cases) and the other three are hemorrhagic. The majority of ischemic strokes are due to atherosclerosis.

Atherosclerotic infarctions are most commonly secondary to a thrombus overlying an atheromatous plaque at the origin of the internal carotid artery. Consequences of atherosclerosis involving the cerebral vessels include cerebral infarction, cerebral atrophy, ischemic encephalopathy (laminar necrosis, watershed infarcts), transient ischemic attacks, and thromboembolism of a portion of atherosclerotic plaque to a distant location. They are usually pale infarcts, because the atherosclerotic plaque occludes most of the lumen and reperfusion of the infarcted area usually does not occur. Grossly, there is softening of the brain after 6 hours, with a visible loss of normal demarcation between the gray and white matter. Microscopically, "red neurons" (i.e., apoptosis of individual neurons), nuclear pyknosis, and degeneration of myelin are present. After 2 to 10 days, the brain tissue is gelatinous. Neutrophils transiently invade the necrotic area but are soon replaced by microglial cells, many of which have engulfed lipid and appear as gitter cells. From 10 days to 3 weeks, liquefactive necrosis produces cystic areas in the brain. The subjacent brain parenchyma contains reactive astrocytes with eosinophilic cytoplasm. Cerebral infarcts present with a gradual onset of symptoms (i.e., transient ischemic attacks; TIAs), followed by localizing neurologic signs of contralateral hemiplegia, aphasia, and visual defects (amaurosis fugax), depending on the site of infarction and whether the dominant hemisphere is involved. The majority of patients recover and regain partial restoration of their initial deficits.

TIAs occur in patients with fixed atherosclerotic disease and are often caused by dislodgment of platelet and/or cholesterol emboli into the peripheral vessels. They generally last a few seconds to a few minutes and, by definition, recovery is within 24 hours. Unilateral symptoms suggest carotid ischemia, whereas bilateral symptoms suggest vertebrobasilar ischemia, especially if accompanied by vertigo, dysarthria, or dysphagia. Ticlopidine, which inhibits the synthesis of adenosine diphosphate, or aspirin, which decreases the synthesis of thromboxane A_2, are commonly used to prevent TIAs.

17. The answer is D. *(Microbiology)*

Klebsiella pneumoniae is more likely than *Escherichia coli* to be associated with lobar pneumonia in an alcoholic. *K. pneumoniae* is a fat, nonmotile, gram-negative rod that is surrounded by a capsule that is responsible for its invasiveness. They characteristically produce moist mucoid colonies on culture. *K. pneumoniae* is a weak pathogen and requires a host with weak defenses (e.g., alcoholics, diabetics) to infect tissue. It is more commonly associated with urinary tract infections than with pneumonia. However, it produces a lobar pneumonia, particularly in alcoholics, diabetics, or those with weakened defenses. The pneumonias are characterized by blood-tinged mucoid sputum, a tendency for lung abscesses, and a mortality in 20% of patients. In general, *K. pneumonia* is susceptible to ceftriaxone.

Escherichia coli is the most common cause of acute cystitis and pyelonephritis, spontaneous bacterial peritonitis in alcoholics, enterotoxigenic strain of traveler's diarrhea, hemolytic uremic syndrome in children caused by eating undercooked hamburgers, endotoxic

shock, and acute cholecystitis. It is a common pathogen in neonatal meningitis, pneumonia in hospitalized patients caused by colonization of the airways by the organism, enteropathogenic gastroenteritis in infants under 2 years of age, enteroinvasive gastroenteritis with bloody diarrhea, peritonitis, wound infections (particularly in diabetics), and septicemia.

18. The answer is A. *(Pathology)*

A 35-year-old woman with a 7-day history of a severe occipital headache has xanthochromia in her cerebrospinal fluid (CSF), indicating the presence of a previous bleed, which, in this patient's history, must be a subarachnoid hemorrhage. This type of hemorrhage is most commonly caused by a ruptured congenital berry aneurysm. The majority of these bleeds (60%) occur in women who are older than 40 years of age. Most congenital berry aneurysms develop at branching points off the circle of Willis in the carotid artery system. The aneurysms lack smooth muscle and the internal elastic lamina, thus making them susceptible to outpouching under normal or increased pressure in the vascular system.

Subarachnoid hemorrhages commonly present as a sudden onset of unconsciousness that improves over the next few hours. There are signs of meningeal irritation (e.g., stiff neck) and increased intracranial pressure (e.g., headache, papilledema). There is a 10% mortality in the first day, and a 25% mortality in the first 3 months. After 1 week, the patient may experience further deficits due to a vasospasm of the cerebral vessels caused by the release of thromboxane A_2 in platelets and associated with resolution of the blood clot and endothelin, a powerful vasoconstrictor released from injured endothelial cells. More than 50% of patients who recover have severe neurologic deficits.

Turbidity of the CSF implies an increase in protein, cellular elements, or the presence of infectious organisms. Bloody CSF taps are most often because of trauma caused by the procedure; or, it may represent a pathologic bleed into the subarachnoid space. A pathologic bleed into this space may be secondary to a ruptured berry aneurysm, bleeding from an arteriovenous malformation, trauma, or a hypertensive, intracerebral bleed that extends into the subarachnoid space. Pathologic bleeds produce a pale pink-to-orange supranate after centrifugation of the CSF. This color is caused by oxyhemoglobin and later, bilirubin, which imparts a yellowish tinge to the fluid called xanthochromia.

A brain tumor, multiple sclerosis, an intracranial hemorrhage, and meningitis do not present with an abrupt onset of symptoms as in this patient. An intracranial hemorrhage may be associated with xanthochromic spinal fluid; however, it is most commonly caused by hypertension, which is not common in a 35-year-old woman. The relatively sudden onset of the findings in this patient in addition to the presence of blood in the CSF essentially exclude a brain tumor or multiple sclerosis.

Viral meningitis has a sudden onset, but the characteristic location of the headache and xanthochromia rule out that diagnosis.

19. The answer is B.   *(Pharmacology)*
Both fenfluramine and phentermine have been successfully used, alone and in combination, for the treatment of obesity. They apparently reduce appetite by affecting the satiety centers in the hypothalamus. Whereas phentermine is a central nervous system (CNS) stimulant related to the amphetamines and is believed to act by releasing norepinephrine from CNS neurons, fenfluramine causes lethargy and sedation and acts by augmenting serotonin neurotransmission. For this reason, the drugs may be used together without causing excessive CNS stimulation or depression.

20. The answer is B.   *(Pathology)*
Laminar necrosis and watershed infarcts characterize disease most likely secondary to atherosclerosis, producing ischemia in the brain. Ischemia is differentiated from hypoxia as a cause of brain damage. Hypoxia is a deprivation of oxygen with maintenance of blood flow; examples include cyanide poisoning, effects of being in a high altitude, carbon monoxide poisoning, methemoglobinemia, and hypoxemia (low arterial PO_2). Ischemia is a reduction in blood flow with associated tissue hypoxia. It may be caused by atherosclerosis, which is the most common cause; compression of vessels by an expanding mass; vasculitis; shock; hyperviscosity; or embolism.

The neurons in the brain withstand hypoxia much better than they do in the presence of ischemia, because blood flow is present in conditions associated with pure tissue hypoxia. However, in ischemia, the accumulation of lactic acidosis in the brain tissue begins

showing deleterious effects within 8 to 10 seconds and irreversible damage after 6 to 10 minutes. Neurons are more sensitive to oxygen deprivation than to lack of glucose, because glucose stores are sufficient for 30 to 60 minutes. Sommer's sector of the hippocampus, the Purkinje cells of the cerebellum, and the third, fifth, and sixth layers of the cerebral cortex (mnemonic: 365 days in a year) are particularly susceptible to ischemia and hypoxia. Chronic ischemia of the brain is most commonly secondary to atherosclerosis involving the internal carotid artery, which may result in cerebral infarction, cerebral atrophy, ischemic encephalopathy (laminar necrosis, watershed infarcts), transient ischemic attacks, and thromboembolism.

Laminar necrosis is apoptosis (i.e., individual cell necrosis) of the neurons in layers 3, 5, and 6 of the cerebral cortex, which leads to cerebral atrophy. Watershed infarcts occur in the ischemia-prone junctional zones between the major arterial territories, such as the junction of the anterior and middle cerebral arteries.

21. The answer is C.   *(Microbiology)*
Staphylococcus aureus, *Bacillus cereus*, and *Clostridium botulinum* all produce food poisoning secondary to ingesting preformed toxins.

S. aureus food poisoning is caused by the presence of preformed heat-stable enterotoxin B that is produced by toxigenic strains of *S. aureus*. It usually grows in custards and cream-filled pastries that have not been refrigerated properly. The disease is an acute, self-limited gastroenteritis that occurs 1 to 6 hours after ingesting the toxin. The food rather than the feces should be cultured, because it is a toxin-induced, not an invasive, gastroenteritis.

B. cereus, a gram-positive rod, produces a self-limited, short incubation type (~ 4 hours) of food poisoning when ingested as a preformed enterotoxin in contaminated fried rice. There is no specific treatment.

C. botulinum produces food poisoning by the proliferation of the organisms in contaminated food, usually canned or preserved food. It produces a powerful preformed neurotoxin, which may be inactivated by heat. The neurotoxin attaches to the synaptic vesicles of cholinergic nerves, where it blocks the release of acetylcholine and causes a descending paralysis from the cranial nerves to the extremities. It requires a neutral or alkaline environment. The onset of disease begins 8 to 36 hours after ingestion of the toxin.

22. The answer is D. *(Pathology)*
Blockage of the arachnoid granulations would most likely cause a communicating, or nonobstructive, hydrocephalus.

Hydrocephalus is an increase in cerebrospinal fluid (CSF) volume with distention of the ventricles. It may be caused by (1) overproduction of CSF, which is uncommon (e.g., in neoplasms of the choroid plexus); (2) decreased absorption of CSF from the arachnoid villi that is caused by an organizing meningitis with fibrosis blocking the arachnoid granulations, dural sinus thrombosis, or organization of blood clot in a subarachnoid hemorrhage; or (3) obstruction of CSF flow within the ventricles with distention of the ventricles proximal to the block, in conditions such as a colloid cyst of the third ventricle, stenosis of the duct of Sylvius, tumor (e.g., ependymoma, medulloblastoma) in the fourth ventricle, or the blockage of flow out of the foramina of Luschka and Magendie by pus (tuberculous meningitis) or blood. Blockage of CSF flow within the ventricles produces an obstructive, or noncommunicating hydrocephalus. Blockage of the resorption of CSF out of the subarachnoid space produces a communicating hydrocephalus, because there is still an open communication between the ventricles and the subarachnoid space. In any of these situations, the ventricles dilate under the increased pressure and are easily identified by computerized tomography scans or magnetic resonance imaging.

23. The answer is A. *(Anatomy)*
The genioglossus muscle is paralyzed on the side of the lesion in the hypoglossal nerve. When the tongue is protruded, the vector of the fully innervated muscles is unopposed by the muscle on the opposite side, thus producing the obvious deviation of the tongue from the midline. Protrusion is still possible due to the normally innervated side. Taste is not related to the muscle innervation of the tongue; it is carried by the trigeminal and glossopharyngeal nerves. Spasticity is a sign of an upper motor neuron lesion. In a lower motor neuron lesion, atrophy of the affected side may be observed by the examiner.

24. The answer is C. *(Pathology)*
Oligodendrocytes in the central nervous system (CNS) share a similar function with Schwann cells in the peripheral nervous system—synthesis of myelin. Oligodendrocytes are small, round, lymphocyte-size cells that produce and maintain CNS myelin, which is primarily located in the white matter. Certain diseases, such as progressive multifocal leukoencephalopathy, caused by a papovavirus, specifically attack oligodendrocytes and produce demyelination. Oligodendrogliomas are malignant tumors that are derived from oligodendrocytes. However, unlike Schwann cells, oligodendrocytes contribute segments of myelin sheaths to more than one axon.

Gemistocytes are reactive astrocytes that have an eosinophilic cytoplasm. They are commonly seen along the periphery of cerebral infarctions. Some astrocytomas have a gemistocytic appearance.

Astrocytes provide the structural framework for the neurons and are analogous to the fibroblasts in connective tissue. However, scarring in the brain is not associated with collagen synthesis but with filling in the defect with the cellular processes of astrocytes. A cerebral abscess is the only example of CNS repair with collagen, which is derived from the blood vessels.

Microglial cells are derived from monocytes. They are the phagocytic cell of the CNS.

Ependymal cells line the ventricles of the brain and the spinal canal. They do not produce CSF nor are they responsible for reabsorption of CSF, a function relegated to arachnoid cells.

25. The answer is C. *(Microbiology)*
Trichuris trichiura (whipworm), primarily produces gastrointestinal disease without lung involvement. It infests humans following ingestion of the eggs, which develop into larvae in the small intestine and then into adults in the cecum and appendix, where they appear to be "sewn into" the mucosa. Clinically, they cause bloody diarrhea with abdominal pain that is often confused with inflammatory bowel disease. In severe infections, particularly in children, there is a potential for rectal prolapse. A peripheral blood eosinophilia is present. The diagnosis is best made by identifying the eggs in the stool (nipples at both ends). Mebendazole is used for treatment.

Ascaris lumbricoides infests humans after ingestion of the eggs, which develop larvae that migrate through the small intestine and pass through the lungs to produce a cough and hemoptysis. They are then swallowed and develop into adults in the small intestine.

Necator americanus (hookworm) has a larval form in soil that penetrates the intact skin of bare feet, usually between the toes. The larvae subsequently migrate through the lungs, are swallowed, and then develop into adults in the small intestine.

Strongyloides stercoralis infects humans through free-living rhabditiform larvae in the soil that metamorphose into infective filariform larvae and penetrate intact skin. The larvae pass through the lungs, and then follow a similar course of events as described for *A. lumbricoides* and *N. americanus*.

Dirofilaria immitis (dog heartworm) is transmitted by a mosquito bite, introducing larvae into the host. The larvae migrate and stay in the lungs. The immune system eventually destroys the parasites. In the dog, adults are formed in the right ventricle. The adults embolize to the lungs where they produce an infarction.

26. The answer is C.   *(Pathology)*

The patient is a 70-year-old man who has transient ischemic attacks that are characterized by vertigo, dysarthria, dysphagia, and numbness of the ipsilateral face and contralateral limbs that lasts for 10 to 15 minutes and then resolves without any deficits. His disease is most likely caused by ischemia involving the vertebral artery. If an infarction occurs in these patients, it usually involves the lateral medulla with or without involvement of the posteroinferior cerebellum (Wallenberg syndrome). Because of the transient nature of the patient's complaints, it is less likely that the lesion is a demyelinating disease, a cerebellar tumor, or a neoplasm involving the brain stem. Parkinson disease, with a deficiency of the neurotransmitter dopamine, is associated with extrapyramidal findings, such as muscle rigidity.

27. The answer is D.   *(Physiology)*

There is a decrease in sodium permeability (inactivation of the sodium channels) and a delayed increase in potassium permeability during the repolarization phase of the action potential. The pump plays no direct role in the action potential.

28. The answer is D.   *(Pathology)*

A frontal headache when waking up in the morning and a computerized tomography (CT) scan showing a frontal lobe mass with focal areas of calcification are characteristic findings in oligodendrogliomas, which commonly involve the frontal lobe. These are tumors derived from oligodendrocytes that frequently locate in the cerebral hemispheres of adults 30 to 50 years of age. Calcifications are visible on routine skull films or CT in 90% of cases. They commonly have an admixture with other types of glial tumors, such as an astrocytoma (50%). Overall, oligodendrogliomas have a good prognosis but a high recurrence rate.

29. The answer is C.   *(Microbiology)*

Mycobacterium tuberculosis is the most common cause of intestinal tuberculosis in the United States; in other countries, *Mycobacterium bovis* is the primary causative agent. The difference in organisms is associated with drinking unpasteurized milk versus pasteurized milk. The organisms gain access to the gastrointestinal tract by being swallowed in the sputum from a primary focus in the lung. They pass into the small bowel and infect Peyer patches in the terminal ileum. Because the lymphatics drain in a circumferential pattern, lymphatic drainage of the organisms with subsequent host reaction to the infection causes a stricture formation and bowel obstruction.

Shigella are highly infectious, gram-negative, nonmotile, lactose-negative organisms that do not produce hydrogen sulfide. *Shigella sonnei* and *Shigella flexneri* are the most frequent cause of bacillary dysentery, or shigellosis, in the United States. The bacteria produce endotoxins and exotoxins that contribute to the toxicity of the disease. Shigellosis is an invasive enterocolitis primarily involving the terminal ileum and the colon. It is transmitted by human contact and the "4 F's": food, fingers, feces, and flies. Unlike salmonellosis, there are no animal reservoirs and a septicemic phase is rare. The diarrheal syndrome is characterized by low volume, painful stools that contain mucous and blood; fecal smears exhibit neutrophils. Pseudomembranes are produced as well as ulcerations, thus simulating antibiotic-induced colitis and amebic dysentery. Bowel obstruction is not a complication of the infection. Ciprofloxacin is the treatment of choice.

Schistosomiasis may involve the bowel and produce a diarrheal state, but bowel obstruction is not a complication.

Taeniasis caused by the tapeworms *Taenia saginata* or *Taenia solium* is primarily associated with anorexia, digestive disturbances, and weight loss. Bowel obstruction is not present.

Typhoid fever caused by *Salmonella typhi* involves the Peyer patches in the terminal ileum, but the ulcers that develop overlying the hyperplastic lymphoid tissue are longitudinally oriented and are not associated with bowel obstruction.

30. The answer is C. *(Pathology)*
The patient is an adult with decreased pain and temperature sensation in the upper extremities, atrophy of the intrinsic muscles of his hand, and brisk deep tendon reflexes in the upper extremity. This constellation of clinical findings strongly suggests syringomyelia, which most commonly affects the cervical spinal cord. Syringomyelia refers to a fluid-filled space within the cervical spinal cord that produces (1) cervical cord enlargement, best visualized with magnetic resonance imaging; (2) cape-like neurologic abnormalities involving the shoulders and upper extremities; (3) decreased pain and temperature sensation from involvement of the crossed lateral spinothalamic tracts, with preservation of light touch and proprioception; (4) atrophy of the small muscles of the hands from anterior horn cell involvement, simulating amyotrophic lateral sclerosis; (5) involvement of the lateral corticospinal tract with upper motor neuron findings; (6) Horner's syndrome, consisting of pupillary constriction, lid lag, and anhidrosis; (7) and associations with Arnold-Chiari malformation and Dandy-Walker cysts.

Regarding the other choices:

- Amyotrophic lateral sclerosis involves motor neurons producing upper and lower motor neuron disease. Sensory findings are not present.
- Multiple sclerosis has sensory and motor deficits.
- Subacute combined degeneration occurs in vitamin B₁₂ deficiency and involves the dorsal columns and the lateral corticospinal tract.
- Guillain-Barré syndrome is an ascending paralysis without the type of sensory deficits described in this patient.

31. The answer is B. *(Anatomy)*
The nucleus ambiguus gives rise to the motor innervation of larynx, pharynx, and palate. The hypoglossal nucleus innervates the tongue muscles. The nucleus solitarius is innervated by visceral sensory neurons

from the viscera. The dorsal motor nucleus of the vagus is comprised of parasympathetic preganglionic neurons that innervate the viscera. The Edinger-Westphal nucleus is comprised of preganglionic parasympathetic neurons that innervate the smooth muscles of the eye (sphincter pupillae and ciliary apparatus).

32. The answer is A. *(Pathology)*
Apoptosis refers to individual cell necrosis and is operative in (1) the normal turnover of cells, (2) programmed cell death in embryogenesis, (3) toxin-induced injury, (4) viral cell death, (5) death of cells secondary to cytotoxic T cells or natural killer cells, (6) atrophy of tissue, and (7) cell death in tumors. A characteristic of apoptosis is densely staining eosinophilic cytoplasm with pyknotic nuclei on hematoxylin and eosin stained tissue plus the lack of inflammation. Chronic ischemia in the brain often produces cerebral atrophy associated with neuron loss, the latter manifested by the presence of red neurons.

33. The answer is D. *(Microbiology)*
The enterotoxigenic strain of *Escherichia coli* secretes a heat-labile toxin that stimulates adenylate cyclase, producing a cholera-like syndrome that is responsible for the majority of cases of traveler's diarrhea. Because the bowel mucosa is not invaded and there is no toxin-induced damage, the fecal smear is negative for leukocytes. *Campylobacter* enteritis, shigellosis, typhoid fever, and amebiasis are all invasive, and infected individuals have stools with inflammatory cells. Typhoid fever is unique because the inflammatory cells are not neutrophils, but mononuclear cells.

34. The answer is C. *(Behavioral science)*
Blood alcohol concentration of 0.08%–0.15% is considered evidence of legal intoxication. The specific percentage depends on individual state regulations.

35. The answer is C. *(Anatomy)*
Shining a light in the right eye would elicit the pupillary reflex in both eyes; even though the optic nerve to the left eye was destroyed, the consensual reflex is intact because the left oculomotor nerve carries the innervation to the pupillary muscles. The stimulus from the right eye crosses to the opposite side at the level of the tectum of the midbrain. However, the

light in the left eye would not produce any effect because the retinal receptor would not carry the information to the brain stem. Permanent dilation would most likely occur only if the oculomotor nerve to the left eye was severed.

36. The answer is D.   *(Pathology)*
The neuropathologist developed a fatal, rapidly progressive dementia associated with a "bubbles and holes" spongiform change on sections of the cerebral cortex. This is consistent with the slow virus disease called Creutzfeldt-Jakob, or subacute spongiform encephalopathy. The infectious agent involved is known as a prion. The characteristic "bubble and holes" spongiform change in the gray matter of the cerebral cortex is associated with little or no inflammatory reaction. It is a health hazard to those who work with brain specimens. Kuru, another spongiform encephalopathy, was seen in New Guinea where the disease was transmitted by the practice of cannibalism; tribe members ate the brains of their enemies. Recently, the disease has been transmitted in beef.

37. The answer is C.   *(Physiology)*
During excitation-contraction coupling in a skeletal muscle fiber, calcium is released from the sarcoplasmic reticiulum (not the sarcolemma) and binds to troponin (not tropomyosin or myosin). The binding of calcium to the troponin causes the troponin to shift the position of the tropomyosin to which it is attached, thus uncovering the actin binding sites for binding with myosin.

38. The answer is E.   *(Pathology)*
The most common central nervous system (CNS) infection is primarily transmitted by the hematogenous route. This infection is called leptomeningitis. Infections of the CNS may occur via (1) the hematogenous route (most common), (2) direct implantation as a result of trauma, (3) local extension from a sinus or ear infection, or (4) ascent up through the peripheral nervous system into the brain (e.g., rabies virus). The layers of the skull from the outside in are skin, skull, dura mater, arachnoid, pia mater, and cerebral cortex of the brain. Four kinds of infection involve the CNS: (1) leptomeningitis (most common), (2) encephalitis (inflammation of the brain), (3) epidural infections

(pachymeningitis involving the dura), and (4) subdural infections. Infections originating from the bloodstream (hematogenous) may result in leptomeningitis (most common form), encephalitis (inflammation of the brain), or a cerebral abscess.

39. The answer is B.   *(Pharmacology)*
The phenothiazines and other traditional neuroleptic drugs are believed to exert their therapeutic effects by blocking dopamine D2 receptors. Clozapine and other new antipsychotic agents may exert their therapeutic effects by selectively blocking dopamine D4 receptors and serotonergic receptors. Several neuroleptics, including thioridazine and clozapine, have more potent antimuscarinic activity, and this may partly account for their lower incidence of extrapyramidal side effects. Phenothiazines also block alpha-adrenergic receptors, causing postural hypotension; some phenothiazines block histamine receptors and are useful in treating allergic reactions.

40. The answer is E.   *(Pathology)*
Krabbe's disease is an autosomal recessive leukodystrophy resulting from a deficiency of lysosomal galactocerebroside β-galactosidase with accumulation of galactocerebroside in large multinucleated, histiocytic cells, called globoid cells. Leukodystrophies are characterized by the synthesis of abnormal myelin.

Regarding the other choices:

- Subacute sclerosing panencephalitis (SSPE) is a slow virus disease associated with rubeola. Intranuclear, eosinophilic inclusions appear in neurons in the gray matter of the cerebral cortex and basal ganglia. This condition is also associated with demyelinization.
- Parkinson's disease is associated with intracytoplasmic Lewy bodies, which are composed of irregular filaments and electron dense granules. The bodies are present in depigmented substantia nigra neurons.
- The intracytoplasmic eosinophilic Negri body is present in neurons (Purkinje cells of the cerebellum, Ammon's horn, and spinal cord) that are infected by the rabies virus.
- Herpes encephalitis is associated with intranuclear, eosinophilic inclusions in neurons and glial cells, particularly those located in the temporal lobe.

41. The answer is C. *(Physiology)*
Control of skeletal muscle stimulation occurs at the anterior gray horn in the spinal cord where numerous excitory postsynaptic potentials (EPSPs) and inhibitory postsynaptic potentials (IPSPs) occur on the alpha motor neurons. The motor neurons cannot inhibit at the neuromusclar junction; they only excite through endplate potentials. There are no synapses at the dorsal root ganglion, just the cell bodies of sensory neurons.

42. The answer is A. *(Pathology)*
An increased spinal fluid protein concentration, obliterative vasculitis, and scarring at the base of the brain are characteristic of tuberculous (TB) meningitis. Tuberculous meningitis is usually a complication of primary TB in the lung in children. In the meninges, it commonly produces postinflammatory scarring with obstructive hydrocephalus. The cerebrospinal fluid (CSF) white blood cell count is usually < 500 cells/μL with a cellular infiltrate consisting predominantly of mononuclear cells. Other findings include a high CSF protein, which forms a pellicle when left overnight in a refrigerator, low glucose levels, and low CSF chloride levels.

Regarding the other choices:

- Guillain-Barré syndrome is a demyelinating type of ascending paralysis which has an immunologic basis. It is associated with high CSF proteins but normal CSF glucose and chloride levels. It does not produce an obliterative vasculitis.
- Neurosyphilis is the tertiary stage of syphilis, which develops in about 10% of patients. The major types are meningitic (25%), paretic, and tabes dorsalis. The meningitic form of neurosyphilis is a chronic low-grade meningitis with vasculitis that frequently presents as a stroke in a young patient in the absence of hypertension. The paretic form of neurosyphilis is characterized by diffuse atrophy of the brain with enormous numbers of organisms present, dementia, and an Argyll Robertson pupil. Tabes dorsalis is a form of neurosyphilis in which the spirochete attacks the posterior columns and the dorsal roots of the spinal cord. Laboratory findings in neurosyphilis include a (1) positive VDRL (25%–50%), (2) positive FTA-ABS (80%–95%), (3) mild lymphocytosis, (4) increased protein, and (5) normal glucose.

- Aseptic meningitis is most commonly due to the enteroviruses, coxsackievirus in particular. It is not associated with low CSF glucose or obliterative endarteritis.
- *Neisseria meningitidis* meningitis is the most common bacterial meningitis in adolescents. It does not produce an obliterative endarteritis, but has CSF findings similar to those in TB meningitis, except for a neutrophil predominant infiltrate and normal chloride levels.

43. The answer is B. *(Behavioral science)*
Desipramine is the least sedating of the antidepressants listed and therefore is best for a patient who must remain very alert on the job. Trimipramine, amitriptyline, and doxepin are strongly sedating antidepressants. Imipramine is less sedating than trimipramine, amitriptyline, and doxepin but more sedating than desipramine.

44. The answer is B. *(Pathology)*
The most common causes of pathologic fractures are metastatic bone disease and primary diseases of bone. They are called pathologic because there is a disease in the bone as opposed to trauma resulting is a fracture of normal bone. Common primary sites that metastasize to bone are tumors arising from the breast (most common), lung (small-cell carcinoma), and thyroid gland (follicular carcinoma). Multiple myeloma is the most common primary malignancy of bone. It is also commonly associated with pathologic fractures due to the presence of lytic lesions secondary to the secretion of osteoclast activating factor by the malignant plasma cells. This explanation would be the most likely for a pathologic fracture in an elderly individual with a lytic lesion. Benign diseases causing pathologic fractures include bone cysts, Paget's disease of bone, osteoporosis, eosinophilic granuloma, and a non-ossifying fibroma (fibrous cortical defect).

Regarding the other choices:

- A fibrous cortical defect (nonossifying fibroma) is a non-neoplastic cystic lesion most commonly seen in children.
- Metastatic prostate cancer to bone is most commonly osteoblastic and is not associated with pathologic fractures.

- Osteochondromas are the most common benign tumor of bone. They are a lobulated outgrowth on bone capped by a zone of benign cartilage. They usually occur in long bones. They are the least likely of the choices to present as a pathologic fracture.
- Osteoporosis is commonly associated with vertebral fractures, but osteopenia is seen on x-ray, not osteolytic areas.

45. The answer is E. *(Physiology)*
Inhibitory postsynaptic potentials (IPSPs) are local potential changes occurring at the cell bodies and dendrites of neurons within the central nervous system. The greater the distance from the site of the synapse, the more the effects of IPSPs diminish. The IPSPs are not propagated; only action potentials are propagated.

46. The answer is A. *(Pathology)*
A fibrous cortical defect (nonossifying fibroma) is a non-neoplastic process that most commonly involves the tibia, fibula, and femur. It creates an irregular, sharply demarcated radiolucent defect in the metaphyseal cortex. It is a frequent cause of a pathologic fracture. The defect characteristically presents with nocturnal pain in the legs.

Fibrous dysplasia refers to a benign, non-neoplastic process of bone (ribs and femur) in which bone is replaced by fibroconnective tissue (woven bone). It may involved a single bone (monostotic) or many bones (polyostotic), the latter often associated with Albright's syndrome. This syndrome consists of abnormal skin pigmentation (cafáe au lait spots), polyostotic fibrous dysplasia, and precocious sexual development, usually in females. Fibrous dysplasia is not associated with nocturnal pain.

An aneurysmal bone cyst is a benign condition (most commonly seen in children) that characteristically causes enlargement of the bone. The femur and the vertebra are most commonly involved. The cyst is composed of hemorrhagic spaces and reactive-appearing giant cells. On x-ray, it appears as a multicystic, radiolucent lesion. It is not associated with nocturnal bone pain.

Enchondromas (chondromas) are benign, generally asymptomatic, solitary or multiple cartilaginous tumors that result from a failure of normal endochondral ossification below the growth plate. They develop within the medullary cavity of the bone. The risk for transformation into a chondrosarcoma is greatest when multiple lesions are present. Ollier's disease refers to multiple enchondromas that most frequently involve the bones of the hands and feet. There is no association with nocturnal pain or pathologic fractures.

An osteoma is a solitary benign tumor usually confined to the skull and facial bones, which may be associated with Gardner's hereditary polyposis syndrome. It is not associated with nocturnal pain or a pathologic fracture.

47. The answer is C. *(Pharmacology)*
Clozapine produces agranulocytosis in 1 to 2 percent of patients, and all patients must have regular blood cell counts so that the drug can be stopped at the first sign of leukopenia. Clozapine is less likely to cause tardive dyskinesia than other neuroleptics. Unlike older phenothiazines, clozapine does not cause jaundice due to cholestatic obstruction.

48. The answer is A. *(Pathology)*
A 65-year-old woman with rheumatoid arthritis who complains of an inability to swallow dry crackers and states that her eyes "feel like they have sand in them" most likely has Sjögren syndrome. This autoimmune disease is characterized by diminished lacrimal and salivary gland secretions, resulting in dry eyes (keratoconjunctivitis) and dry mouth (xerostomia). The majority are women with rheumatoid arthritis. Xerostomia is the most common initial symptom accompanying the complaint of not being able to eat dry crackers. Proximal renal tubular acidosis and an increased incidence of malignant lymphoma are possible complications. The laboratory findings include a (1) positive antinuclear antibody (50%–80%), (2) a positive anti-SS-A/Ro and anti-SS-B/La (more specific than anti Ro) in approximately 60%, and (3) a positive rheumatoid factor (75%–90%). The confirmatory test for Sjögren syndrome is a lip biopsy of a minor salivary gland demonstrating lymphocytic destruction of the glands.

Regarding the other choices:

- A positive anti-Smith (Sm) antibody is present in systemic lupus erythematosus.

- An abnormal esophageal motility study is most commonly associated with CREST syndrome and progressive systemic sclerosis.
- A positive anti-centromere antibody is noted in CREST syndrome.
- A history of night blindness indicates vitamin A deficiency.

49. The answer is B. *(Physiology)*
The A band is the width of the column of thick myosin filament, which does not change size during a contraction. The thin, actin-rich filaments also do not change size during the contraction. However, the I band refers only to that portion of the thin filaments that extends outside the A band, and during a contraction, as the thin filaments slide between the thick filaments, the part of the thin filaments that extends outside the A band gets smaller. Therefore, the I band gets narrower. The H zone is the center portion of the A band where the thin filaments do not extend. As the muscle shortens, the thin filaments extend further into the A band; therefore, the H zone gets narrower.

50. The answer is D. *(Anatomy)*
The medial longitudinal fasciculus (MLF) is a bilateral bundle of myelinated fibers connecting several levels of the brain stem. Its fibers connect the nuclei associated with extraocular muscle innervation, mainly the abducens, trochlear, and oculomotor nuclei. The medial lemniscus represents the axons of the second neurons in the dorsal column-medial lemniscal system. It ascends through the brain stem to synapse in the thalamus (ventral posterolateral nucleus).

The corticobulbar tract is comprised of axons that arise from the cerebral cortex (face area of the motor cortex) and descend into the brain stem. In the brain stem, these axons synapse on nuclei of cranial nerves involved in innervating skeletal muscles of the orofacial region (V, VII, IX, X, and XII). The dorsal longitudinal fasciculus is a descending bundle of fibers in the brain stem arising from the hypothalamus. It influences the activity of autonomic nuclei (parasympathetic) in the brain stem. The stria terminalis is a fiber connection between the amygdala and the hypothalamus.

51. The answer is E. *(Pharmacology)*
Both succinylcholine and mivacurium are completely and rapidly eliminated by plasma cholinesterase. Other nondepolarizing neuromuscular blockers, such as tubocurarine, pancuronium, and atracurium, are eliminated by renal or hepatic mechanisms or by spontaneous hydrolysis (atracurium). Patients with genetically determined atypical cholinesterase may be detected by measuring the inhibition of cholinesterase by dibucaine, a local anesthetic. Dibucaine inhibits the normal enzyme about 80%, but the abnormal variant is inhibited only 20%.

52. The answer is B. *(Pathology)*
A young woman with photophobia, morning stiffness in her hands, and an unexplained pericardial effusion most likely has systemic lupus erythematosus (SLE). She would most likely have a positive test for serum antinuclear antibodies. SLE is a connective tissue disorder resulting from an immunoregulatory disturbance of multifactorial etiology. It is thought to be the result of an interplay of genetic, hormonal, and environmental factors. The disturbance in immune regulation manifests itself in polyclonal activation of B cells, with the production of autoantibodies. Environmental factors that trigger attacks include sunlight and drugs. Arthritis is the most common presenting symptom of SLE (95%). Similar to rheumatoid joint disease, it has symmetrical involvement of both large and small joints and morning stiffness; but unlike rheumatoid arthritis, the joint involvement in SLE is usually less destructive. The skin is involved in 80% of patients and is either localized (discoid lupus erythematosus) or part of a systemic disease. The skin lesion in SLE is due to immune complex deposition along the basement membrane (basis for the band immunofluorescent test); but unlike discoid lupus, these deposits are also present in normal appearing skin as well. The classic butterfly rash of lupus occurs in 50% of cases. Serositis, or inflammation of the pericardium and pleura, occurs in 30% to 50% of patients. Pericarditis is the most common cardiovascular manifestation of SLE. Any unexplained pleural or pericardial effusion in a young woman is suspect for SLE. Other autoimmune diseases associated with SLE include autoimmune hemolytic anemia (Coombs' positive), thrombocytopenia, and leukopenia. Renal disease occurs in 50% to 60% of cases. The most common type is

diffuse proliferative glomerulonephritis. It is characterized by subendothelial deposition of immune complexes. Renal failure is the most common cause of death. The laboratory findings include (1) a positive serum antinuclear antibody test in 95% to 99% of patients; (2) a positive double-stranded DNA, which has a high specificity for renal disease; (3) a positive anti-Sm; (4) a positive anti SS-A (anti Ro), which may be responsible for complete heart block in newborns of women who have SLE; (5) a positive LE prep (50%–80%); and (6) low C3 complement levels when the disease is active.

Regarding the other choices:

- An HLA-B27 haplotype is most commonly associated with ankylosing spondylitis and its variants.
- Antistreptolysin (ASO) antibodies are primarily increased in group A streptococcal infections and rheumatic fever.
- A rheumatoid factor may be positive in SLE, but not as commonly as a positive antinuclear antibody (ANA) test.
- A positive syphilis serology is also possible in SLE, due to the presence of anti-cardiolipin antibodies, which cross-react with the cardiolipin antigen in the test system of the RPR and VDRL. The FTA-ABS, however, is negative, thus making this a false-positive syphilis serology. This finding is not as common as a positive ANA.

53. The answer is B. *(Anatomy)*
The concept of circuits of neuronal systems within the limbic system is best illustrated by the "Papez circuit." In order, beginning with the cingulate cortex, neuronal communication proceeds as follows: the cingulate cortex projects to the parahippocampal gyrus; which projects to the hippocampus; which via the fornix projects to the hypothalamus; which via the mamillothalamic tract projects to the thalamus (anterior nucleus); which projects back to the cingulate cortex.

54. The answer is B. *(Pathology)*
Anti-Smith (Sm) and anti–double-stranded DNA antibodies are both used in the diagnosis of systemic lupus erythematosus (SLE). Anti-Sm (Smith) antibodies are less sensitive (30%) than anti–double-stranded DNA (60% to 70%), but are more specific (100%).

Regarding the other choices:

- Anti-SS-A (Ro) antibodies are positive in Sjögren syndrome and anticentromere antibodies are positive in CREST syndrome.
- Anti-ribonucleoprotein has a high specificity for mixed connective tissue disease.
- Anti-histone antibodies have a high specificity (> 95%) in drug-induced SLE.
- Anti-SS-B (La) antibodies have a high specificity (60%–90%) for Sjögren syndrome.
- Anti–single-stranded DNA antibodies are commonly seen in drug-induced SLE.
- Anti-mitochondrial antibodies have a high specificity for primary biliary cirrhosis.
- Anti-microsomal antibodies are seen in Graves disease and Hashimoto's thyroiditis.

55. The answer is E. *(Pharmacology)*
Succinylcholine, a depolarizing neuromuscular blocking agent, causes transient muscle fasciculations in nonmedicated patients. The fasciculations, which primarily involve the chest and abdomen, occur as the muscle is initially depolarized. Persistent depolarization of the motor end plate leads to the onset of muscle paralysis.

56. The answer is C. *(Pathology)*
A bitemporal hemianopia is represented by blindness in the peripheral fields of vision. Compression of the crossing fibers in the optic chiasm produces this deficit because the crossing fibers represent retinal ganglion cell axons carrying information from the peripheral aspects of the visual fields. The location of the pituitary gland ventral to the optic chiasm places the chiasm in jeopardy if a tumor of the gland occurs. A tumor in the orbit would produce deficits related to one eye, perhaps blindness. An aneurysm of the posterior cerebral artery may compress the optic tract, encroach upon the lateral geniculate, or produce ischemia in the occipital visual cortex. In all of these cases, the visual deficit would be related to a homonomous half of the visual field. Transverse sinus thrombosis could compress the visual cortex. Again, the resulting deficit would most likely be of a homonomous nature. Uncal herniation of the medial aspect of the temporal lobe could compress the optic tract and produce homonomous visual field deficits. It is more likely to

compress the oculomotor nerve and produce eye movement and pupillary innervation abnormalities.

57. The answer is E.   *(Pharmacology)*

The miotic effect of morphine is caused by activation of the Edinger-Westphal nucleus of the third cranial nerve, which activates the parasympathetic outflow to the iris sphincter muscle, causing pupillary constriction. This effect can be antagonized by muscarinic antagonists such as atropine. Atropine has no effect on the other central nervous system or peripheral actions of opiates.

58. The answer is E.   *(Pathology)*

A 42-year-old woman with clinical features that suggest combinations of systemic lupus erythematosus, progressive systemic sclerosis, and polymyositis without any evidence of renal disease most likely has mixed connective tissue disease (MCTD). Anti-ribonucleoprotein antibodies are specific for MCTD (> 95% of cases). MCTD follows a more benign course than the other autoimmune diseases, mainly because of the lack of renal involvement.

Regarding the other antibodies:

- Anti–double-stranded DNA antibodies are specific for systemic lupus erythematosus.
- Anti–single-stranded DNA antibodies are commonly seen in drug-induced lupus.
- Anti–Scl-70 antibodies are noted in 70% of cases of progressive systemic sclerosis.
- Anti-Jo-1 antibodies are present in 10% to 30% of cases of dermatomyositis.

59. The answer is D.   *(Behavioral science)*

This patient probably has generalized anxiety disorder. This condition usually starts during the third decade of life and develops more frequently in women than in men. In contrast to panic disorder, generalized anxiety disorder cannot be linked to a specific situation. Instead, the patient has persistent anxiety, with sympathetic and parasympathetic symptoms, including gastrointestinal problems. Treatment of generalized anxiety disorder includes relaxation therapy and antianxiety agents, for example, diazepam and buspirone.

60. The answer is A.   *(Behavioral science)*

A stuporous patient shows little or no response to environmental stimuli. In clouding of consciousness, the patient cannot respond normally to external events; somnolence involves abnormal sleepiness. The delirious patients show confusion, restlessness, and disorientation.

61. The answer is B.   *(Behavioral science)*

Bipolar disorder has a strong genetic component. The illness is more common in higher socioeconomic groups, and its prognosis is worse than the one for major depressive disorder. Bipolar disorder shows no racial, cultural, or gender differences and is characterized by return to normal functioning between episodes.

62. The answer is C.   *(Pathology)*

The patient is an acutely ill child with a history of blunt trauma to the right upper thigh and evidence of an inflammatory reaction in the area of trauma, associated with systemic signs and symptoms. This constellation of findings is most consistent with an early acute osteomyelitis. Infection of the bone marrow is referred to as osteomyelitis. The three most serious infections of bone include pyogenic osteomyelitis, tuberculosis, and syphilis. Pyogenic osteomyelitis occurs most frequently in children and young adults and is most commonly due to *Staphylococcus aureus,* which reaches the bone via the hematogenous route. Other routes of infection are trauma (open fractures) and direct extension from subjacent tissue. In children, it characteristically involves the metaphyseal area of the long bones (diaphysis in adults) of the extremities where vascularity is most prominent. Infants show subperiosteal spread and extension into the joint space resulting in suppurative arthritis and permanent damage to the joint. In acute osteomyelitis, the marrow cavity is filled with acute inflammatory cells, which enzymatically destroy bone and leave devitalized portions of bone (called sequestra) floating in a sea of pus. The patient presents with high fever, chills, and localized pain in the affected bone. An absolute neutrophilic leukocytosis and positive blood cultures occur in approximately 70% of cases. Initial x-rays usually reveal soft tissue swelling and a periosteal reaction after approximately 10 days. Lytic changes and loss of bone occur 2–6 weeks later, when 50%–75% of the bone is lost. However, in 95% of cases, a technetium radionuclide scan is positive within 24 hours of symptoms and reflects osteoblastic activity and skeletal vascularity. It cannot distinguish osteomyelitis from a fracture, tumor, or avascular necrosis, so the clinical context must be taken into account. Children with sickle cell anemia commonly develop osteomyelitis secondary to *Salmonella* species. If not properly treated, it may progress into a chronic osteomyelitis, where there is a mixture of both acute and chronic inflammatory cells with extensive reactive bone formation in the periosteum, called involucrum. Complications of osteomyelitis include (1) chronic osteomyelitis (10%), (2) draining sinus tracts to the skin, (3) reactive amyloidosis (chronic disease), (4) squamous cell carcinoma developing within the sinus tract (chronic disease), (5) a focus for continued bacteremia with the potential for metastatic abscesses, and (6) a Brodie's abscess. The latter complication refers to an osteomyelitis that becomes encapsulated, thus forming a well-demarcated abscess that contains pus which is often surrounded by sclerotic bone. The other choices in the question, including tumor, avascular necrosis, fracture, and autoimmune disease, do not present with acute illness and systemic signs and symptoms as noted in this child.

63. The answer is C. *(Anatomy)*
The ulnar nerve lies within the medial intermuscular septum of the arm and then passes behind the medial epicondyle of the humerus, crosses the elbow, and enters the anterior compartment of the forearm. The region where the ulnar nerve is posterior to the medial epicondyle is the "funny bone." In this region, the nerve is subcutaneous and is subject to injury.

64. The answer is A. *(Pathology)*
Pemphigus vulgaris, vitiligo, bullous pemphigoid, and dermatitis herpetiformis are all immunologic diseases. Pityriasis rosea is an eruption that develops in children and young adults in the spring and fall. The cause is unknown, but it is often associated with a recent upper respiratory infection or flu. It first presents as a single, scaly pink plaque on the trunk, called a "herald patch." Days to weeks later, an eruption of rose-colored papules follows the lines of cleavage in a "Christmas tree" distribution. It typically resolves in 4–6 weeks.

Vitiligo is an autoimmune destruction of melanocytes resulting in areas of depigmentation. It is commonly associated with other autoimmune diseases such as pernicious anemia, Addison's disease, and thyroid disease. It is frequently observed in the black population. Unlike albinism, an autosomal recessive disease, the melanocytes are destroyed along with the pigment.

Pemphigus vulgaris, bullous pemphigoid, and dermatitis herpetiformis are autoimmune diseases associated with vesicles (fluid filled blister < 5 mm) and bullae (> 5 mm). The classification of these diseases is based on location of bullae into subcorneal, suprabasal, and subepidermal. In pemphigus vulgaris (PV), large, flaccid bullae filled with fluid occur on the skin and within the oral mucosa (very common). It is characterized by the presence of IgG antibodies against the intercellular attachment sites between keratinocytes, which is an example of a cytotoxic antibody, type II hypersensitivity reaction. The vesicle in PV is intraepidermal and has a suprabasal location, which is just above the basal cell layer, thus resembling a row of "tombstones." Scattered keratinocytes are present in the fluid as a result of acantholysis, which refers to the separation of epidermal cells, usually as a result of an immunologic destruction of the intercellular bridges. PV bullae exhibit Nikolsky's sign, where the epidermis slips when touched with the finger. PV is a fatal disease if the patient is not treated with systemic corticosteroids.

Bullous pemphigoid (BP) is an immunologic vesicular disease in which vesicles are in a subepidermal location. A circulating IgG antibody against antigens in the basement membrane makes this disease another example of a cytotoxic antibody, type II hypersensitivity reaction.

Unlike PV, (1) oral lesions are infrequent, (2) Nikolsky's sign is negative, (3) patients are less sick than in PV, and (4) the vesicles are subepidermal rather than suprabasilar in location.

Dermatitis herpetiformis is an immunologic vesicular lesion characterized by the presence of IgA immune complexes (type III hypersensitivity). These lesions are located at the tips of the dermal papilla at the dermal/epidermal junction, which produces a subepidermal vesicle filled with neutrophils. There is a strong association with gluten-sensitive enteropathy, or celiac disease.

65. The answer is B. *(Behavioral science)*
The area of the brain most closely associated with mood and affect is the frontal lobe.

66. The answer is C. *(Pathology)*
A keratoacanthoma most closely resembles a well-differentiated squamous cell carcinoma in gross and histologic appearance. The carcinomas commonly occur on sun-exposed areas in white patients over 50 years of age. It is characterized by the rapid growth of a crateriform lesion in 3–6 weeks, usually on the face or upper extremity. Histologically, it is composed of glassy appearing squamous cells associated with islands of keratin debris. It eventually regresses and involutes with scarring.

An actinic (solar) keratosis is a premalignant skin lesion induced by ultraviolet light damage. It occurs on sun-exposed areas (face, hands, and forearms). Hyperkeratosis (increases thickness of the stratum corneum, parakeratosis (persistence of nuclei in the stratum corneum layer), cytologic atypia (dysplasia) of the keratinocytes, and basal cell hyperplasia are noted. There is solar damage to underlying elastic and collagen tissue (solar elastosis). These conditions may regress, remain stable, or progress into squamous carcinoma in situ (Bowen's disease) or invasive cancer.

Lichen planus is characterized by intensely pruritic, scaly, violaceous, flat-topped papules on the wrists, lower back, legs and scalp. It may occur in the oral mucosa (50%), where is has a fine white net-like appearance (called Wickham's striae). Its pathogenesis may relate to increased epidermal proliferation or an immunologic reaction initiated by epidermal injury from drugs, viruses, or topical agents. The characteristic histologic features include hyperkeratosis, the absence of parakeratosis, a prominent stratum granulosum (granular cell layer), and irregular "saw-toothed" accentuation of the rete pegs (accentuation of the basal cell layer), and a dermal–epidermal junction obscured by a band-like infiltrate of lymphocytes. Civatte bodies, which are eosinophilic, hyaline bodies, are noted in the epidermis and papillary dermis.

Ichthyosis vulgaris is a genetic disease characterized by increased cohesiveness of the cells in the stratum corneum; thus, the skin resembles the scales of a fish.

Erythema nodosum is the most common cause of inflammation of subcutaneous fat (panniculitis). It is associated with tuberculosis, leprosy, drugs (sulfonamides), coccidioidomycosis, and sarcoidosis. It usually presents with multiple exquisitely tender, raised, erythematous nodular lesions located on the lower extremities.

67. The answer is B. *(Pharmacology)*
Although the etiology of dementia is unknown, a reduction in brain level of choline acetyltransferase (needed to synthesize acetylcholine) and aluminum toxicity, as well as genetic factors have been implicated in Alzheimer disease. Long-term alcohol abuse results in Korsakoff syndrome, a form of dementia caused in part by thiamine deficiency. Folic acid deficiency is a somatic cause of dementia.

68. The answer is E.   *(Pathology)*
A 42-year-old man with recurrent development of vesicular and bullous lesions in sun-exposed areas, which appear to have a relationship with alcohol intake, is strongly suspect for porphyria cutanea tarda. One would expect the patient to have a decrease in red blood cell uroporphyrinogen decarboxylase. The classification for porphyria may be based on the tissue of origin of excess metabolites or on the clinical manifestations of the disease. The two most common porphyrias in the United States are acute intermittent porphyria (AIP) and porphyria cutanea tarda (PCT). Recall that porphyrins are involved in oxidative or oxygen-transferring functions. They are also precursors for heme synthesis. Enzyme defects in the heme synthesis pathway account for the clinical porphyrias (refer to the chart).

$$
\begin{array}{c}
\text{ALA synthetase (}\uparrow\text{ AIP)} \\
\text{glycine + succinyl CoA} \xrightarrow{\hspace{3cm}} \delta\text{-aminolevulinic acid (ALA)} \\
\uparrow \\
\downarrow \text{ ALA dehydrase} \\
\text{Porphobilinogen} \\
\downarrow \\
\downarrow \text{ Uroporphyrinogen synthetase (}\downarrow\text{ AIP)} \\
\downarrow \\
\downarrow \text{ Uroporphyrinogen isomerase} \\
\text{Uroporphyrinogen III} \\
\downarrow \textbf{ Uroporphyrinogen decarboxylase (}\downarrow\textbf{ PCT)} \\
\text{Coproporphyrinogen III} \\
\downarrow \\
\text{Protoporphyrinogen IX} \\
\downarrow \\
\text{Protoporphyrin IX} \\
\downarrow \text{ + iron} \\
\text{Heme (negative feedback on ALA synthetase)}
\end{array}
$$

ALA synthetase is the rate-limiting enzyme in heme synthesis and has a negative feedback with its end product, heme. When drugs are being metabolized in the liver by the cytochrome P-450 system (e.g., alcohol, phenobarbital), heme is used in the process. When the heme levels drop, ALA synthetase activity increases; this change may precipitate an acute porphyria attack if enzymes along the pathway are deficient. Porphyrinogen compounds, or reduced porphyrin compounds, are colorless and not fluorescent in the reduced state. However, when "oxidized" in voided urine upon exposure to light, they become "porphyrins," which have a wine-red color. Oxidized porphyrins under ultraviolet (UV) light have an intense reddish orange fluorescence. In certain porphyrias (PCT), porphyrins in the peripheral circulation absorb UV light near the skin surface, and become photosensitizing agents, which may damage the skin and produce vesicles and bullae.

Porphyria cutanea tarda (PCT) is the most common of the porphyrias and is due to decreased activity of uroporphyrinogen decarboxylase in the liver (most common type) or the red blood cells (less common type). In the liver type of PCT, there is an autosomal recessive inheritance. The net result of the enzyme defect is an increased excretion of uroporphyrin (resulting in a wine-red urine), a slight increase in formation of coproporphyrins, and normal urine porphobilinogen levels. It is often precipitated with drugs, the two most common being alcohol and oral contraceptives. There is also a relationship between increased hepatic stores of iron and reduced enzyme levels. The clinical features include (1) photosensitive skin lesions in sun-exposed areas, (2) hyperpigmentation, (3) fragile skin, and (4) increased hair (hypertrichosis), the latter findings often exaggerated in the numerous werewolf horror stories on television. The treatment is with phlebotomy to reduce iron levels. Chloroquine is also used, since it binds excess porphyrins and increases their excretion.

Acute intermittent porphyria (AIP) has two basic defects, (1) an increased activity of ALA synthetase and (2) a decreased activity of uroporphyrinogen synthetase. The net effect of the two defects in AIP is an excessive quantity of δ-aminolevulinic acid (ALA) and porphobilinogen (PBG) in the urine. It is an autosomal dominant disease characterized by intermittent exacerbations of neurologic dysfunction, including psychosis, neuropathy, severe colicky abdominal pain, with the latter often mistaken for a surgical emergency necessitating an operation. Many patients with AIP presenting with abdominal pain have the classic "bellyful of scars" from previous surgeries. Similar to PCT, AIP is often precipitated by drugs that induce hepatic ALA synthetase activity by the mechanisms previously discussed. Laboratory findings in AIP include (1) a colorless fresh-voided urine, which—when left standing in light—will turn a wine-red color (windowsill test); (2) low RBC uroporphyrinogen synthetase activity even when the patient is asymptomatic; and (3) increased amounts of porphobilinogen in the urine, as well as increased amounts of ALA. Patients commonly have inappropriate antidiuretic hormone syndrome with hyponatremia. This combination is related to central nervous system damage and the organic brain syndrome. Intravenous infusion of heme is considered the treatment of choice for acute attacks, rather than intravenous infusion of glucose.

69. The answer is E. *(Anatomy)*
Opposition of the thumb is performed by the opponens pollicis, which is innervated by the recurrent branch of the median nerve, which arises distal to the carpal tunnel. Adduction of the thumb is performed by the adductor pollicis, which is innervated by the ulnar nerve. Extension of the thumb is performed by the extensor pollicis longus and brevis, both of which are innervated by the radial nerve. The recurrent branch of the median nerve also innervates the flexor pollicis brevis and the abductor pollicis brevis, which flex and abduct the thumb. However, these functions are also served by the flexor pollicis longus, which is innervated by the median nerve proximal to the carpal tunnel, and the abductor pollicis longus, which is innervated by the radial nerve.

70. The answer is B. *(Behavioral science)*
In delirium, illusions and hallucinations, often visual, occur. The hallucinations associated with delirium also

are less organized than those associated with schizophrenia.

71. The answer is B. *(Anatomy)*
A flattening of the thenar eminence is caused by atrophy of the thenar muscles secondary to their denervation. The thenar muscles are innervated by the recurrent branch of the median nerve. The thenar eminence may be flattened as a result of a lesion of the recurrent branch of the median nerve, the median nerve within the carpal tunnel, or the median nerve at a more proximal position. The anterior interosseous nerve is a branch of the median nerve, but it innervates the deep anterior forearm muscles, not the thenar muscles of the hand.

72. The answer is E. *(Pathology)*
Lepromatous leprosy is characterized by poor cellular immunity, so the organisms of *Mycobacterium leprae* are easily demonstrated in tissue. Biopsies of the skin in these patients reveal macrophages in the underlying dermis, with numerous organisms. There is a lack of involvement (sparing) of the dermis directly beneath the basal cell layer which is called the Grentz zone.
   Regarding the other choices:

- Psoriasis is associated with collections of neutrophils in the epidermis, called Munro's abscesses. Pautrier's microabscesses are collections of malignant helper T-cells in mycosis fungoides.
- Urticaria pigmentosum is associated with mast cell infiltration (not eosinophils) in the superficial dermis. These cells contain histamine, which when released produce pruritic urticarial lesions. Mast cells stain positive with Giemsa and toluidine blue.
- Molluscum contagiosum is due to a poxvirus and is associated with molluscum bodies in the crater that contains the virus. Civatte bodies are eosinophilic, hyaline bodies located in the epidermis in lichen planus.

73. The answer is C. *(Behavioral science)*
A teenage marriage is a high-risk factor for divorce. Risk factors for divorce also include a short courtship, premarital pregnancy, differences in socioeconomic background, and differences in religion.

74. The answer is A. *(Pathology)*
Systemic lupus erythematosus is associated with decreased thickness of the epidermis (atrophy), follicular plugs, liquefactive degeneration of the basal cells at the junction (immunologic destruction), and a lymphoid infiltrate at the dermal–epidermal junction. Chronic eczema, lichen planus, psoriasis, and ichthyosis vulgaris are all associated with hyperkeratosis, or thickening of the stratum corneum.

75. The answer is D. *(Anatomy)*
The muscles capable of supinating the forearm are the biceps brachii muscle, supinator muscle, and brachioradialis muscle. The biceps brachii is innervated by the musculocutaneous nerve. The supinator and brachioradialis muscles are innervated by the radial nerve. The biceps is the strongest supinator but is most effective only when the elbow is flexed to about 90 degrees. The supinator is an effective supinator regardless of the position of the elbow. The brachioradialis is an effective supinator only when the forearm is fully pronated.

76. The answer is E. *(Behavioral science)*
Anhedonia is the lack of any ability to feel pleasure. Euthymia is the normal mood, with no significant depression or elevation of mood. Dysphoria is a subjectively unpleasant feeling, whereas euphoria is a strong feeling of elation. In irritability, the patient is easily bothered and quick to anger.

77. The answer is E. *(Anatomy)*
The A1 segment of the anterior cerebral artery follows the contour of the corpus callosum. Angioradiographically this landmark is helpful.

The middle cerebral artery runs laterally in the lateral fissure before turning horizontally on the lateral brain surface.

The vertebral vessels run along the ventral surface of the medulla.

The posterior cerebral artery passes around the region of the cerebral peduncles of the midbrain and courses along the ventral surface of temporal and occipital lobes.

The course of the superior cerebellar artery is similar to that of the posterior cerebral artery except that the superior cerebellar artery passes under the tentorium cerebelli to the dorsal surface of the cerebellum.

78. The answer is B. *(Anatomy)*
The unreactive dilated pupil in a patient with a known cerebral mass most likely indicates medially directed pressure that has produced an uncal herniation. The uncus on the medial surface of the temporal lobe compresses the oculomotor nerve against the tentorium cerebelli. If the condition is not relieved, the brain stem and associated ascending reticular activating system can be depressed, leading to coma and perhaps death.

79. The answer is D. *(Anatomy)*
The vertebral–basilar arterial system supplies the neural structures in the posterior cranial fossa. Compromise of this vessel produces the generalized findings of "posterior fossa syndrome." Segmental radicular arteries supply the spinal cord. Carotid or anterior circulation is primarily to neural structures above the posterior cranial fossa. Anterior cerebral artery aneurysm or rupture would most likely affect eye movement or vision because either condition would compress the extraocular nerves or optic nerve. Death can be the outcome if bleeding is severe.

80. The answer is E. *(Behavioral science)*
Heroin addicts more commonly live in large cities, are usually in their 20s, and are more likely to be men. Although withdrawal is dramatic and uncomfortable, death from withdrawal of the drug is rare. Methadone is a synthetic opioid that suppresses the heroin withdrawal symptoms but also causes physical dependence and tolerance. Unlike heroin, methadone can be obtained legally. In addition, methadone can be administered orally and results in less euphoria and drowsiness than taking heroin produces.

81. The answer is A. *(Anatomy)*
The ulnar nerve innervates all seven interosseous muscles, which are represented for abduction and adduction of digits II through V. The ulnar nerve also innervates the lumbrical muscles to digits IV and V. Paralysis of the interosseous and lumbrical muscles results in clawing of the digits. Because the lumbrical

and interosseous muscles of digits IV and V are paralyzed, the clawing is most prominent in these digits. The median nerve innervates the lumbricals to digits II and III. The radial nerve does not innervate any intrinsic muscle of the hand.

82. The answer is D. *(Behavioral science)*
Most patients in pain are undermedicated in the United States, primarily because of doctors' fears of causing addiction. However, patients in pain do not become addicted the way that addicts do. Therefore, pain medication should be given at high enough doses to be effective and given before the patient experiences severe distress. Although analgesia is the first line of treatment for pain caused by cancer, behavior modification is also useful for patients in pain.

83. The answer is B. *(Anatomy)*
The two major flexors of the wrist are the flexor carpi radialis and the flexor carpi ulnaris. The flexor carpi radialis is innervated by the median nerve and permits flexion and lateral deviation. The flexor carpi ulnaris is innervated by the ulnar nerve and permits flexion and medial deviation. When both muscles act together, flexion without deviation occurs. If the median nerve is injured and the flexor carpi radialis is paralyzed, wrist flexion occurs with only the flexor carpi ulnaris, and medial deviation accompanies the wrist flexion.

84. The answer is B. *(Behavioral science)*
Weight gain is associated with withdrawal from nicotine. Delirium tremens is associated with withdrawal from alcohol. Euphoria and excitability may occur with use of nicotine. Long-term abstinence is difficult to achieve after withdrawal from nicotine; most patients return to smoking within 2 years after withdrawal.

85. The answer is B. *(Physiology)*
Calcitonin, which is secreted by the parafollicular cells of the thyroid gland, produces a quiescent effect on the ruffled border of the osteoclast, the resorptive cell of bone. Ruffled borders are essential for the activity of osteoclasts. Serum calcium and phosphate levels are lowered because the resorptive abilities of the osteoclast

have been stymied. The ruffled border creates an environment for lysosome release and an increase in surface area. In osteopetrosis, which is characterized by dense, heavy bones, the osteoclasts lack ruffled borders.

Calcification of the osteoid depends on seeding by matrix vesicles of the osteoblasts. Calcitonin does not directly affect this process.

Processes of the osteocyte extend through bone to meet other osteocytes and connect to the nutrient source at the haversian canal. Calcitonin does not affect these processes.

Acid phosphate is present in matrix vesicles and produces phosphate for hydroxyapatite formation.

The concise arrangement of hydroxyapatite crystals along collagen is important in the calcification process and is not affected by calcitonin.

86. The answer is B. *(Pathology)*
Brodmann classification of cerebral cortex areas is a helpful and quick way to refer to specific functional areas. Brodmann area 4 is the precentral gyrus of the frontal lobe and is the primary motor cortex contributing to the corticospinal tract. Area 6 is the premotor area and the frontal eye field area. Area 3,1,2 is the postcentral gyrus and is the primary somatosensory cortex. Area 17 is located along the banks of the cerebral cortex on either side of the calcarine fissure and represents the primary visual cortex. Finally, area 41 is located in the temporal lobe and is the primary auditory cortex.

87. The answer is D. *(Anatomy)*
The long thoracic nerve innervates the serratus anterior muscle, which inserts along the medial border of the anterior surface of the scapula. The origin of this muscle is on the anterolateral chest wall. Contraction of this muscle pulls the medial border of the scapula against the chest. Paralysis of this muscle results in "winging," which is a posterior protrusion of the medial border of the scapula.

88. The answer is B. *(Microbiology)*
The induction of apoptosis, also referred to as "programmed cell death" and "induced suicide," is one of the two mechanisms by which cytotoxic T lymphocytes (CTLs) destroy target cells. CTLs can program their targets to die within 5 minutes, although the

dying process usually takes several hours. Since the programming period is so short, it is believed that preformed effector molecules released by the CTL activate an endogenous self-destructive pathway within the target cell.

A hallmark of apoptosis is the fragmentation of target cell DNA into 200 base pair segments by activated endogenous nucleases. The disruption of the nucleus is followed by "blebbing" of the cytoplasmic membrane, cell shrinkage, and degradation into small, membrane-enclosed pieces that can be readily ingested by phagocytes. The endogenous nucleases that are activated in the target cell will also degrade viral DNA. Thus, the induction of apoptosis in a virally infected cell can serve to limit the spread of the virus to other cells in the vicinity.

Natural killer (NK) cells are also able to induce apoptosis in target cells. NK cells kill target cells via mechanisms very similar to those of CTLs. However, they are nonspecific and not major histocompatibility (MHC) class I (or II) restricted.

Tumor necrosis factor-β (TNF-β), which is produced by CTLs, and TNF-α, a major macrophage cytokine, can induce apoptotic death in target cells. Receptors for TNF are expressed on virtually all nucleated cells, and cross-linkage of the receptors can initiate the apoptotic process. However, this has been observed primarily with tumor cells.

89. The answer is C. (Anatomy)

While numerous cortical functions would also be tested, given this site of the suspected epileptic focus, motor skills of speech would be evaluated. Broca's motor speech center is located within this part of the frontal lobe. While this is a generalized location in most humans, extensive brain mapping must be done to determine individual variation in the location and extent of this critical functional area of cerebral cortex. Visual fields would be a concern if the epileptic area was in the occipital cortex. Somatosensory testing would be done to evaluate localization within the postcentral gyrus of the parietal lobe. Word association would be used to test the parietotemporal cortex associated with Wernicke's area, and distal extremity movement would evaluate the precentral gyrus of the frontal lobe.

90. The answer is E. (Pathology)

Uncal herniation at the edge of the incisure results in compression of the ipsilateral third nerve. This produces an ipsilateral dilated pupil, thus disrupting the pupillary light reflex, and ipsilateral third nerve palsy. The sixth nerve, which follows a long intradural course along the floor of the cranial cavity, is not anatomically related to the incisure and would not be affected by this trauma.

91. The answer is C. (Physiology)

Although stimulation of skeletal muscle contraction involves an alteration of the actin-rich thin filaments by calcium binding to the troponin, the major mechanism for initiating smooth muscle contraction does not involve troponin and does not alter the actin filaments. In smooth muscle, phosphorylation of the light chain portion of the thick myosin filaments initiates contraction, and myosin light chain kinase (MLCK) is the enzyme that catalyzes the phosphorylation. Intracellular calcium and cyclic adenosine monophosphate (cAMP) regulate MLCK through opposing effects. MLCK is activated when increasing levels of inositol triphosphate increase the intracellular ionized calcium concentration. However, increasing levels of cAMP induce an inactivation as MLCK.

92. The answer is A. (Pharmacology)

Bupropion is a structurally and pharmacologically unique antidepressant that appears to act by blocking the neuronal reuptake of dopamine without affecting serotonin or norepinephrine reuptake or metabolism. It has a low incidence of side effects, with few adverse autonomic or cardiovascular effects, and it appears safe for use in the elderly. Bupropion may cause central nervous system stimulation and seizures, and it is contraindicated in patients with a history of seizures or in those taking drugs that lower the seizure threshold.

93. The answer is A. (Physiology)

The chloride concentration inside cells is quite low, perhaps 5 to 10 mEq/L, which creates a large concentration gradient that tends to move chloride into the cell. The membrane potential (MP) creates an electrical gradient that tends to move Cl^- out. When the two gradients balance each other, there is electrochemical equilibrium for Cl⁻. If the Cl⁻ concentration inside the cell is reduced, as it is in many nerve cells, then there is a greater concentration gradient, which requires a greater (more negative) electrical gradient for electrochemical equilibrium. If the intracellular Cl⁻ concentration is elevated. This decreases the concentration gradient which requires a lower MP for electrochemical equilibrium. The cell's resting MP is then greater than the value for electrochemical equilibrium. If Cl⁻ permeability is increased, the MP will go toward the Cl⁻ electrochemical equilibrium, resulting in depolarization.

94. The answer is E.   *(Anatomy)*

With no loss of sensation or motor control below the arms and upper chest, it is unlikely that ascending and descending tracts in the white matter of the cord have been cut. The retention of touch (a sensation that is largely uncrossed in the cord) but the loss of pain (a sensation that crosses in the cord) in the affected region suggests that the injury does not involve the spinal nerves; rather, it most likely involves the area of decussation within the cord, as in syringomyelia.

95. The answer is D.   *(Pathology)*

Arboviruses are carried by arthropod vectors (e.g., mosquitoes, ticks) and produce encephalitis. Arboviruses are in two families: (1) the Togaviridae family, which is responsible for Eastern and Western equine encephalitis, St. Louis encephalitis, yellow fever, and dengue and (2) the Bunyavirus family, which is responsible for the California encephalitis virus.

Arboviruses do not produce disease in the vector or the vertebrate animal that is the natural host (e.g., wild birds) of the virus. Infections primarily occur in humans, who are dead-end hosts. The term *dead-end host* refers to the fact that the viral concentration in the patient's blood stream is of such low concentration, that another mosquito feeding on the patient is not likely to pick up the virus and spread it to another person.

St. Louis encephalitis is the most common encephalitis in the United States and may occur in city dwellers; English sparrows serve as the reservoir. Eastern equine encephalitis is associated with the highest mortality. The mosquitoes are located in swamp and rural areas.

Wild birds are the reservoir for the virus. Both humans and horses are dead-end hosts. Western equine encephalitis occurs west of the Mississippi. The reservoir for the virus is wild birds. In California encephalitis, small mammals (e.g., forest rodents) are the reservoir for the virus.

96. The answer is E.   *(Microbiology)*

The patient has most likely contracted plague from the bite of a flea. *Yersinia pestis*, a gram-negative rod, causes the plague. The primary animal reservoir is ground squirrels in the Southwest. It is transmitted by (1) the bite of infected rat fleas that have bitten infected rodents, (2) contact with an infected rodent, or (3) droplet infection from a patient with the disease.

There are three main types of plague in humans: bubonic, which is the most frequent form, pneumonic, and septicemic plague. *Y. pestis* is inoculated into the skin by a rat flea bite and from there it enters the regional lymph nodes, where organisms proliferate without being killed by neutrophils. The capsular fraction 1 envelope antigen prevents phagocytosis of the organism by neutrophils, and the V and W antigens protect the bacteria from destruction by macrophages. The infected lymph nodes, which are usually in the groin, enlarge, mat together, and drain to the surface (buboes). Patients with pneumonia may transmit the disease to others by droplet infection. If left untreated, 50% to 100% of patients will die, whereas 95% of cases recover with early treatment. Cultures of blood or aspirate material from the nodes and serologic tests secure the diagnosis. Streptomycin is the treatment of choice.

97. The answer is D.   *(Pathology)*

Herpes encephalitis most commonly involves the temporal lobes, where it produces a hemorrhagic necrosis. Dystrophic calcification is not a feature of the inflammatory process.

In cysticercosis, where the larval form of *Taenia solium* embeds in tissues (e.g., the brain, eye, muscle, subcutaneous tissue), dystrophic calcification frequently develops in the surrounding tissue. Trichinosis, which is caused by *Trichinella spiralis*, is associated with dystrophic calcification in muscle tissue, where the larval forms encyst.

In both congenital cytomegalovirus and toxoplasmosis in newborns, periventricular dystrophic calcification is frequently present on skull radiographs.

98. The answer is B. *(Microbiology)*
Mycoplasma pneumoniae is the most common cause of atypical pneumonia. Atypical pneumonia is characterized by low-grade fever; an insidious onset; constitutional symptoms such as malaise, headache, and anorexia; a nonproductive cough; a gram-negative sputum stain; a patchy, interstitial infiltrate on a chest radiograph; and myalgias and arthralgias.

A *Streptococcus pneumoniae* (Pneumococcus) pneumonia would most likely present with sudden onset; chills and high fever; a gram-positive sputum stain; a parenchymal or lobar consolidation on a chest radiograph; and a cough that produces rust-colored sputum. Pneumococcus is the most common cause of community acquired pneumonia and offers considerable risk for patients (1) who are ≥ 65 years of age, (2) who have symptomatic or asymptomatic human immunodeficiency virus infection, (3) who have alcoholic cirrhosis, (4) who have nephrotic syndrome, (5) who have sickle cell disease, (6) who are asplenic, (7) who have chronic cardiovascular or respiratory disease, (8) who have cerebrospinal fluid leaks, and (9) who are diabetic. These patients should receive Pneumovax. The vaccine has a protective efficacy of approximately 60%. It should be given after 2 years of age.

99. The answer is B. *(Microbiology)*
The p24 antigen is the best marker of disease activity in patients who are HIV positive. HIV contains reverse transcriptase, which allows the virus genome to integrate itself into the host's DNA by the viral RNA serving as the template for DNA synthesis. The virus is covered by a membrane derived from the host cell. The membrane contains the viral glycoproteins gp120 and gp41. The core of the virus contains RNA and proteins p18 and p24. The CD_4 molecule on the T helper cells is the receptor for the virus and first attaches to the gp120 glycoprotein. The CD_4 molecule is also on monocytes and macrophages. Following this high affinity binding, gp41 fuses with the host cell membrane, and the HIV genomic RNA is uncoated and internalized. Reverse transcriptase then converts the viral RNA into double-stranded DNA, which becomes integrated into the host DNA with the help of

an integrase enzyme coded for by the virus. The proviral DNA is either locked in the host DNA for months to years (latent infection) or is transcribed by the host genome into a complete virus, which is cytolytic to the T cell.

To be transcribed, the T helper cell must be activated by an antigen (e.g., cytomegalovirus, herpes simplex, hepatitis B, herpes virus 6) or cytokines. Antigenic stimulation of the T helper cell causes activation of the genes that transcribe interleukin-2 (IL-2) and its receptor as well as activation of the HIV genome. CD_4 T helper cells are lost by (1) direct cytolysis by the virus, (2) destruction of precursor T helper cells in the thymic progenitor cells, (3) fusion with infected and uninfected cells to form multinucleated giant cells that later die, and (4) antibody-dependent cytolysis by cytotoxic T cells. T helper cells with latent infection do not function properly; they have impaired production of IL-2 and gamma interferon to activate natural killer cells. Macrophages also have CD_4 molecules on their surface and are infected by HIV. However, unlike T helper cells, the virus proliferates in the macrophage without killing the cell, so that the macrophage acts as a reservoir for the virus and also transmits it to other sites, most importantly, the brain. The viral particles are located in vacuoles in the cytoplasm. Other cells, like astrocytes, lack the CD_4 molecule, so other receptors for gp120 must be involved. The first antibodies to appear are directed against products of the gag gene, mainly p17 and p24, which decreases the level of their free antigens in serum. Antibodies then develop against the envelope proteins gp120 and gp41. Finally, antibodies form against products of the pol gene (p31, p51). Increased free levels of p24 antigen correlate with reduced levels of antibody against p24 antigen. The p24 antigen is elevated at the beginning of the infection and when the patient develops AIDS. Patients who are in latent disease who demonstrate a rise in p24 antigen have a three times greater risk for developing AIDS. In addition, patients receiving antiretroviral therapy exhibit a decline in circulating p24 antigen levels. A p24 capture assay is used to detect the antigen.

100. The answer is A. *(Microbiology)*
Disseminated strongyloidiasis is sometimes seen in immunocompromised hosts. Loss of host immunity, malnutrition, or malignancy leads to a hyperinfectious

strongyloidiasis, generating large numbers of filariform larvae. Larvae invade the bowel, lungs, central nervous system, and kidneys. Penetration of the bowel mucosa allows other pathogens to complicate the infection.

Strongyloides stercoralis is a nematode that infects humans through penetration of unprotected skin by free-living filariform larvae in the soil. Similar to hookworm and ascaris larvae, they pass through the lungs, are swallowed, and then develop into adults after the larvae penetrate the mucosa of the duodenum. Adult worms in the duodenal mucosa copulate, and the females lay eggs that hatch into rhabditiform larvae, which pass out of the mucosa and into the lumen. From this location, they may reinfect the mucosa and pass through the lung, penetrate the perianal skin, and pass through the lung again; or, they may pass out of the body and live in the soil as free-living filariform larvae. Clinically, patients present with cough, epigastric pain, diarrhea, and peripheral blood eosinophilia. The diagnosis is made by finding rhabditiform larvae in the stool, duodenal aspirates, or by the string test (Enterotest). Thiabendazole is the treatment of choice.

Ancyclostoma duodenale (hookworm), *Enterobius vermicularis* (pinworm), *Ascaris lumbricoides,* and *Trichuris trichiura* (whipworm) are not associated with disseminated diseases in immunocompromised patients.

101. The answer is D. *(Pathology)*
Bee and wasp envenomations may produce a fatal anaphylactic, type I, immunoglobulin E–mediated hypersensitivity reaction in susceptible individuals. Bees and wasps are responsible for most deaths in the United States due to envenomation.

The black widow spider *(Latrodectus mactans)* has a red "hourglass" on the undersurface of the thorax. The spider is common in the Southern states, Arizona, and California. They construct their webs in wood piles, sheds, and basements and are active in April to October. They have a neurotoxic venom, which produces swelling and intense pain in the area of the bite, followed by intense abdominal contractions that simulate an acute appendicitis. Other possible sequelae include hemoglobinuria, glomerulonephritis, and hypertension. Treatment is intravenous calcium gluconate and methocarbamol. An antivenom is available.

The brown recluse spider (*Loxosceles reclusa,* or violin spider) is common in the Midwest and Southwest. They are hunting spiders (no webs), so they are most active during the night and they frequently end up under the sheets or tangled in clothes. The spiders are glossy brown and have a prominent violin (no stripes) on their dorsum. They possess a powerful necrotoxic venom. The initial bite is associated with a mild stinging sensation, which is followed in a few hours by intense pain and erythema, with a breakdown of the tissue and ulcer formation. Lymphangitis is common. Treatment includes the use of corticosteroids, debridement, colchicine, and dapsone.

Only two species of scorpions, both of which are located in Arizona deserts, cause fatalities in the United States. Scorpion venom is neurotoxic and in the nonlethal varieties, which are most common, the envenomation is associated with an immediate burning sensation, followed by paresthesias and numbing of the bite site. The poisonous species may have an ascending motor paralysis, which may lead to death. Cryotherapy and constriction bands are primarily used for therapy.

Mites include chiggers and the human itch mite (scabies, or Sarcoptes scabiei). Chiggers produce a pruritic dermatitis best treated with topical antipruritic agents (e.g., crotamiton, calamine lotion). In adults, scabies is limited to the intertriginous areas and spares the soles, palms, face, and head. In infants, there are no burrows and the palms, soles, face and head are involved. Treatment is topical benzene hexachloride (lindane) and permethrin dermal cream.

102. The answer is A. *(Microbiology)*
The most common bacterial infections associated with intravenous drug abuse are skin and soft-tissue infections. The high incidence of infection is caused by many factors, including "skin popping" (injecting drugs subcutaneously); extravasation of drugs into soft-tissue intravenous injection; adulterants present in the injection material; sharing contaminated needles; and the presence of pathogenic organisms on the skin. Group A streptococci and *Staphylococcus aureus* are the most commonly isolated organisms.

Other infections that are common in this high-risk group are hepatitis B with hepatitis D as a coinfection (same needle) or superinfection (after the patient already has hepatitis B); AIDS; acute endocarditis, which is most commonly caused by

S. aureus involving the tricuspid and/or aortic valve; pneumonia caused by *Streptococcus pneumoniae, Haemophilus influenzae, Mycobacterium tuberculosis,* or *Pneumocystis carinii*; osteomyelitis, which is most commonly caused by *Staphylococcus* and less commonly caused by other organisms (e.g., *Pseudomonas aeruginosa, Serratia marcescens,* fungi); and central nervous system complications (e.g., embolic strokes caused by valvular vegetations).

103. The answer is A.   *(Pathology)*
Carbon monoxide poisoning is associated with necrosis of the globus pallidus and degeneration in the substantia nigra. This condition is the result of severe hypoxic damage to the brain because of a reduction in the oxygen saturation and oxygen content of hemoglobin. Involvement of the substantia nigra produces an acquired Parkinson's disease.

Regarding the other choices:

- Wernicke's encephalopathy is associated with neuronal loss and ring hemorrhages primarily in the mamillary bodies and around the ventricles. This disease is most commonly associated with thiamine deficiency in alcoholics. The clinical findings include the acute onset of confusion, ataxia, and nystagmus (mnemonic CAN: C for confusion, A for ataxia, and N for nystagmus).
- Huntington's disease is characterized by a severe loss of neurons in the caudate nucleus and putamen in the neostriate. The tail of the caudate is often missing. The globus pallidus is affected to a lesser extent. The loss of the neostriatal neurons in the caudate, putamen, and globus pallidus interrupts the striatal loop for voluntary movement, resulting in chorea, extrapyramidal signs, and dementia. Huntington's disease is an autosomal dominant trait with a delayed appearance of symptoms until a mean age of 35 to 45 years. It is an example of a genetic defect associated with triplet repeats of CAG on chromosome 4. There is a decrease in γ-aminobenzoic acid (GABA), a false neurotransmitter, and a decrease in acetylcholine and substance P. The CAG repeat lengths on the abnormal gene are readily detected with polymerase chain reactions, which are more sensitive than the restriction fragment length polymorphism method.

- Alzheimer's disease is associated with senile plaques, which consist of a core of amyloid β (Aβ) protein polymerized into fibrils that are surrounded by dystrophic neurites. The Aβ peptide is derived from amyloid precursor protein (APP), which is coded for on chromosome 21, thus the relationship with Down syndrome. In high concentration, the Aβ peptide is toxic to mature neurons.
- Wilson's disease is an autosomal recessive disease with a defect in excreting copper in bile. Chronic liver disease and degeneration of the lenticular nuclei eventually occur because of the toxic damage by free copper.

104. The answer is C.   *(Anatomy)*
The nucleolus is the site of ribosomal RNA synthesis and remains the same size or becomes larger during axonal injury. New proteins are produced as the new nerve cell processes regenerate.

The perikaryon is the cell body of the neuron. Swelling of the perikaryon is one of the first responses to injury of the axon.

Nissl substance (rough endoplasmic reticulum) is lost from the cell body after injury. This loss is called chromatolysis.

The dissolution or loss of the Nissl substance would decrease basophilia because ribosomes are basophilic.

The axonal nucleus is displaced to one side after injury.

105. The answer is B.   *(Pathology)*
Tetanus toxoid is recommended for nonimmunized patients who have clean minor wounds that have been properly cleaned and débrided. An individual with complete immunization has received at least the three diphtheria-pertussis-tetanus (DTP) shots at 2, 4, and 6 months of age. Another DTP booster is given at 15 to 18 months of age and between 4 and 6 years of age. A tetanus toxoid booster is administered between 14 to 16 years of age, or before entering college. Tetanus toxoid is active immunization, because the patient must make antibodies against the toxin; the immune globulin is passive immunization, because the antibodies are already in the preparation. The following chart describes the recommended guidelines for tetanus prophylaxis.

| History | Clean minor wounds | | Dirty wounds | |
	Give Td toxoid	Give immune globulin	Give Td toxoid	Give immune globulin
Unknown or < 3 doses	Yes	No	Yes	Yes
≥ 3 doses	No, if last booster was < 10 years ago; yes if >10 years ago	No	No, if last booster ≤ 5 years ago; Yes, if > 5 years since last dose	No

Td = tetanus toxoid

106. The answer is D. *(Physiology)*
Skeletal muscle fibers can be divided into two major groups; fast and slow, based on the speed of their adenosine triphosphatase (ATPase) activity. All fast fibers have fast ATPase. However, fast fibers can be further subdivided based on their ability to sustain contractions. Some fatigue more quickly, have less myoglobin (which makes them white), and have fewer mitochondria and capillaries. The fatigue-resistant fast fibers have a reddish color due to more myoglobin, and they have more mitochondria and capillaries. The slow fibers are similar to the fatigue-resistant fast fibers except they have slower ATPase activity.

107. The answer is C. *(Pathology)*
A supracondylar fracture in children may be associated with a compartment syndrome (compartment hypertension), which refers to a buildup of pressure in a closed muscle compartment, with subsequent decrease in perfusion and the potential for permanent ischemic contractures of the muscle. Venous flow is first affected, followed by arterial flow. The tibial and the forearm muscle compartments are prone to this injury. Supracondylar fractures of the humerus in children predispose to possible entrapment of the brachial artery and median nerve. There is danger of developing Volkmann's ischemic contracture of the forearm muscles due to loss of the brachial artery blood supply.

Fractures of bone may occur in previously normal bone from external trauma or from a preexisting disease in the bone that produces a pathologic fracture (e.g., metastatic disease, bone cysts, and osteoporosis).

Fractures may be (1) complete or incomplete (green stick); (2) closed (simple) with intact overlying tissue; (3) comminuted, when the bone has been splintered; or (4) compound, when the fracture site communicates with the skin surface.

The three distinct stages of bone healing are (1) organization of a hematoma at the fracture site, (2) conversion of the organized hematoma (procallus) to a fibrocartilaginous callus, and (3) replacement of the fibrocartilaginous callus by mature bone, with eventual remodeling along the lines of weight-bearing to complete the repair.

A greenstick fracture is commonly seen in children and refers to a break in the cortex on the convex side of the shaft, but an intact concave side.

A Colles' fracture involves the distal end of the radius at the suprastyloid level, plus a fracture of the styloid process of the ulnar. It produces a dinner-fork deformity in that the radial fragment is displaced upward and backward. The fractures commonly occur when a person falls on an outstretched hand.

Clavicular fractures are the most common fracture noted in newborns. They occur in breech deliveries, newborns who are large for gestational age, or those situations that involve difficulty in delivering the shoulder.

The rotator cuff of the shoulder includes the following muscles: (1) supraspinatus, (2) infraspinatus, (3) teres minor, and (4) subcapsularis. These muscles keep the humeral head in the glenoid fossa to allow abduction of the arm by the deltoid muscle. Acute tears may be associated with anterior dislocation or fracture of the greater tuberosity. Other conditions are pain over the tip of the shoulder, weakness, and inability to abduct the arm.

108. The answer is D. *(Anatomy)*
In a lesion of the oculomotor nerve, the pupil would be dilated due to the unopposed contraction of the dilator pupillae muscle, which is innervated by the sympathetic nervous system. The eye would be in lateral and inferior (down and out) position as a result of an oculomotor nerve lesion due to the unopposed influence on the eyeball of the superior oblique muscle, which is innervated by the trochlear nerve, and the lateral rectus muscle, which is innervated by the abducens nerve. The pupillary light reflex is disrupted, and the pupil will not constrict when the examiner shines a light into the affected eye. A lesion of the oculomotor nerve would cause a ptosis of the eyelid because the levator palpebrae muscle is motor innervated by the oculomotor nerve. All muscles of the eye would show flaccid paralysis except the lateral rectus and superior obliques muscles, which are the only extraocular muscles not innervated by fibers in the oculomotor nerve.

109. The answer is E. *(Pathology)*
The x-ray appearance of bone lesions is often characteristic enough to warrant a diagnosis. Avascular necrosis, which is an infarction of bone, is associated with reactive bone formation and increased density of bone. Avascular necrosis of the femoral head due to long-term steroid usage is the most common cause.

Regarding the other choices:

- Osteogenic sarcomas are the second most common overall primary malignancy of bone (multiple myeloma is the most common). They occur around the knee in adolescents. They begin in the metaphysis of bone and spread out through the periosteum into the surrounding tissue. Portions of tumor-making bone produce densities in the subjacent tissue, giving a sunburst appearance. Lifting up of the periosteum by a tumor simulates a triangle, thus the term Codman's triangle.
- Ewing's sarcoma is another common primary malignancy of bone in children. When it spreads out of bone into the surrounding tissue, it produces an onion-skin appearance on x-ray.
- An osteoid osteoma is a benign neoplasm presenting with a distinctive radiographic pattern of a small radiolucent focus (nidus) surrounded by densely sclerotic bone. Males are more frequently involved than

females. The osteomas are characteristically associated with extreme pain in the favorite sites of involvement, which include the femur, tibia, and humerus. The pain is usually nocturnal and is due to excess production of prostaglandin E_2. As expected, the pain diminishes rapidly in response to aspirin. The treatment is en bloc resection.

110. The answer is C. *(Pharmacology)*
Unlike the tricyclic antidepressants (TCAs), the selective serotonin reuptake inhibitors (SSRIs), such as fluoxetine, sertraline, and paroxetine, tend to cause nervousness and anxiety rather than sedation. SSRIs are usually taken in the morning, whereas TCAs are often taken at bedtime. Unlike TCAs, SSRIs often cause weight loss rather than weight gain. SSRIs are generally less toxic in overdose and have less effect on autonomic and cardiovascular function than do the TCAs. However, SSRIs may be more likely to cause gastrointestinal and sexual dysfunction. Whereas fluoxetine and its metabolite have long half-lives (several days), the half-life of sertraline is about 24 hours.

111. The answer is B. *(Pathology)*
A 65-year-old man with a progressive increase in hat size, pain in the pelvic bones, an elevated serum alkaline phosphatase and thickened bone in the skull and pelvic areas has Paget's disease. Paget's disease of bone (osteitis deformans) refers to an abnormal thickening and architecture of bone that primarily occurs in elderly men. The cause is unknown, although slow virus infection and the measles virus have been implicated. The bone changes begin with an initial period of excessive osteoclastic resorption of bone followed by excessive bone formation with haphazard arrangement of the new bone into what is called mosaic bone. Despite its thickness, the bone is extremely soft. The excessive osteoblastic activity is responsible for the markedly elevated alkaline phosphatase levels in these patients. Complications include (1) arteriovenous fistulas within bone, with the potential for high-output cardiac failure as blood bypasses the microcirculation and returns quickly to the heart; (2) pathologic fractures; (3) enlargement of the head and increase in hat size; and (4) an increased risk for developing osteogenic sarcoma and chondrosarcoma. The only other condition with an increase in hat size is acromegaly, which

is due to a pituitary adenoma secreting excess growth hormone. Enlargement of the sella turcica is commonly present in this condition, but not in Paget's disease of bone.

112. The answer is D. *(Physiology)*
Nerve fiber conduction refers to the propagation of an action potential, which requires the influx of sodium ions through voltage-gated sodium channels in order to produce the depolarization phase of the action potential. Replacing extracellular sodium with potassium or an impermeate cation, or blocking sodium channels with tetrodotoxin will prevent the action potential. At a very low resting membrane potential, the sodium channels are inactivated and unable to produce an action potential. Momentarily stopping the pump does not interfere with the action potential or its propagation because it takes some time for the transmembrane concentration gradients to be destroyed, and the pump plays no other role in the action potential.

113. The answer is A. *(Pathology)*
Eczema includes a large category of skin lesions characterized by pruritus and distinctive gross and microscopic features. Dermatitis is a less specific term than eczema and indicates "inflammation of the skin." Eczema is divided into acute, subacute, and chronic stages. Acute eczema is characterized by a weeping, erythematous rash with vesiculation. Subacute eczema is acute eczema that lasts more than week and has crusts over the ruptured vesicles, erythema, and some scaling of the epidermis. Chronic eczema (lichen simplex chronicus) involves lichenification (thickening due to hyperkeratosis from constant scratching), scaling, hyperpigmentation, and less erythema than in the previous stages.

Acne rosacea is an inflammatory disease of the skin on the face. It is characterized by flushing, telangiectasia, papules and pustules, and sebaceous gland hyperplasia, the latter often called rhinophyma. It is treated with antibiotics.

Acanthosis nigricans is a pigmented skin lesion commonly present in the axilla. It is a phenotypic marker for gastric adenocarcinoma as well as an insulin receptor abnormality associated with diabetes mellitus.

Chronic discoid lupus is primarily limited to the skin, whereas systemic lupus erythematosus (SLE) may involve the skin and other systems. In either case, there is a deposition of DNA (planted antigen) and/or immune complexes in the basement membrane, with destruction of the basal cell layer (liquefactive degeneration), including the hair shaft, the latter resulting in alopecia. There is also a lymphocytic infiltrate at the dermal–epidermal junction, in the papillary dermis, around the adnexa, and around vessels (vasculitis). Immunofluorescent studies reveal a band of immunofluorescence (band test) in the involved skin of chronic discoid lupus or the involved and uninvolved skin of SLE.

Merkel cell carcinoma is a malignant tumor derived from neural crest–derived Merkel cells, which are thought to have a tactile function. The cells resemble those seen in a small cell carcinoma of the lung, which are also derives from the neural crest.

114. The answer is A. *(Anatomy)*
The skin of the lateral side of the hand is in the C_6 dermatome. The ventral side of the lateral hand is innervated by the median nerve, and the dorsal side is innervated by the radial nerve. The C_6 nerve fibers enter the median nerve through its lateral root. The lower trunk of the brachial plexus contains anterior ramus fibers from C_8 and T_1. These nerve fibers do not go to the lateral side of the hand; they go to the medial side of the hand and forearm.

115. The answer is B. *(Pharmacology)*
Phenylzine and tranylcypromine are the monoamine oxidase inhibitors (MAOIs) currently used for treating mood depression. These drugs inhibit both the A and B forms of monoamine oxidase (MAO), but the effect on MAO-A is believed responsible for their antidepressant effects because it metabolizes norepinephrine and serotonin. Like other antidepressants, the therapeutic effect is usually not observed for 2 to 3 weeks after starting treatment, whereas inhibition of MAO occurs shortly after beginning therapy. These drugs may cause a number of unpleasant and serious adverse effects, including orthostatic hypotension, weight gain, ejaculatory delay, hyperprexia, and hypertension. Dietary tyramine and dopamine are ordinarily degraded by MAO, and MAO inhibition may enable them to exert an indirect-acting sympathomimetic effect by causing the release of norepinephrine from sympathetic nerve terminals.

116. The answer is D.   *(Behavioral science)*
Decreased social contact and avoidance of social activities characterize the premorbid personality of the person with schizophrenia. The prodromal signs of schizophrenia include somatic problems such as back pain, headache, and digestive difficulties. The prodromal signs also include strange perceptions, peculiar behavior, and new interest in the occult, philosophy, or religion.

117. The answer is D.   *(Pharmacology)*
Drugs that are well known to lower the seizure threshold include the antipsychotics, such as chlorpromazine and loxapine (which is especially prone to cause seizures in epileptic patients). Tricyclic antidepressants, such as amitriptyline, and the fluoroquinolone antimicrobial agents also cause seizures. Lorazepam, a benzodiazepine, increases the seizure threshold and is an alternative to diazepam for the treatment of status epilepticus.

118. The answer is B.   *(Anatomy)*
The radial nerve innervates the major extensors of the arm, forearm, hand, and digits. A radial nerve injury therefore results in wristdrop and a loss of thumb extension. The long thumb abductor is also innervated by the radial nerve, but the short thumb abductor is innervated by the median nerve. To make a tight fist, the wrist must be stabilized by wrist extensors while the digits are flexed with digital flexors; a radial nerve injury prevents this action. Supination of the forearm can be performed by the biceps brachii, which is innervated by the musculocutaneous nerve. When the supinator muscle is denervated, supination is still possible.

119. The answer is D.   *(Pharmacology)*
Acute ethanol administration may inhibit the metabolism of other drugs, such an benzodiazepines, and contribute to their potentiation of central nervous system (CNS) depression. Chronic ethanol induces cytochrome P450 enzymes and thereby enhances drug elimination. Valproate inhibits the metabolism of other drugs and may increase their serum levels, whereas carbamazepine and phenytoin induce hepatic drug-metabolizing enzymes. The depressant effects of ethanol are potentiated by all other CNS depressants. Levodopa, or dihydroxyphenylalaine, is an amino acid

and is transported into the brain by amino acid transport systems. Amino acids derived from dietary proteins may compete with levodopa and reduce its brain uptake. Pyridoxine, a cofactor for the decarboxylation of levodopa to dopamine, can reduce the therapeutic effect of levodopa by stimulating its conversion to dopamine in the periphery.

120. The answer is E.   *(Behavioral science)*
Sensitivity to rejection, timidity, and social withdrawal are characteristic of avoidance personality disorder. Peculiar appearance is characteristic of schizotypal personality disorder.

121. The answer is E.   *(Pharmacology)*
Overuse of sedative-hypnotic drugs, including benzodiazepines, is a common cause of delirium and confusion in elderly patients. Elderly are more sensitive to central nervous system (CNS) depressants, and doses equal to about half of those used in younger patients are usually sufficient in the elderly.

122. The answer is E.   *(Anatomy)*
A lesion of the upper trunk of the brachial plexus results in Erb palsy. This palsy is characterized by adduction of the upper limb, which is extended at the side and internally rotated, resulting in the "porter's tip" sign. The muscles innervated by nerve fibers in the upper trunk (C_5 and C_6) include the major abductors of the shoulder (deltoid and supraspinatus), the major flexors of the shoulder (anterior deltoid, brachioradialis, and biceps brachii), and the major external rotators of the shoulder (infraspinatus and teres minor). Pronation of the forearm is accomplished primarily by the pronator teres (innervated by C_6 and C_7) and the pronator quadratus (innervated by C_7 and C_8).

123. The answer is A.   *(Pharmacology)*
The amphetamines have never been used in treating respiratory depression, though analeptics, another class of central nervous system (CNS) stimulants, have historically had limited use for this indication. The analeptics, including doxapram, nikethamide, picrotoxin, and pentylenetetrazole, are seldom used today because their toxicity is often greater than their efficacy. Doxapram and nikethamide may still be used rarely to counteract postanesthetic respiratory depression,

where they act by stimulating the brain stem respiratory and vasomotor centers. Narcolepsy, characterized by uncontrolled sleep at frequent intervals during the daytime, can be improved with the use of amphetamines, methylphenidate, or pemoline. Children and adults with attention deficit disorder or hyperkinetic syndrome may also benefit from the amphetamines. These drugs also reduce appetite and may be used in the management of obesity.

124. The answer is C.   *(Anatomy)*
All of the intrinsic muscles of the hand are innervated by nerve fibers in the lower trunk. Some of these nerve fibers travel in the median nerve and some in the ulnar nerve. Abduction and adduction of digits II through V are performed by the interosseous muscles, which are innervated by the ulnar nerve. Clawing of the digits is primarily a result of paralysis of the lumbrical muscles. The lumbricals to digits II and III are innervated by the median nerve. The lumbricals to digits IV and V are innervated by the ulnar nerve. Adduction of the thumb is performed by the adductor pollicis, which is innervated by the ulnar nerve. Opposition of the thumb is performed by the opponens pollicis, which is innervated by the median nerve. The entire dorsal and ventral surfaces of the hand include dermatomes C_6–C_8. A sensory deficit in this entire region would require injury to these nerves.

125. The answer is A.   *(Pharmacology)*
Psychotomimetic and hallucinogenic drugs have less dependence liability than other abused central nervous system agents, including the opiates, cocaine, and nicotine. Phencyclidine has a moderate dependence liability that appears to be greater than that of lysergic acid diethylamide (LSD), mescaline, or cannabis (marijuana). Drugs that have a strong dependence liability, but one that is less than that of heroin, cocaine, and nicotine, include ethanol, the solvents, barbiturates, and amphetamines. The dependence liability of benzodiazepines and methaqualone is considered to be moderate.

126. The answer is C.   *(Anatomy)*
The abductor pollicis brevis muscle (one of the thenar muscles) is innervated by the recurrent branch of the median nerve, which contains nerve fibers from spinal

cords levels C_8 and T_1. The medial root of the median nerve is the contribution to the median nerve from the lower trunk and contains fibers from C_8 and T_1. The anterior interosseous nerve is a branch of the median nerve that arises from the median nerve in the proximal forearm and innervates the deep muscles of the anterior compartment of the forearm. This nerve does not innervate muscles of the hand.

127. The answer is D.   *(Pharmacology)*
Pancuronium is a highly ionized derivative that acts as a neuromuscular blocking agent by competing with acetylcholine for nicotinic receptors in skeletal muscle. Unlike tubocurarine, it does not block autonomic ganglia significantly or release histamine. Pancuronium is administered parenterally and is eliminated by renal excretion.

128. The answer is E.   *(Anatomy)*
The infraspinatus muscle is innervated by the suprascapular nerve, which arises from the upper trunk of the brachial plexus. The teres minor is innervated by the axillary nerve, which arises from the posterior cord. The teres major is innervated by the lower subscapular nerve, which arises from the posterior cord. The latissimus dorsi is innervated by the middle subscapular nerve, which arises from the posterior cord. The subscapularis is innervated by the upper and lower subscapular nerves, which both arise from the posterior cord.

129. The answer is B.   *(Pharmacology)*
The neuromuscular blockade produced by the nondepolarizing blockers such as tubocurarine can be rapidly reversed by a cholinesterase inhibitor such as neostigmine. Tubocurarine acts by competing with acetylcholine for nicotinic receptors at the motor end plate, and this effect can be surmounted by increasing acetylcholine concentrations via cholinesterase inhibition. Neostigmine augments the Phase I neuromuscular blockade of succinylcholine, whereas the nondepolarizing blockers are antagonistic to Phase I succinylcholine blockade.

130. The answer is C.   *(Anatomy)*
The upper trunk of the brachial plexus consists of an anterior division, which contributes to the lateral cord,

and a posterior division, which contributes to the posterior cord. The lateral pectoral nerve and the musculocutaneous nerve arise from the lateral cord and contain upper trunk fibers. The axillary nerve and the radial nerve arise from the posterior cord and contain upper trunk fibers. The median nerve arises in part from the lateral cord and in part from the medial cord. Whereas the median nerve contains upper trunk fibers, the recurrent branch of the median nerve (which innervates the thenar muscles of the hand) contains only lower trunk fibers.

131. The answer is A.   *(Pharmacology)*
Inhalational anesthetics, particularly halogenated agents such as isoflurane, augment the neuromuscular blockade of nondepolarizing muscle relaxants. Local anesthetics, such as lidocaine, and numerous antibiotics, particularly aminoglycosides such as gentamicin, also augment neuromuscular blockade. Patients with myasthenia gravis are extremely sensitive to neuromuscular blocking agents. The loop diuretic furosemide has no significant effect on neuromuscular function or the response to blocking agents.

132. The answer is B.   *(Anatomy)*
The lateral pectoral nerve, a branch of the lateral cords of the brachial plexus, contains nerve fibers from spinal cord segments C_5 and C_6 and innervates the upper portion of the pectoralis major muscle. All nerves that innervate muscles of the hand contain nerve fibers from C_8 and T_1. Therefore, this group of nerves includes the recurrent branch of the median nerve and the superficial and deep branches of the ulnar nerve.

133. The answer is D.   *(Pharmacology)*
Tubocurarine is more likely to cause hypotension, primarily through release of histamine, than other nondepolarizing neuromuscular blockers. Ganglionic blockade may contribute to hypotension after higher doses of tubocurarine. Tubocurarine does not increase intraocular pressure, which is an adverse effect of succinylcholine.

134. The answer is E.   *(Anatomy)*
The medial pectoral nerve is a branch of the medial cord of the brachial plexus, which contains only anterior division nerve fibers. The thoracodorsal (middle

subscapular) nerve and lower subscapular nerve are branches of the posterior cord, which contains only posterior division fibers. The axillary nerve is also a branch of the posterior cord. The posterior interosseous nerve is a branch of the radial nerve, which is a branch of the posterior cord.

135. The answer is B.   *(Pharmacology)*
Halogenated anesthetics are respiratory depressants and decrease arterial blood pressure, by depressing cardiac output and/or causing peripheral vasodilation. Anesthetics relax skeletal and smooth muscle, though additional muscle relaxants are usually required during surgery. While these agents produce some analgesia, they have less analgesic activity than diethylether and nitrous oxide. For these reasons, halogenated agents are often combined with analgesics, benzodiazepines, nitrous oxide, and muscle relaxants in an approach called balanced anesthesia, thereby reducing the amount of halogenated agent required for complete surgical anesthesia and muscle relaxation.

136. The answer is D.   *(Anatomy)*
The superior temporal gyrus is generally part of the temporal lobe and is involved in associative functions of auditory origin.

The cingulate gyrus, hippocampus, parahippocampal gyrus, and hypothalamus make up the functional lobe called the limbic system.

137. The answer is C.   *(Pharmacology)*
Opiates may reduce urine output both by decreasing renal plasma flow and GFR as well as by stimulating the release of antidiuretic hormone. Opiates produce respiratory depression, primarily by reducing the hypercapnic drive in the brain stem. Constipation results from stimulation of opiate receptors in gastrointestinal smooth muscle that increase muscle tone but not propulsive motility. Nausea and vomiting are produced primarily through activation of dopaminergic receptors in the chemoreceptor trigger zone in the medulla. Pruritus and flushing are due primarily to the release of histamine, which may be triggered by morphine and other opiates.

138. The answer is E. *(Behavioral science)*
Patients taking lithium are no more likely to experience food intolerance than are patients on other medications. However, patients taking lithium are more likely to experience hypothyroidism, gastric distress, tremor, and mild cognitive impairment.

139. The answer is E. *(Pharmacology)*
Repeated administration of opiates usually results in the development of tolerance to most of the central nervous system effects of these drugs, accompanied by the onset of physical dependence. Tolerance also develops to the antidiuretic effect of opiates. However, the miotic and constipative effects are relatively stable during chronic administration.

140. The answer is E. *(Anatomy)*
Rough endoplasmic reticulum is restricted from the axon. Most if not all protein is synthesized near the nucleus and transported down the axon and dendrites.

Vesicles contain material moving from the cell body to the axon end (anterograde flow) and from the axon terminal to the cell body (retrograde flow). Cytoskeletal proteins move by anterograde flow as neurotransmitters, amino acids, nucleotides, calcium, and sugars. Retrograde flow carries endocytosed material from the terminal end as well as many of the elements carried by anterograde flow.

Neurotubules or microtubules are present in the axon, providing the structural framework of the axon and serving as a system of railroad tracks for the transport of vesicles. Dynein and kinesin are two proteins that interact with tubulin to produce this vesicle movement.

Mitochondria are present along the axon, providing energy for vesicle and other organelle transport.

Neurofilaments provide structural stability for the axon; therefore, they are evident in almost any cross-sectional profile of the axon.

141. The answer is D. *(Pharmacology)*
Lithium has a low therapeutic index of about 3, and elevated serum levels (above 2.5 mEq/L) may precipitate serious toxicity (seizures, coma, and death). Common adverse effects with therapeutic levels include sedation, a fine tremor, weight gain, polyuria/polydipsia, and gastrointestinal symptoms. Chronic therapy

may lead to hypothyroidism. Lithium's mechanism is not fully understood, but it appears to act by altering G-protein function so as to diminish receptor and G-protein coupling, and it also appears to interfere with phosphoinositol metabolism and the production of second messengers (inositol triphosphate and diacylglycerol). Lithium is used almost exclusively in the chronic treatment of bipolar disorder. It is most effective against the manic phase, though it exerts a mild antidepressant effect. Lithium is eliminated in the urine and is actively reabsorbed in the proximal tubule at sites ordinarily utilized by sodium. Sodium depletion, due to dietary restriction of diuretics, promotes lithium reabsorption and increases serum levels and the potential for toxicity. Sodium loading decreases lithium reabsorption and serum levels.

142. The answer is C. *(Anatomy)*
The femoral nerve is outside of and lateral to the femoral sheath. Within the femoral sheath at the proximal portion of the thigh, the femoral artery is lateral to the femoral vein. The floor of the femoral; triangle in the region of the femoral nerve is the iliopsoas muscle. The neurovascular structures that pass behind the inguinal ligament are, from lateral to medial, the femoral nerve, femoral artery, femoral vein, and inguinal lymphatics. A femoral nerve block can be accomplished by injecting the anesthetic agent lateral to the femoral pulse immediately below the inguinal ligament.

143. The answer is B. *(Pharmacology)*
The mu and delta receptors are both found in the spinal cord, supraspinal structures, and peripheral smooth muscle, where they mediate analgesia, euphoria, sedation, respiratory depression, miosis, and increased smooth muscle tone, causing constipation and biliary spasm. Kappa receptors are primarily located in the spinal cord and mediate analgesia, sedation, and dysphoria. Sigma receptors do not mediate analgesia, but they are believed to cause the dysphoria and hallucinations associated with some partial/mixed opiate agonists. Sigma receptors are not true opioid receptors and are activated by other psychotomimetics, such as phencyclidine. They may be associated with glutamate-activated ion channels.

144. The answer is D.   *(Physiology)*
Smooth muscle stimulation can occur through an action potential or through excitation of membrane receptors without an action potential. Both methods involve an increase in intracellular calcium ion concentration, and a significant amount of this calcium may come from the extracellular space. The calcium ions bind to calmodulin, and the calcium-calmodulin complex activates (it does not inhibit) myosin light chain kinase so that an adenosine triphospate-dependent actin-myosin contraction can occur.

145. The answer is A.   *(Anatomy)*
The pathway for unconscious proprioception (the spinocerebellar tract) ascends to the cerebellum without crossing to the other side of the brain. Therefore, choice C would be lost. Voluntary movement descends from the contralateral side and crosses in the medulla to descend on the same side as the muscle to be stimulated; therefore, choice D would be lost. The other sensations (pain, touch, temperature) ascend to the thalamus and cerebral cortex on the contralateral side of the brain. The key is the point at which these tracts cross. Touch (vibratory and 2-point discrimination) ascends on the same side of the cord and crosses in the medulla. As a result, choice B would be lost. Pain and temperature cross at the level where they enter the cord to ascend on the contralateral side. Therefore, choice E would be lost, but choice A would remain intact.

146. The answer is E.   *(Pathology)*
In bites from wild animals suspected of being rabid, thorough cleansing of the wound site with quaternary ammonium compounds (1% to 4% benzalkonium chloride or 1% cetrimonium chloride) and water, injection with half of the dose of the rabies immune globulin (not the vaccine) to the wound site, and active immunization with human diploid vaccine are recommended.

The rabies virus is an RNA virus in the Rhabdoviridae family. In nature, it is primarily found in skunks, foxes, bats, and raccoons. In the United States, humans contract rabies by the bite of a rabid skunk, fox, raccoon, or bat, whereas in third-world countries, 75% of rabies cases are caused by bites from rabid dogs. It is also possible to contract rabies from aerosolization in bat infested caves. The virus is in the saliva of the rabid animal and enters through a bite or scratch in the skin.

Bites by bats or from animals such as skunks, coyotes, foxes, or raccoons are considered rabid, and full immunization is recommended. The incubation period for the virus is usually 30 to 90 days. Areas of the body with a greater nerve supply (e.g., the fingers, face, genitalia) have a shorter incubation period. Children are also affected earlier than adults.

The virus enters the central nervous system (CNS) by ascending along peripheral nerves. In the brain, it produces an encephalomyelitis. The prodrome includes fever, headache, malaise, excitability, and paresthesias around the wound site in more than 50% of patients (diagnostic finding). Approximately 80% of patients enter an extraordinary CNS excitability stage with (1) the slightest touch evoking tremendous pain, (2) convulsions, (3) autonomic excitability, (4) frothing of the mouth, (5) hydrophobia, because drinking water stimulates muscular spasms, and (6) flaccid paralysis occurs, which progresses to coma and respiratory failure. "Dumb" rabies is a predominantly paralytic form of rabies, which occurs in 15% to 20% of patients. Neurons, particularly in the Purkinje cells of the cerebellum, contain pathognomonic intracytoplasmic inclusions called Negri bodies in 70% of patients. The diagnosis of rabies is established by serologic tests, culture of infected material (brain biopsy), or direct immunofluorescent techniques on corneal smears, saliva, or skin. Human rabies immune globulin is available for passive immunity and human vaccine is available for active immunization. Full immunization is not necessary in domestic dog or cat bites if the animals show no signs of rabies after 10 days of observation. However, if the animal does show signs of the disease, it should be killed and the brain examined by direct immunofluorescence techniques.

147. The answer is E.   *(Anatomy)*
The synovial membrane lines the inner surface of the articular fibrous capsule and the intra-articular surface of the bone. It does not line the articular cartilage. Articular cartilage is directly in contact with the synovial fluid within the synovial cavity. The cartilages of the two articulating bones contact one another with a thin film of synovial fluid between them.

148. The answer is A. *(Microbiology)*
In the elderly population, influenza vaccination is only 30% to 40% effective in preventing influenza, but it is 80% effective in preventing death. In young people, the vaccine is 70% to 90% effective in preventing the disease. The vaccine contains only noninfectious viruses, so it does not produce a weak type of influenza. It protects the patient against influenza type A but not type B. It is indicated for all high-risk patients, including patients who have acquired or congenital heart disease, are diabetic, have sickle cell disease, have chronic lung, cardiac, liver, or renal disease, and those who are immunocompromised. Health care workers and everyone more than 65 years of age should also receive the vaccine. Patients who have an anaphylactic reaction to eggs should not receive the vaccine, because it is an egg-based vaccine.

Influenza viruses are RNA viruses in the Orthomyxoviridae family. They are a significant cause of mortality, especially among individuals older than 55 years of age who have underlying renal, cardiac, liver, or lung problems. Influenza virus type A produces pandemics and epidemics; type B is associated with epidemics; and type C is involved in sporadic cases. Hemagglutinins bind the virus to cell receptors in the nasal passages. Antibodies against hemagglutinins provide protective immunity, so when point mutations occur in hemagglutinins, antigenic shifts resulting in pandemics occur and require a new vaccine. Neuraminidase aids viral entry into the cell by breaking down the protective mucus, thus exposing viral receptor sites on the mucosa and also facilitates the release of the virus particles from infected cells. Local epidemics, called antigenic drifts, result from minor changes in the antigenicity of the organisms caused by point mutations. Influenza viruses produce respiratory disease, ranging from a mild cold to bronchitis to severe pneumonias.

149. The answer is C. *(Anatomy)*
A motor unit is a single efferent neuron and all the muscle fibers innervated by that neuron. When a motor neuron depolarizes, all the muscle cells innervated by it depolarize. When a muscle cell depolarizes, it contracts maximally. Gradation of muscle contraction occurs by varying the number of motor units that depolarize simultaneously. All the motor units in a muscle do not depolarize simultaneously. Maximal contraction of a muscle takes place by asynchronous depolarization of the motor units in the muscle. The position of the muscle cells within the muscle determines the function of those muscle cells. Therefore, different motor units within a muscle can perform different functions.

150. The answer is A. *(Pathology)*
Central nervous system calcifications are least likely to be associated with an astrocytoma. Disorders associated with calcifications that are evident on a plain film of the skull include (1) the normal dystrophic calcification of the pineal gland in the elderly, (2) calcification of the basal ganglia in hypoparathyroidism, (3) the cyst wall in cysticercosis, (4) meningiomas, (5) cytomegalovirus involving the newborn (periventricular calcifications), (6) congenital toxoplasmosis (periventricular calcifications), (7) tuberous sclerosis, (8) the abnormal vessels in arteriovenous malformations, (9) craniopharyngiomas, (10) oligodendrogliomas, and (11) pinealomas.

151-155. The answers are: 151-C, 152-E, 153-A, 154-D, 155-B. *(Pharmacology)*
Opiate analgesics differ in their potency, efficacy, oral bioavailability, and receptor selectivity. Propoxyphene and methadone have a relatively high oral to parenteral potency ratio, whereas morphine has a lower ratio due to first-pass metabolism. Propoxyphene is a weak agonist, whereas methadone is a full agonist with a long duration of action and is well suited for substitution therapy in heroin addicts. Fentanyl is a very short-acting and highly potent opiate that can be administered intravenously for surgical procedures, where it produces less cardiac depression than most other drugs. A sustained-release transdermal system is also available for fentanyl administration in the treatment of severe pain in ambulatory patients. Dextromethorphan lacks most of the central nervous system effects of the levorotatory isomer, but it retains good antitussive activity and is available without a prescription in many cough and cold preparations. Butorphanol is a mixed agonist/antagonist opiate that has reduced drug dependence liability and causes less respiratory depression in overdose. It is available for parenteral administration and recently became available in a transnasal formulation for the short-term management of moderately severe pain.

156-159. The answers are: 156-D, 157-B, 158-A, 159-C. *(Pharmacology)*

Were it not for its flammability, disagreeable odor, and high blood-gas partition coefficient, diethylether would be an ideal anesthetic. It can be used with little or no drug supplementation, and it stimulates respiration and increases blood pressure, thereby increasing its margin of safety. For these reasons, ether is still widely used in parts of the world where expensive monitoring equipment (and anesthetics) are not available. Halothane is nonflammable and has a relatively low blood-gas partition coefficient, but it sensitizes the heart to catecholamine and may cause considerable hypotension. Nitrous oxide is an excellent analgesic, but it is a relatively weak anesthetic and must be combined with other agents for major surgery. Ketamine produces so-called dissociative anesthesia, in which the patient appears to be awake but is dissociated from sensory stimulation. Ketamine increases muscle tone and stimulates cardiovascular function.

160-164. The answers are: 160-B, 161-D, 162-E, 163-C, 164-A. *(Anatomy)*

The spinal cord lesion in figure B has affected the lateral funiculus, damaging the descending lateral corticospinal tract and producing a loss of voluntary motor skills. The dorsal (posterior) spinocerebellar tract has been damaged, and a loss of the ascending unconscious proprioception to the cerebellum results in an ataxia, especially of lower extremities.

The spinal cord lesion in D represents a loss of blood supply in the distribution of the anterior spinal artery. The infarcted tissue is the ventral white commissure and the ventral horn tissue of the gray matter. Fibers associated with pain and temperature cross in the ventral white commissure. Loss of these fibers often produces aberrant tingling and numbness in the area of distribution. The loss of the ventral horn neurons produces a weakness in the voluntary skeletal muscles innervated at this segmental level.

The spinal cord lesion in E represents demyelinization of fibers in the dorsal columns. These axons are the first order neurons in the ascending system serving the function of 2-point discrimination, vibratory sensation, and conscious proprioception. Romberg's sign is elicited by having a patient stand with eyes closed and feet together. Posture maintenance requires an intact dorsal column-medial lemniscal system; if this pathway is lesioned, the patient will not be able to maintain a standing position, will begin to drift, and may fall to the side.

The spinal cord lesion in C represents a loss of the neuronal population in the ventral horn of the gray matter. This may result from loss of blood supply, metabolic disorders, disease, such as amyotrophic lateral sclerosis, or viral infection.

The spinal cord lesion in A represents a hemisected spinal cord from a traumatic injury, such as from a gunshot, knife wound, or bone fragments. The constellation of neurological deficits produced from this type of injury is referred to as a Brown-Sequard syndrome. These deficits include ipsilateral upper motor neuron findings below the level of the lesion; ipsilateral loss of 2-point touch, vibratory sensation, and conscious proprioception; and contralateral loss of pain and temperature below the level of the lesion. The key to understanding these findings is recognizing where these pathways cross along the longitudinal axis of the spinal cord and brain stem.

165-169. The answers are: 165-C, 166-A, 167-E, 168-B, 169-D. *(Pharmacology)*

Clozapine and risperidone are newer drugs that appear to be more effective in treating resistant schizophrenic patients and do not appear to cause as many extrapyramidal side effects or tardive dyskinesia. Whereas clozapine may cause agranulocytosis, risperidone seems to be free of this adverse effect. In contrast, haloperidol is associated with a high frequency of extrapyramidal side effects. While both haloperidol and fluphenazine are high-potency neuroleptics that cause considerable extrapyramidal side effects, haloperidol is a benzophenone and fluphenazine is a phenothiazine. Long-acting injectable fluphenazine preparations may be useful in the chronic management of schizophrenic patients, particularly those who are noncompliant.

170-174. The answers are: 170-B, 171-C, 172-D, 173-A, 174-D. *(Anatomy)*

The first case represents a pontine lesion producing an alternating hemiplegia. Localization to the pons is possible due to a knowledge or the origin of the abducens nerve from the abducens and of the nerve fibers from the pons.

The seventh and eighth cranial nerves exit the brain stem at the cerebellopontine angle. Compression of both nerves at this site would produce the ipsilateral signs and symptoms and auditory dysfunction and paralysis of the muscles of facial expression displayed in the second case.

Regarding the third case, partial paralysis of the face affecting only the lower half is indicative of an upper motor neuron lesion affecting facial nucleus innervation. The lesion is most likely in the internal capsule of the hemisphere on the opposite side of the neurological findings.

Lesions of the ipsilateral pontine tegmentum would affect the abducens nucleus and the internal genu of the facial nerve as it courses dorsally to the abducens nucleus, resulting in the symptoms indicated in the fourth case.

Regarding the fifth case, the lesion is most likely in the left hemisphere because Broca's speech center is located in the left hemisphere; weakness in the right upper extremity would be evident in a lesion of the opposite cerebral hemisphere.

175-178. The answers are: 175-E, 176-A, 177-D, 178-C. *(Pharmacology)*

Dantrolene is the only skeletal muscle relaxant that acts directly on skeletal muscle to block excitation-contraction coupling by inhibiting the release of calcium from the sarcoplasmic reticulum. Besides its use in treating spasticity, dantrolene is effective in malignant hyperthermia, a disorder that may be triggered in genetically predisposed patients by general anesthetics and neuromuscular blocking agents and is characterized by a profound release of calcium from the sarcoplasmic reticulum. Baclofen and benzodiazepines both work by augmenting GABA neurotransmission, but baclofen produces less sedation than diazepam at doses required to treat spasticity. Cyclobenzaprine, orphenadrine, chlorzoxazone, and carisoprodol are all centrally acting muscle relaxants whose effects may be partly attributed to sedation. All are used in the short-term treatment of muscle spasm resulting from minor trauma. Diazepam is an alternative to dantrolene and baclofen for the treatment of muscle spasm and spasticity resulting from spinal cord injuries and other neurological or neuromuscular conditions. Pancuronium is a nondepolarizing neuromuscular blocker that must be given parenterally and is primarily used as an adjunct to general anesthesia.

179-180. The answers are: 179-C, 180-B. *(Pathology)*

The figure in question 179 is a cross-section of brain that shows a dark area in the thalamus, representing an intracerebral hemorrhage that has shifted the structures across the midline. Because an intracerebral hemorrhage is most commonly caused by hypertension, the most likely patient is a 55-year-old black man with essential hypertension who presented with a sudden onset of hemiplegia.

The figure of the gross specimen of brain in question 180 exhibits a large black mass, representing a blood clot located on top of the dura. This represents an epidural hematoma, which would most likely occur in a major league baseball player who was hit on the side of the head with a baseball bat and developed signs of increased intracranial pressure. Traumatic intracranial hemorrhage is most often manifested as an epidural hematoma or a subdural hematoma. An acute epidural hematoma results from trauma to the side of the head with fracture of the temporoparietal bone and severance of the middle meningeal artery (which should not be confused with the middle cerebral artery), which lies between the dura and the inner table of the bone. Normally, the dura is tightly adherent to the periosteum of bone; however, the pressure generated by an arterial bleed creates an epidural space between the calvarium and dura. The patient is initially rendered unconscious and then regains consciousness (i.e., lucid interval). After 4 to 8 hours, when there is approximately 30 to 50 ml of blood in the space, the patient develops increased intracranial pressure and may die of herniation unless the blood is removed. There is a 20% mortality rate.

Test 3

DIRECTIONS:

Each of the numbered items or incomplete statements in this section is followed by answers or by completions of the statement. Select the ONE lettered answer or completion that is BEST in each case.

1. A structure that passes through the adductor hiatus of the thigh is the

(A) femoral nerve
(B) femoral artery
(C) profunda femoral artery
(D) posterior tibial artery
(E) saphenous nerve

2. This figure represents a gross specimen of brain from a 58-year-old man who was a heavy smoker. A few days before his death, he had projectile vomiting, lid lag, ophthalmoplegia, and mydriasis. Which cause of death would be expected?

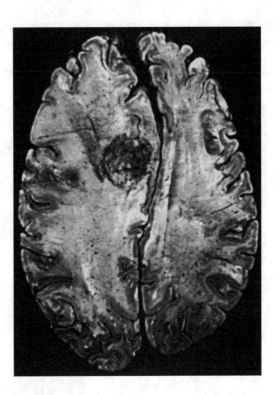

(A) A glioblastoma multiforme resulting in cerebral edema and herniation of the cerebellar tonsils into the foramen magnum

(B) Metastatic cancer from the lung to the brain resulting in cerebral edema and uncal herniation

(C) A hemorrhagic infarction of the brain with edema leading to uncal herniation

(D) A cerebral abscess from a primary site in the lungs with hematogenous spread to the brain resulting in cerebral edema and herniation of the cerebellar tonsils into the foramen magnum

(E) A low-grade astrocytoma resulting in cerebral edema and uncal herniation

3.   Which of the following organisms cause conjunctivitis and pneumonia in a newborn?

(A) Parainfluenza virus
(B) *Streptococcus agalactiae*
(C) *Neisseria gonorrhoeae*
(D) *Chlamydia trachomatis*
(E) Respiratory syncytial virus

4.   An adverse reaction after receiving recombinant hepatitis B vaccine would most likely occur in a patient who is/has

(A) pregnant
(B) lactating
(C) a history of anaphylaxis to baker's yeast
(D) a history of anaphylaxis after eating eggs or egg products
(E) AIDS

5.   Greenish discoloration of the sputum in a febrile 4-year-old with cystic fibrosis is most likely caused by which of the following organisms?

(A) *Staphylococcus aureus*
(B) *Serratia marcescens*
(C) *Pseudomonas aeruginosa*
(D) *Hemophilus influenzae*
(E) *Bacteroides melaninogenicus*

6.   A 46-year-old man has atrophy of the intrinsic muscles of both hands and absent deep tendon reflexes in the upper extremity. Muscle fasciculations are also noted in the affected muscles. These findings are most likely related to

(A) a reduction in the synthesis of dopamine
(B) a defect in the reabsorption of vitamin B_{12}
(C) a reduction in superoxide dismutase
(D) an HLR-DR2 haplotype
(E) the presence of nucleotide triplet repeats in DNA

7.   In the figure below, which curve represents the time course of the distribution of thiopental in skeletal muscle and skin?

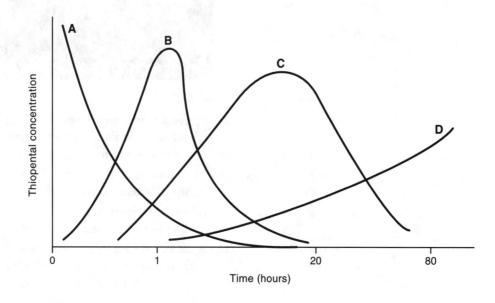

8. In adults, the most common location for a primary brain tumor is the

(A) cauda equina
(B) cerebellum
(C) brain stem
(D) cerebral cortex
(E) fourth ventricle

9. Which of the following diseases is most commonly transmitted by a mosquito bite?

(A) Tularemia
(B) Plague
(C) Yellow fever
(D) African sleeping sickness
(E) Leishmaniasis

10. Which of the following vaccines is contraindicated in a patient who is HIV positive?

(A) Hemophilus influenzae biotype II
(B) Diphtheria-pertussis-tetanus (DPT)
(C) Bacille Calmette-Guérin (BCG)
(D) Influenza
(E) Measles-mumps-rubella (MMR)

11. Which of the following pathogens is easily identified with the standard Gram stain?

(A) *Nocardia asteroides*
(B) *Legionella pneumophila*
(C) *Pneumocystis carinii*
(D) *Afipia felis*
(E) *Chlamydia trachomatis*

12. A midline, lobulated, mucoid mass occurring in the sphenoccipital or sacrococcygeal region is most likely derived from

(A) ependymal cells
(B) astrocytes
(C) notochord
(D) microglial cells
(E) oligodendrocytes

Questions 13-19

A 29-year-old man goes to the emergency room because of a severe headache. The patient says that the headache, which seems localized to the area behind his ears, has been intermittent but persistent since he was involved in a beach volleyball game while on vacation. Shortly after he returned from his vacation, he made an appointment with his family physician because he was worried about the headache and the fact that he had developed noticeable clumsiness. An avid fitness enthusiast, he noted his performance was awkward and uncoordinated. When questioned, he mentioned unusually frequent bouts of nausea and vertigo. Physical examination reveals an alert, oriented, thin man with mild hoarseness and some difficulty swallowing oral secretions. The left side of his face is affected by Horner's syndrome, and he has pronounced bilateral rotatory nystagmus in the primary position with all directions of gaze. He has decreased sensitivity to light touch on the left side of his face, flattening of the left nasolabial fold, and paresis of the left soft palate. Finger to nose testing shows left-sided dysmetria. When asked to walk across the examining room, his gait is ataxic and he deviates to the left. There is diminished pain and thermal sensation on the right side. Reflexes are symmetric. There is no Babinski reflex, and the remainder of the motor and sensory examination is normal.

13. The attending and resident physicians suspect a vascular occlusion or rupture. Which one of the following vessels should be the primary suspect? The

(A) middle cerebral artery
(B) internal carotid artery at the cavernous sinus
(C) superior cerebellar artery
(D) posterior inferior cerebellar artery
(E) anterior communicating artery

14. What is the most likely cause of the patient's Horner's syndrome?

(A) Descending autonomic innervation from the hypothalamus
(B) Parasympathetic dystonia
(C) Compression of the sympathetic chain and superior cervical ganglion in the neck as a result of torticollis
(D) A reactive conjunctivitis caused by sand in the patient's eyes
(E) A hypothalamic cyst

15. Which brain stem pathway affected by the lesion is responsible for the findings of diminished pain and thermal sensation on the right side?

(A) Dorsal column–medial lemniscus
(B) Anterolateral system (spinothalamic tract)
(C) Dorsal spinocerebellar tract
(D) Pontocerebellar tract
(E) Periaqueductal gray pathway

16. This patient's dysmetria is indicative of a problem associated with the

(A) extrapyramidal descending motor systems
(B) lateral lemniscus
(C) dorsal longitudinal fasciculus
(D) cerebellum
(E) pyramidal tract

17. The lack of a Babinski reflex indicates that which one of the following pathways is intact?

(A) Anterolateral system (spinothalamic tract)
(B) Pyramidal (corticospinal) tract
(C) Dorsal column–medial lemniscal system
(D) Auditory system
(E) Olivocerebellar tract

18. Involvement of which one of the following cranial nerves is responsible for the findings of hoarseness and difficulty swallowing?

(A) Glossopharyngeal nerve
(B) Hypoglossal nerve
(C) Vagus nerve
(D) Spinal accessory nerve
(E) Trigeminal nerve

19. What is the most likely diagnosis?

(A) Wernicke's syndrome
(B) Klüver-Bucy syndrome
(C) Weber's syndrome
(D) Locked-in syndrome
(E) Wallenberg's syndrome

20. A tumor in an adult that involves the optic nerve, spinal cord, or skull bone and is associated with new onset seizure activity would most likely have which of the following histologic features?

(A) Antoni A and B areas
(B) Psammoma bodies
(C) Physaliphorous cells
(D) Vascular proliferation and necrosis
(E) Perivascular pseudorosettes

21. A 65-year-old man, who recently moved to Phoenix, Arizona, presents with fever, flu-like symptoms, a nonproductive cough, and painful red nodules on the anterior aspect of his lower left leg. A solitary coin lesion with an egg shell-like cavity is noted in the upper portion of his left lower lobe on a chest radiograph. A biopsy of this lung lesion would be expected to show which of the following disorders?

(A) Metastatic disease
(B) Spherules with endospores
(C) Narrow angled septate hyphae with fruiting bodies
(D) Budding yeasts with pseudohypha
(E) A hemorrhagic infarction secondary to a pulmonary embolus

22. The most common source of gram-negative bacteremia in hospitalized patients is related to

(A) pneumonia
(B) intravenous catheters
(C) right upper quadrant surgery
(D) indwelling urinary catheters
(E) septic thrombophlebitis

23. An asymptomatic, afebrile 48-year-old black man, who has lived all of his life in Ohio, has multiple calcifications throughout both lung fields and in the spleen. The patient is expected to have which of the following disorders?

(A) Histoplasmosis
(B) Blastomycosis
(C) Metastatic osteogenic sarcoma
(D) Cryptococcosis
(E) Sarcoidosis

24. A tumor of the filum terminale in an adult is most likely derived from

(A) ependymal cells
(B) notochord
(C) astrocytes
(D) microglial cells
(E) arachnoid granulations

25. Which one of the following statements regarding the normal human eye is true?

(A) There are more cones than rods in the retina
(B) There are more photoreceptors than ganglion cells in the retina
(C) There are more afferent fibers in the optic nerve than ganglion cells in the retina
(D) The optic disk contains more cones than rods
(E) The lens has a greater refractive power than the cornea

26. Which of the following actions is more likely to be a purely bacterial mechanism for killing host cells rather than a viral mechanism for killing host cells?

(A) Inhibit host cell DNA, RNA, or protein synthesis
(B) Lyse host cells
(C) Damage host cell membranes
(D) Alter class I antigens, leaving them susceptible to CD 8 cytotoxic T-cell destruction
(E) Elaboration of toxins

27. Botulinum toxin is now used to treat spasm of the extraocular muscles because of its ability to

(A) block choline transport into motor neurons
(B) inhibit acetylcholine (ACh) synthesis
(C) block storage of ACh in neuronal vesicles
(D) inhibit the release of ACh from cholinergic nerves
(E) compete with ACh for nicotinic receptors in skeletal muscle

28. Which of the following uses a mechanism other than impairing mucociliary clearance in producing disease in the lungs?

(A) Smoking
(B) Kartagener syndrome
(C) Influenza virus
(D) *Bordetella*
(E) *Mycobacterium tuberculosis*

29. In patients with multiple sclerosis, areas of demyelinated axon membrane may have potassium channels but lack voltage-gated sodium channels. Electrical stimulation of such a membrane should cause

(A) a normal action potential
(B) a larger than normal action potential
(C) hyperpolarization or no response
(D) an excitatory postsynaptic potential (EPSP)
(E) an inhibitory postsynaptic potential (IPSP)

30. Asthma, massive hemoptysis, and external otitis are most closely associated with infections caused by which of the following organisms?

(A) *Pseudomonas aeruginosa*
(B) *Candida albicans*
(C) *Aspergillus fumigatus*
(D) *Streptococcus pneumoniae*
(E) *Staphylococcus aureus*

31. A 34-year-old woman is brought to the community clinic by her neighbor. The patient is alert and cooperative now, but the neighbor says that she had acted like she had had some kind of seizure. Upon questioning, the patient reveals that she has been experiencing tingling, numbness, and some brief episodes of sharp facial pain. The pain radiates into the temporal and lower jaw region. A thorough neurologic examination, including cranial nerve testing, shows no other apparent neurologic problems. What do these initial findings suggest?

(A) A meningioma within the tentorium
(B) Trigeminal neuralgia
(C) Alternating hemiplegia
(D) Bell's palsy
(E) Aneurysm of the posterior cerebral artery

32. Which one of the following diseases would most likely have an interstitial pneumonia rather than a cavitary lesion on a chest radiograph?

(A) Pneumonia caused by *Chlamydia pneumoniae*
(B) Reactivation tuberculosis
(C) Primary squamous carcinoma of the lung
(D) Histoplasmosis
(E) Lung abscess

33. Which one of the following agents would be most likely to increase a patient's heart rate?

(A) A muscarinic cholinergic blocker
(B) A β-adrenergic blocker
(C) An α-adrenergic agonist
(D) A nicotinic cholinergic blocker

34. *Mycobacterium tuberculosis* and sarcoidosis are both associated with which of the following disorders?

(A) Granulomatous hepatitis
(B) A positive Kveim test
(C) Constrictive pericarditis
(D) Caseous necrosis
(E) Restrictive lung disease

35. Positive symptoms of schizophrenia include

(A) flattening of affect
(B) hallucinations
(C) poverty of speech
(D) blocking
(E) social withdrawal

36. Which of the following disorders would most likely be associated with *Hemophilus ducreyi* rather than *Hemophilus influenzae?*

(A) Osteomyelitis
(B) Painful ulcer on the penis
(C) Otitis media
(D) Chronic bronchitis
(E) Epiglottitis

37. Which one of the following adrenergic receptors is considerably less sensitive to the stimulating effects of norepinephrine?

(A) α_1
(B) α_2
(C) β_1
(D) β_2

38. Which of the following disorders would more likely be associated with *Staphylococcus saprophyticus* rather than *Staphylococcus aureus?*

(A) Osteomyelitis
(B) Tension pneumothorax
(C) Burns
(D) Acute cystitis
(E) Furuncles

39. Climbing fibers arise from the

(A) inferior olivary nucleus
(B) motor cortex
(C) vestibular nuclei
(D) Ia muscle afferents
(E) spinocerebellar tract

40. Progressive degeneration of neurons rather than demyelination is associated with which of the following disorders?

(A) Progressive multifocal leukoencephalopathy
(B) Pick's disease
(C) Tabes dorsalis
(D) Subacute sclerosing panencephalitis
(E) Adrenoleukodystrophy

41. Which one of the following neurotransmitters, released from the neurons of the sympathetic nervous system, stimulates the cells of the adrenal medulla?

(A) Epinephrine
(B) Norepinephrine
(C) Dopamine
(D) Glutamate
(E) Acetylcholine (ACh)

42. This figure represents a skull film from a child with frontal headaches, growth retardation, and bitemporal hemianopia. The lesion that is producing these clinical findings most likely derives from

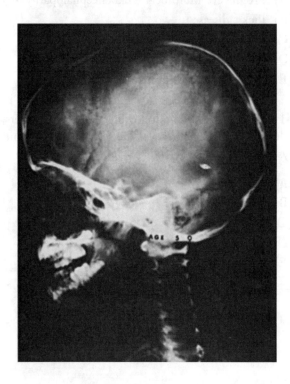

(A) ependymal cells
(B) oligodendrocytes
(C) astrocytes
(D) Rathke's pouch
(E) the arachnoid granulations

43. Within the motor circuits of the central nervous system, convergence of the cerebellum and basal ganglia occurs at which one of the following structures?

(A) Cerebral cortex
(B) Thalamus
(C) Brain stem
(D) Spinal cord
(E) Contralateral basal ganglia

44. Which of the following disorders is characterized by extrapyramidal signs and autonomic system failure with severe postural hypotension and urinary incontinence?

(A) Wilson disease
(B) Idiopathic Parkinson disease
(C) Wernicke encephalopathy
(D) Shy-Drager syndrome
(E) Huntington disease

45. Which one of the following autonomic functions would most likely be blocked by atropine?

(A) Inhibition of gastrointestinal motility
(B) Stimulation of the sweat glands
(C) Enhancement of cardiac muscle contractility
(D) Dilation of the bronchioles
(E) Dilation of the pupil of the eye

46. An alcoholic develops an acute onset of confusion, ataxia, and nystagmus after receiving an intravenous of 5% glucose and isotonic saline. The most likely cause of this patient's condition is

(A) excess copper levels
(B) thiamine deficiency
(C) direct toxic effect of alcohol on the brain
(D) niacin deficiency
(E) vitamin B_{12} deficiency

47. The lentiform nuclei consist of the

(A) subthalamic nucleus and substantia nigra
(B) caudate nucleus and putamen
(C) putamen and the globus pallidus
(D) caudate nucleus, putamen, and globus pallidus
(E) ventral anterior and ventral lateral thalami

48. Which of the following sites in the brain is a favored location for ischemic damage, rabies virus infestation, and toxic damage resulting from alcohol?

(A) Nucleus basalis of Meynert cell
(B) Purkinje cells of cerebellum
(C) Third, fifth, and sixth cortical layers of neurons in cerebral hemispheric grey matter
(D) Ammon's horn of the hippocampal gyrus
(E) Watershed zones

49. The use of a concave lens is likely to improve vision in which one of the following conditions?

(A) Presbyopia
(B) Hyperopia
(C) Myopia
(D) Astigmatism
(E) Emmetropia

50. A 65-year-old man has broad-based ataxia, loss of pain, and temperature sensation in the lower extremities with lightening pains. His pupils accommodate but do not constrict with direct light stimulation. The spinal fluid would be expected to exhibit

(A) encapsulated yeast cells
(B) a neutrophil-dominant cell count
(C) a positive VDRL (test for syphilis)
(D) *Toxoplasma* cysts
(E) malignant cells

51. Which of the following is true about infantile autism?

(A) More females are affected than males
(B) There is usually a family history of schizophrenia
(C) The onset is after 6 years of age
(D) There is no evidence of neurologic abnormality
(E) It is a pervasive development disorder of childhood

52. A 3-year-old girl presents with fever, nuchal rigidity, and seizure activity. The spinal fluid reveals neutrophils and decreased glucose. Which of the following Gram stain results would be most likely?

(A) Gram-negative diplococci
(B) Gram-positive diplococci
(C) Gram-negative rods
(D) Gram-positive rods
(E) Gram-positive cocci in chains

53. In response to light on the retina, the major difference between "on" and "off" centers is

(A) the receptor cells in "on" centers depolarize and the receptor cells in "off" centers hyperpolarize in response to light
(B) bipolar cells in "on" centers depolarize and the bipolar cells in "off" centers hyperpolarize in response to light
(C) ganglion cells in "on" centers hyperpolarize and ganglion cells in "off" centers depolarize in response to light
(D) rods stimulate "on" centers while cones stimulate "off" centers
(E) rods stimulate "off" centers while cones stimulate "on" centers

54. A patient with AIDS has multiple space-occupying lesions in the brain that are visible on a computerized tomography scan. The patient most likely has

(A) a primary malignant lymphoma arising in the brain
(B) multiple abscesses secondary to *Cryptococcus neuformans*
(C) cerebral toxoplasmosis
(D) metastatic Kaposi sarcoma to the brain
(E) cerebral involvement with cytomegalovirus

55. When a patient sticks his tongue out, it deviates to the left side. The muscles on the left side of the tongue demonstrate flaccid paralysis and are atrophied. The most likely cause for these symptoms would be

(A) a lesion involving corticobulbar fibers in the internal capsule on the right side
(B) injury to the right hypoglossal nerve
(C) a lesion involving corticobulbar fibers in the internal capsule on the left side
(D) a lesion involving the left hypoglossal nerve
(E) a lesion involving the left nucleus ambiguus

56. A patient with AIDS is developing blindness in both eyes. Cotton-wool exudates, necrotizing retinitis, and perivascular hemorrhages are noted on a funduscopic exam. The etiology of the complication is most closely related to

(A) oxygen-free radical damage
(B) optic neuritis secondary to demyelinating disease
(C) retinitis caused by cytomegalovirus
(D) cerebral edema secondary to ecephalitis
(E) retinitis caused by *Candida albicans*

57. The bone of the tarsus that articulates with the tibia is the

(A) talus
(B) calcaneus
(C) cuboid
(D) navicular
(E) cuneiform

58. A 25-year-old woman has fever, pain in her face when leaning forward, pain in her upper teeth, and a chronic cough. A physical exam reveals halitosis, a greenish-yellow postnasal discharge, boggy nasal mucosa bilaterally, and bilateral percussion tenderness over the zygomatic arch area. The patient most likely has

(A) orbital cellulitis
(B) acute ethmoiditis
(C) acute maxillary sinusitis
(D) erysipelas
(E) a frontal lobe abscess

59. After talking at length with a patient, it becomes apparent to the physician that the patient is using inappropriate words to refer to objects and circumstances in his daily life. However, he is fluent. Further evaluation shows foci of abnormal brain wave activity in the left temporal lobe over the supramarginal and angular gyri. What type of disorder does this patient have?

(A) Jacksonian aphasia
(B) Wernicke's aphasia
(C) Parkinsonian aphasia
(D) Alzheimer's aphasia
(E) Broca's aphasia

60. This figure represents a histologic section taken during an autopsy from necrotic areas in the frontal lobe of a 38-year-old man who had diabetic ketoacidosis. The findings are compatible with

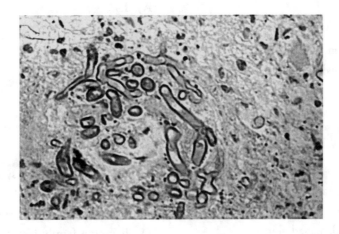

(A) aspergillosis

(B) mucormycosis

(C) candidiasis

(D) cryptococcosis

(E) histoplasmosis

61. Episodes of depression in major depressive disorder tend to

(A) increase in frequency with age

(B) decrease in length with age

(C) last for about 9 months when treated

(D) have a rapid onset

(E) occur an average of 2 to 3 times over a 20-year period

62. Which of the following auditory or visual disorders would more likely occur in children?

(A) Glaucoma

(B) Otosclerosis

(C) Strabismus

(D) Cataracts

(E) Macular degeneration

63. The neurons found in the nucleus ambiguus are similar in function to the neurons found in the

(A) dorsal root ganglia

(B) dorsal motor nucleus of the vagus

(C) sympathetic chain ganglia

(D) otic ganglia

(E) ninth lamina of the spinal cord

64. A 32-year-old woman has muscle weakness and drooping eyelids. An anterior mediastinal mass is noted on a chest radiograph. This patient most likely has

(A) antismooth muscle antibodies

(B) autoantibodies to acetylcholine receptors

(C) a sex-linked recessive disease

(D) lower motor neuron disease

(E) toxin blockade of acetylcholine release

65. The cerebellum is distinguished by

(A) six layers
(B) satellite cells
(C) pyramidal cells
(D) Purkinje cells between two evident layers
(E) a distinctly staining white matter with evident glial cells

66. What do melanomas, squamous cell carcinomas, and basal cell carcinomas have in common? They are all

(A) associated with metastasis
(B) only present on skin
(C) associated with sun-damaged skin
(D) nodular tumors
(E) pigmented tumors

67. A 43-year-old female patient, who has sustained a head injury in a fall, has significant problems with memory. Her brain injury is most likely to the

(A) temporal lobe
(B) frontal lobe
(C) parietal lobe
(D) occipital lobe
(E) cerebellum

68. Immunosuppression is most likely associated with which of the following skin cancers?

(A) Basal cell carcinoma
(B) Malignant melanoma
(C) Squamous cell carcinoma
(D) Merkel tumor
(E) Lymphoma cutis

69. The segmental innervation of the tibialis anterior muscle is from spinal cord segment

(A) L_2
(B) L_4
(C) S_1
(D) S_3
(E) S_5

70. A risk factor for the development of malignant melanoma is

(A) the basal cell nevus syndrome
(B) young age
(C) the dysplastic nevus syndrome
(D) having a family history of breast cancer
(E) African-American ethnicity

71. A 54-year-old patient who has suffered a stroke shows reduced motivation and depression. Damage to his brain is most likely to the

(A) frontal lobes
(B) temporal lobes
(C) parietal lobes
(D) occipital lobes
(E) basal ganglia

72. A 30-year-old woman with a long history of alcohol and barbiturate abuse presents with diffuse colicky abdominal pain. Examination reveals numerous surgical scars on the abdomen. There is no history of photosensitivity or increased facial hair. The patient's urine would probably

(A) contain an increase in uroporphyrin
(B) contain an increase in coproporphyrin
(C) be positive with a dipstick for blood
(D) have an excess amount of urobilinogen
(E) turn a port-wine color after sitting on a window sill for a short time

73. A physician asks his 63-year-old patient to turn her hand palm up, then palm down, rapidly, twenty times in a row. The patient pauses for approximately 1 minute and then begins the task slowly. As she concentrates on the task, her persistent (resting) tremor subsides. This suggests a deficit in the

(A) auditory cortex
(B) dentate nucleus of the cerebellum
(C) substantia nigra
(D) red nucleus
(E) post-central gyrus

74. A 45-year-old African-American man has widespread metastatic malignant melanoma. Which of the following areas would most likely have the primary lesion?

(A) Subungual area
(B) Anterior chest
(C) Face
(D) Anterior thigh
(E) Scalp

75. Inhalation of carbon dioxide is most useful in the diagnosis of

(A) major depression
(B) organic brain syndrome
(C) malingering
(D) panic disorder
(E) conversion disorder

76. The figure shows the lips of a 68-year-old wheat farmer. The patient does not drink, smoke, or chew tobacco. The lesion is most likely associated with

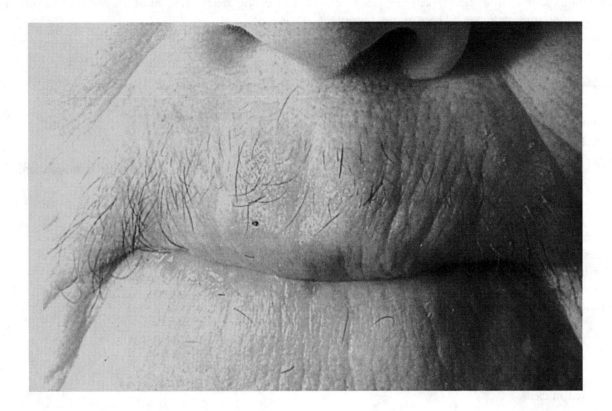

(A) hamartomatous polyps in the small intestine
(B) actinic damage
(C) autoimmune disease
(D) a viral infection
(E) inflammation of the minor salivary glands

77. The deep cerebellar nuclei have their effect on other brain centers by

(A) comparison of inhibitory effects by Purkinje cells and excitatory effects of afferent collateral axons
(B) summation of mossy fibers and climbing fibers synapsing on deep cerebellar nuclei
(C) temporal synaptic effects of granular and parallel fiber input
(D) excitatory Purkinje influences and inhibitory granule cell input
(E) inhibitory granule cell influences and inhibitory Purkinje cell input

78. The figure shows erythematous, pruritic lesions on a 38-year-old man. The pathogenesis of these lesions most closely resembles

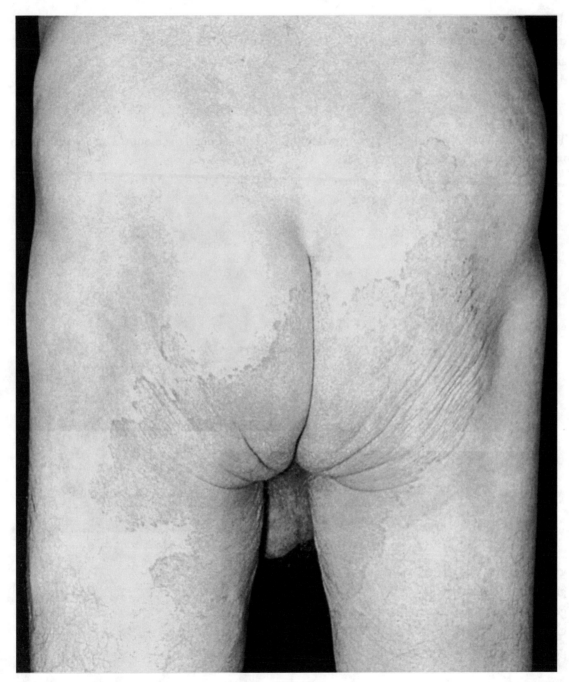

(A) a superficial dermatophyte infection
(B) contact dermatitis
(C) an autoimmune reaction
(D) a bacterial infection
(E) a type I hypersensitivity reaction

79. A 50-year-old California woman whose husband died two weeks previously in an automobile accident wakes up in Texas and does not know how she got there. This patient is probably suffering from

(A) depersonalization disorder
(B) dissociative identity disorder
(C) anterograde amnesia
(D) dissociative amnesia
(E) dissociative fugue

80. The figure shows a 2-year-old child with a yellow, crusty lesion around the mouth. The organism responsible for this lesion is probably a

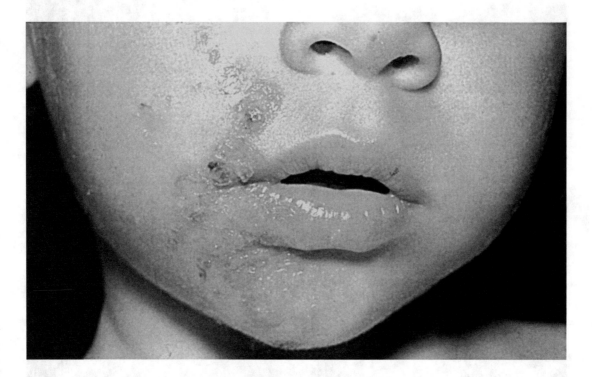

(A) gram-negative rod
(B) gram-positive diplococcus
(C) gram-positive streptococcus
(D) gram-negative diplococcus
(E) gram-positive filamentous bacteria

81. What changes will occur in both the near point of vision and the size of the pupil in the eye of a normal subject following the application of atropine to that eye?

(A) The near point and the size of the pupil will increase
(B) The near point and the size of the pupil will decrease
(C) The near point will decrease but the pupil size will increase
(D) The near point will increase but the pupil size will decrease
(E) The near point will not change but the pupil size will increase

82. The photograph shows nonpruritic, pearl-colored papules on the upper arm of a 25-year-old homosexual patient who has a positive antibody test for the human immunodeficiency virus. The pathogenesis of these lesions is most closely related to

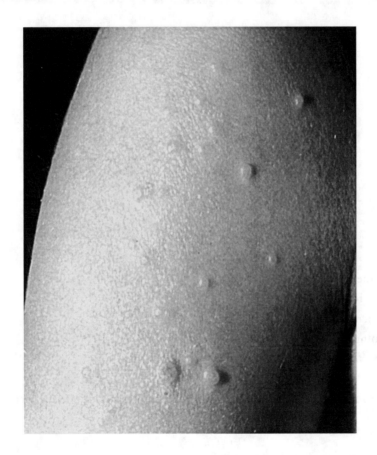

(A) a neoplasm
(B) a virus
(C) ultraviolet light
(D) a bacteria
(E) autoimmune disease

83. The substantia nigra participates in movement by its major connection to which one of the following brain nuclei?

(A) Subthalamic nucleus
(B) Globus pallidus
(C) Caudate nucleus
(D) Cerebral cortex
(E) Thalamus

84. The figure shows a Gram stain of one of three pustular lesions on the wrist of a febrile 25-year-old woman. Her right knee is swollen, feels hot, and contains an effusion with similar findings on Gram stain. The findings are most consistent with

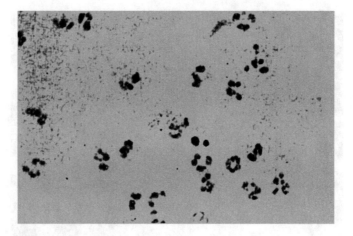

(A) multiple abscess due to *Staphylococcus aureus*
(B) a cellulitis due to group A streptococcus
(C) disseminated gonococcemia
(D) disseminated meningococcemia
(E) a cellulitis due to *Haemophilus influenzae*

85. Which one of the following is most likely to produce considerable drug dependence?

(A) Buprenorphine
(B) Pentazocine
(C) Meperidine
(D) Nalbuphine
(E) Butorphanol

86. The pathogenesis of this lesion on the left calf of a 35-year-old man who also has non-tender inguinal adenopathy on the ipsilateral side is most closely associated with

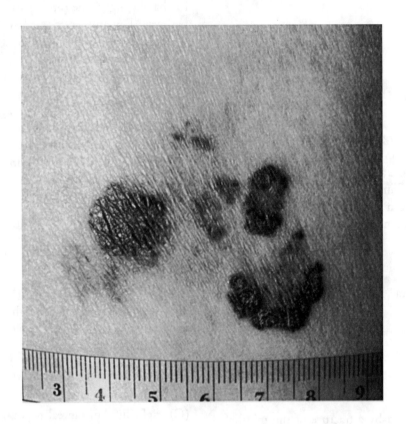

(A) squamous epithelium
(B) fibroblasts
(C) endothelial cells
(D) melanocytes
(E) adnexal structures

87. At the wrist, the ulnar pulse is palpable

(A) immediately medial to the tendon of the flexor carpi ulnaris
(B) immediately lateral to the tendon of the flexor carpi ulnaris
(C) immediately lateral to the tendon of the flexor digitorum superficialis
(D) immediately medial to the tendon of the palmaris longus
(E) immediately lateral to the tendon of the palmaris longus

88. Which one of the following effects is common to both isoproterenol and atropine?

(A) Increased ventricular contractility
(B) Decreased diastolic blood pressure
(C) Decreased heart rate
(D) Bronchodilation
(E) Relaxation of the detrusor muscle

89. At the wrist joint, a bone that articulates with the radius is the

(A) pisiform
(B) hamate
(C) capitate
(D) lunate
(E) trapezium

90. A patient undergoes transection of the spinal cord. The patient develops hypertonus and hyper-reflexia distal to the transection that is attributed, in part, to the loss of inhibitory influence exerted by descending tracts from the brain. Axons that form the descending tracts are most likely to originate from the

(A) cerebellum
(B) neostriatum
(C) substantia nigra
(D) globus pallidus
(E) reticular formation

91. Which of the following is not true of a lesion of the radial nerve?

(A) it may be caused by a fracture of the midshaft of the humerus
(B) it may be caused by a dislocation of the head of the humerus
(C) it may be caused by a deep laceration on the anteromedial surface of the arm overlying the medial epicondyle of the humerus
(D) it may cause paralysis of the extensor digitorum communis muscle
(E) it may cause anesthesia on the dorsal surface of the proximal phalanx of the second digit

92. Dopaminergic neurons from the substantia nigra influence two efferent pathways of the neostriatum of the basal ganglia: the direct pathway and the indirect pathway. Dopaminergic regulation of both pathways is necessary for appropriate feedback to the motor areas of the cerebral cortex and normal motor function. Dopamine excites the direct pathway via D_1 receptors and inhibits the indirect pathway via D_2 receptors. Which one of the following agents (administered orally) would be most likely to restore normal motor function in a patient with Parkinson's disease who has sustained loss of most of the dopaminergic neurons?

(A) The dopamine precursor L-dopa
(B) A D_2 antagonist
(C) A D_1 agonist
(D) A combination D_1 agonist/D_2 antagonist
(E) Dopamine

93. While standing on the right foot, the left side of your patient's hip drops. The nerve that is most likely lesioned is the

(A) right superior gluteal nerve
(B) left superior gluteal nerve
(C) right inferior gluteal nerve
(D) left inferior gluteal nerve
(E) left obturator nerve

94. Damage to the optic tract (but not the optic nerve) on the right side of the brain would interfere with nerve impulses from the

(A) nasal portion of the retina of the right eye and the temporal portion of the retina of the left eye
(B) nasal portion of the retina of the right eye and the temporal portion of the retina of the right eye
(C) temporal portion of the retina of the right eye and the nasal portion of the retina of the left eye
(D) temporal portion of the retina of the right eye and the temporal portion of the retina of the left eye
(E) nasal portion of the retina of the right eye and the nasal portion of the retina of the left eye

95. The ligament that is most effective in resisting extension of the hip joint is the

(A) pubofemoral ligament
(B) iliofemoral ligament
(C) ligament of the head of the femur
(D) sacrospinous ligament
(E) sacrotuberous ligament

96. Which one of the following statements is true of both aspirin and acetaminophen?

(A) Both exert antiinflammatory activity in patients with rheumatoid arthritis
(B) Both inhibit platelet aggregation
(C) Both lower elevated body temperature
(D) Both may cause hepatic necrosis after an overdose
(E) Both have been associated with Reye's syndrome

97. The medial meniscus of the knee is attached to the

(A) lateral meniscus of the knee
(B) anterior cruciate ligament of the knee
(C) posterior cruciate ligament of the knee
(D) medial collateral ligament of the knee
(E) popliteus tendon

98. Which of the following skin or hair disorders would most likely have a negative Wood's lamp evaluation?

(A) Tinea versicolor
(B) Pityriasis rosea
(C) Erythrasma
(D) Tinea capitis caused by *Microsporum canis*
(E) Tinea capitis caused by *Microsporum audouinii*

99. The posterior cruciate ligament of the knee

(A) is injured more frequently than the anterior cruciate ligament of the knee
(B) is within the synovial cavity of the knee
(C) resists anterior displacement of the femur
(D) resists anterior displacement of the tibia
(E) attaches to the lateral femoral condyle

100. Infections associated with prosthetic heart valves, intravenous catheters, and intracranial shunts characterize which of the following bacterial pathogens?

(A) *Escherichia coli*
(B) *Streptococcus pyogenes*
(C) *Pseudomonas aeruginosa*
(D) *Staphylococcus epidermidis*
(E) *Actinomyces israelii*

101. In the region of the knee, popliteus muscle

(A) assists in extension of the knee
(B) medially rotates the femur upon the tibia
(C) is part of the quadriceps femoris muscle
(D) lies between the lateral collateral ligament and the lateral meniscus
(E) is innervated by the obturator nerve

102. In a patient with cyanotic congenital heart disease and focal neurologic deficits, a contrast-enhanced computerized tomography scan of the brain is reported to have multiple ring-enhancing lesions with associated edema. In the unlikely situation that a spinal tap could be done safely in this patient, the spinal fluid would be expected to have a

(A) normal glucose
(B) normal protein
(C) normal cell count
(D) positive Gram stain
(E) low chloride

DIRECTIONS:

Each of the numbered items or incomplete statements in this section is negatively phrased, as indicated by a capitalized word such as NOT, LEAST, or EXCEPT. Select the ONE lettered answer or completion that is BEST in each case.

103. An injury to the median nerve proximal to the elbow may result in all of the following findings EXCEPT

(A) loss of pronation of the forearm
(B) loss of flexion of the thumb
(C) loss of flexion of the forearm at the elbow
(D) loss of opposition of the thumb
(E) loss of sensation of the lateral portion of the palm

104. Which of the following is LEAST likely to contribute to weakening of the normal host defenses against pathogens in the gastrointestinal tract?

(A) Achlorhydria
(B) Vegan diet
(C) Antibiotics
(D) Lack of peristalsis
(E) Immunoglobulin A deficiency

105. All of the following mechanisms may contribute to the beneficial effects of gold compounds in patients with rheumatoid arthritis EXCEPT

(A) inhibition of the release of mediators of inflammation
(B) inhibition of cyclooxygenase
(C) inhibition of lysosomal activity
(D) suppression of macrophage activity
(E) suppression of leukocyte phagocytosis

106. Central nervous system disease in AIDS is clinically similar to all of the following disorders EXCEPT

(A) dementia
(B) Guillain-Barré syndrome
(C) subacute combined degeneration
(D) aseptic meningitis
(E) glioblastoma multiforme

107. A female patient begins to experience episodes of sweating, chest pain, and feelings that she is about to die. Physical examination is normal. Which of the following is LEAST likely to be true about this patient?

(A) Her attacks commonly occur twice per week
(B) Her attacks commonly last 2 to 3 days
(C) Her attacks can be precipitated by carbon dioxide inhalation
(D) She is 20 to 30 years of age
(E) She has mitral valve prolapse

108. A 65-year-old man is noted to have a progressive loss of recent memory and an onset of increased agitation and depression. There are no focal neurologic signs, and he is not on any medications. Which of the following histologic abnormalities in the central nervous system would be least expected of this patient?

(A) Neurofibrillary tangles
(B) Senile plaques
(C) Decreased number of neurons in the locus ceruleus
(D) Decreased number of neurons in the nucleus basalis of the Meynert cell
(E) Granulovacuolar degeneration

109. The slow-acting antirheumatic drugs include all of the following EXCEPT

(A) auranofin
(B) penicillamine
(C) levamisole
(D) hydroxychloroquine
(E) prednisone

110. Which of the following associations is NOT correct?

(A) Dandy-Walker syndrome—noncommunicating hydrocephalus and failure of development of the cerebellar vermis

(B) Anencephaly—polyhydramnios and increased maternal α-fetoprotein

(C) Meningocele—protrusion of meninges through a vertebral arch defect

(D) Sturge-Weber syndrome—cerebellar hemangioblastoma and secondary polycythemia

(E) Arnold-Chiari malformation—elongation of the medulla oblongata and cerebellar tonsils through the foramen magnum, hydrocephalus, and meningomyelocele

111. Muscles innervated by the tibial nerve include all of the following EXCEPT

(A) semimembranosus

(B) semitendinosus

(C) popliteus

(D) long head of the biceps femoris

(E) short head of the biceps femoris

112. How does pityriasis rosea differ from tinea versicolor? Pityriasis rosea

(A) is diagnosed with a KOH preparation of skin scrapings

(B) first presents with a herald patch

(C) is caused by *Malassezia furfur*

(D) has areas of hypo- and hyperpigmentation

(E) is treated with topical antifungal agents

113. All of the following statements are correct concerning aspirin toxicity EXCEPT

(A) zero-order elimination of aspirin after large doses may contribute to aspirin toxicity

(B) tinnitus and vertigo are early signs of aspirin toxicity and may occur in elderly patients taking aspirin for arthritis

(C) patients who are allergic to aspirin may develop nasal polyps, bronchoconstriction, and shock

(D) aspirin may increase bleeding in patients with hemophilia

(E) metabolic acidosis is the earliest acid–base disturbance observed in patients with aspirin overdose

114. Which of the following skin carcinomas is least likely to metastasize?

(A) Squamous cell carcinoma

(B) Basal cell carcinoma

(C) Nodular melanoma

(D) Acral lentiginous melanoma

(E) Superficial spreading malignant melanoma

115. All of the following are true about the etiology of alcoholism EXCEPT

(A) it is more common in the children of alcoholics than in the children of nonalcoholics

(B) it has a higher concordance rate in monozygotic than in dizygotic twins

(C) female children are more at risk than male children

(D) genetic factors are involved in its development

(E) environmental factors are involved in its development

116. Which of the following statements about estrogen supplementation after menopause is NOT correct?

(A) Decreases the risk for death due to coronary artery disease
(B) Decreases the risk for developing osteoporosis-related fractures
(C) Decreases vasomotor symptoms
(D) Decreases urinary urgency, incontinence, and frequency
(E) Adding progestin protects against developing endometrial and breast carcinoma

117. Autonomic ganglia contain all of the following EXCEPT

(A) satellite cells
(B) Schwann cells
(C) unipolar neurons
(D) lipofuscin pigment
(E) synaptic connections

118. A teenager who has abused drugs in the past is arrested for attacking another teenager. Which of the following drugs is the LEAST likely to have just been taken?

(A) Cocaine
(B) Heroin
(C) Amphetamines
(D) PCP
(E) Marijuana

119. All of the following tendons contribute to the extensor expansion of the third digit EXCEPT

(A) extensor digitorum communis
(B) second lumbrical
(C) second dorsal interosseous
(D) second palmar interosseous
(E) third dorsal interosseous

120. All of the following are true about the epidemiology of alcoholism EXCEPT

(A) it is more common in Asian Americans than in European Americans
(B) of the children of alcoholics, sons are more vulnerable than daughters
(C) life expectancy is reduced by about 10 years
(D) it is more common in the Northeastern states

121. The boundaries of the popliteal fossa include all of the following EXCEPT

(A) semimembranosus
(B) soleus
(C) biceps femoris
(D) lateral head of the gastrocnemius
(E) medial head of the gastrocnemius

122. All of the following structures contain neuronal cell bodies or axons that participate in the fine motor movements of the fingers EXCEPT the

(A) crus cerebri
(B) lateral hemisphere of the cerebellum
(C) cervical enlargement of the spinal cord
(D) ventral anterior and ventral lateral thalamic nuclei
(E) genu of the internal capsule

123. All of the following movements can be caused by contraction of the flexor digitorum superficialis EXCEPT

(A) flexion of the distal interphalangeal joint
(B) flexion of the proximal interphalangeal joint
(C) flexion of the metacarpophalangeal joint
(D) flexion of the midcarpal joint
(E) flexion of the radiocarapal joint

124. All of the following may contribute to the analgesic effect of morphine EXCEPT

(A) activation of brain stem neurons that project to the spinal cord and release inhibitory enkephalins
(B) activation of the spinal cord opioid receptors that mediate inhibition of ascending pain transmission
(C) induction of euphoria and sedation
(D) interruption of pain transmission by primary afferent neurons projecting from peripheral tissues to the spinal cord
(E) inhibition of substance P release from dorsal horn neurons in the spinal cord

125. Muscles that can cause external rotation of the hip include all of the following EXCEPT

(A) sartorius
(B) obturator internus
(C) obturator externus
(D) gluteus maximus
(E) gluteus minimus

126. All of the following are characteristic signs of acute opiate withdrawal EXCEPT

(A) hypothermia
(B) piloerection
(C) mydriasis
(D) yawning
(E) nausea and diarrhea

127. Muscles that can extend the hip joint include all of the following EXCEPT

(A) semimembranosus
(B) semitendinosus
(C) gluteus maximus
(D) long head of the biceps femoris
(E) short head of the biceps femoris

128. All of the following agents can counteract opiate withdrawal syndrome in opiate addicts EXCEPT

(A) clonidine
(B) methadone
(C) nalbuphine
(D) morphine
(E) heroin

129. Parasympathetic ganglia in the head include all of the following EXCEPT

(A) otic
(B) ciliary
(C) trigeminal
(D) submandibular
(E) pterygopalatine

130. Administration of atropine may cause all of the following effects EXCEPT

(A) contraction of the lower esophageal sphincter
(B) bronchodilation
(C) decreased intestinal motility
(D) relaxation of the ciliary muscle
(E) relaxation of the detrusor muscle

131. Which one of the following statements is NOT true concerning the crystalline lens?

(A) Its maximum degree of curvature increases with age
(B) It is suspended by zonule fibers attached to the ciliary body
(C) Contraction of the ciliary muscles increases its refractory power
(D) It is avascular
(E) It develops some degree of opacity in most people older than 65 years of age

132. All of the following statements regarding activity at the neuromuscular junction are true EXCEPT

(A) action potentials on the the alpha motor neuron release acetylcholine (ACh) from the axon terminal
(B) ACh stimulates nicotinic cholinergic receptors on the muscle endplate
(C) cholinergic receptors on the muscle endplate are cation channels
(D) alpha motor neurons excite, and Renshaw cells inhibit, the muscle endplate
(E) each action potential produces a contraction of the muscle fiber

133. Muscles innervated by the deep peroneal nerve include all of the following EXCEPT

(A) tibialis anterior
(B) peroneus longus
(C) peroneus tertius
(D) extensor hallucis longus
(E) extensor digitorum longus

134. Which of the following individuals is the LEAST likely to be at great risk for contracting hepatitis B (HBV)?

(A) Prostitute
(B) Blood bank technologist
(C) Homosexual with multiple partners
(D) Down syndrome patient in a long-term care facility
(E) Child living with a mother who has chronic hepatitis B and who is negative for both DNA and E antigen

DIRECTIONS:

Each set of matching questions in this section consists of a list of four to twenty-six lettered options (some of which may be in figures) followed by several numbered items. For each numbered item, select the ONE lettered option that is most closely associated with it. To avoid spending too much time on matching sets with a large number of options, it is generally advisable to begin each set by reading the list of options. Then for each item in the set, try to generate the correct answer and locate it in the option list, rather than evaluating each option individually. Each lettered option may be selected once, more than once, or not at all.

Questions 135-138

Each of the following drugs affects the intraocular pressure. For each mechanism of action, select the appropriate drug.

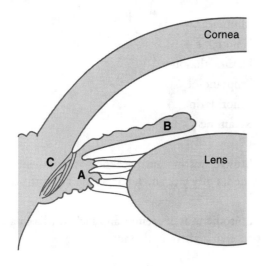

(A) Epinephrine
(B) Acetazolamide
(C) Pilocarpine
(D) Atropine
(E) Timolol

135. Increases the intraocular pressure by relaxing muscle B

136. Decreases the intraocular pressure by contracting muscle C

137. Decreases the intraocular pressure by blocking receptors at site A

138. Decreases the intraocular pressure by inhibiting bicarbonate formation at site A

Questions 139-143

Match the deficit with the most closely associated brain region.

(A) Nondominant parietal lobe
(B) Dominant occipital lobe
(C) Dominant temporal lobe
(D) Dominant frontal lobe
(E) Dominant parietal lobe

139. A 55-year-old male stroke patient, who is a college graduate, cannot add the numbers 5, 2, and 3.

140. A 54-year-old female patient with a head injury can follow spoken instructions but is unable to express herself verbally.

141. A 62-year-old male patient who was involved in a serious automobile accident seems alert and oriented but does not seem to understand what is being said to him.

142. A 48-year-old stroke patient is unable to copy completely a simple drawing of a clock face.

143. A 45-year-old male patient who suffered a stroke can write a sentence that is dictated to him but he is unable to read the sentence aloud.

Questions 144-147

For each mechanism of action, select the appropriate drug.

(A) Sulfinpyrazone
(B) Acetaminophen
(C) Allopurinol
(D) Colchicine
(E) Indomethacin

144. Increases uric acid excretion by blocking its reabsorption from renal tubules

145. Potent inhibitor of prostaglandin synthesis

146. Inhibits xanthine oxidase and the synthesis of uric acid from hypoxanthine

147. Inhibits leukocyte migration and phagocytosis secondary to inhibition of tubulin polymerization

Questions 148-152

Match the patient description with the most closely associated personality disorder.

(A) Schizoid
(B) Schizotypal
(C) Paranoid
(D) Antisocial
(E) Avoidant

148. A 35-year-old female patient dresses strangely, behaves oddly, and has peculiar ideas.

149. A 54-year-old computer programmer is distant and isolated, prefers to work at home alone, and has shown little interest in others throughout life.

150. A 50-year-old male patient is hostile and angry, insists that it is your fault that he became ill, and threatens to file a malpractice suit against you.

151. A 32-year-old female patient tells you that, though she would like to have friends, she feels very self-conscious and shy and is afraid to make social contact with others.

152. A 44-year-old male patient brags to you that he just bought a car with someone else's credit card and that he has done this before.

Questions 153-156

For each clinical scenario, select the drug most likely to cause it.

(A) Albuterol
(B) Halothane
(C) Dexamethasone
(D) Propranolol
(E) Thioridazine
(F) Ketamine

153. Muscle wasting and weakness in a patient with a rounded, puffy face and fat deposition over the trunk

154. Episodic muscle tremor and tachycardia in a patient receiving chronic therapy

155. Muscle rigidity accompanied by fever, involuntary movements, and cardiovascular instability in a patient receiving chronic therapy

156. Muscle rigidity with tachycardia, hypertension, and hyperthermia in a surgical patient

Questions 157-158

For each drug, identify the mechanism of action.

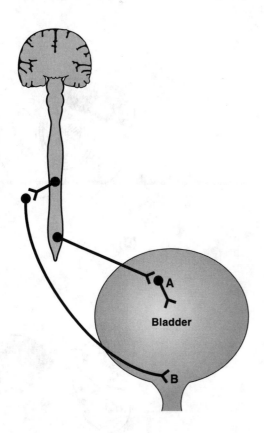

(A) Activates muscarinic receptors at site A
(B) Activates muscarinic receptors at site B
(C) Blocks α_1 receptors at site A
(D) Blocks α_1 receptors at site B
(E) Blocks α_2 receptors at site B

157. Terazosin (facilitates bladder emptying)

158. Bethanechol (counteracts postoperative urinary retention)

Questions 159-162

For each drug, identify its site of action on the diagram below.

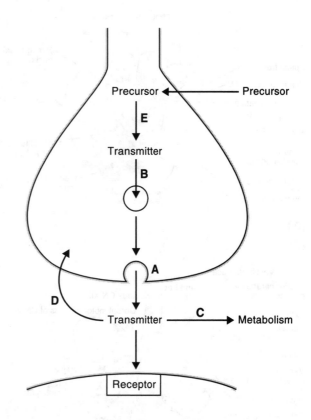

159. Cocaine

160. Guanethidine

161. Methyltyrosine

162. Reserpine

Questions 163-177

Use the figures showing brain-stem lesions to answer the following questions.

(A)

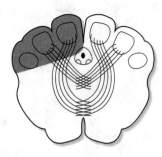

(B)

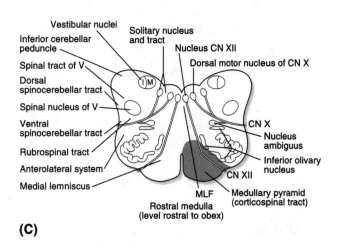

(C)

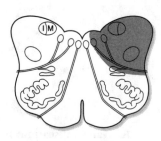

(D)

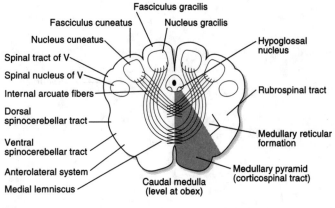

(E)

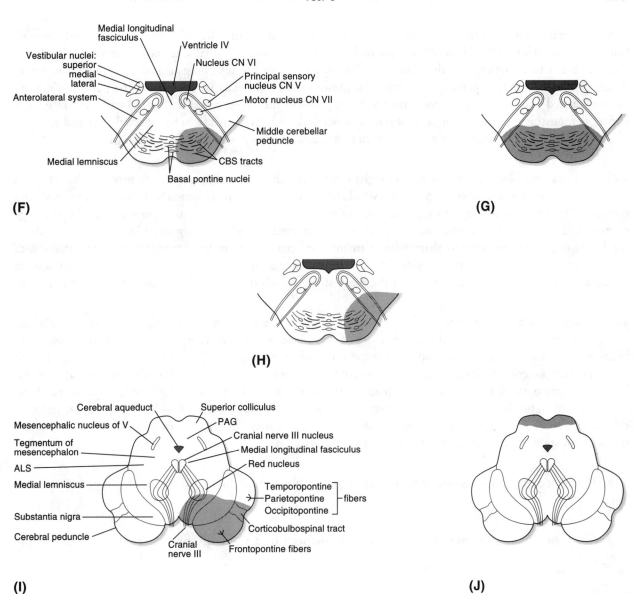

(F)

Medial longitudinal
fasciculus
Ventricle IV
Nucleus CN VI
Vestibular nuclei:
superior
medial
lateral
Principal sensory
nucleus CN V
Anterolateral system
Motor nucleus CN VII
Middle cerebellar
peduncle
Medial lemniscus
CBS tracts
Basal pontine nuclei

(G)

(H)

(I)

Cerebral aqueduct
Superior colliculus
Mesencephalic nucleus of V
PAG
Tegmentum of
mesencephalon
Cranial nerve III nucleus
Medial longitudinal fasciculus
ALS
Red nucleus
Medial lemniscus
Temporopontine
Parietopontine   fibers
Occipitopontine
Substantia nigra
Cerebral peduncle
Corticobulbospinal tract
Cranial
nerve III
Frontopontine fibers

(J)

163. Which figure shows an infarction produced by cerebrovascular disease that has affected the basilar artery?

164. A 42-year-old athletic man noticed a pain behind his ear after playing a vigorous squash match. Over the next several days, certain neurologic symptoms began to appear. Eventually, the pain and the symptoms led him to a physician. The history and physical examination included the following findings: an alert athletic man with normal reflexes, and good control and strength in muscles of extremities; however, his gait was distinctively ataxic on the right. Sensory testing of the body and face showed diminished response to sharp touch and temperature on the left side of the body and numbness with some paresthesia of the face on the right side. In addition, signs of a Horner's syndrome were noted on the right side. Questioning of the patient determined that episodes of dizziness and nausea had occurred over the past several days. Computed tomography scan of the cranial contents was ordered and an infarction of the brain stem was found. Which figure shows a similar situation?

165. A 56-year-old woman with hypertension was swimming with friends when discomfort in her head preceded brief loss of consciousness. When revived, she had blurred vision and was unable to move one side of her body. She was taken to an emergency department where on admission the following neurologic profile was noted: patient was alert; diplopia; paralysis of extraocular muscles with right external strabismus; the pupil of the right eye was dilated and sluggish-to-unresponsive to light; ptosis of the upper eyelid on the right; the left face, arm, and leg demonstrated signs of an upper motor neuron paralysis. Which figure might be expected on the admission's files as the most likely location of a cerebrovascular accident (CVA) producing these findings?

166. A 14-year-old boy was seen by a neurologist several months after a diving accident in which he fractured cervical vertebrae. The orthopedic procedures stabilized the patient, and most neural function had returned with therapy. The rehabilitation report suggested that the residual neurologic deficits were permanent. The discharge neurological examination showed loss of two-point discrimination and vibratory sensation on the left side of the body, decreased sensation to sharp stimuli in the orofacial region on the left side, and slight ataxia with certain motor activity, also on the left side. The neurologist suggested that compression injury from the fractured vertebrae permanently destroyed an area of the brain stem. Which one of the figures shows a similar situation?

167. A patient has had continuing difficulty using his hands. Subsequent visits to the physician's office indicated the following: an alert 35-year-old man with loss of two-point touch, vibration, and conscious proprioception bilaterally and involving the upper and lower extremities. The patient noted that his job as an assembler of small electronic components had become virtually impossible. A complete neurologic workup showed decreased motor control and strength of the left limbs compared with the right. There was a Babinski reflex, spastic paralysis, difficulty with rapid independent finger movement, and ankle clonus on the left side. The physician referred this patient to a neurologist due to suspicion of either a demyelinizaton problem or an ischemia in the region of the brain stem. Which of the figures shows a similar situation?

168. Which one of the figures shows an infarction of the brain stem due to occlusion of the posterior spinal artery?

169. Which figure shows a lesion site that could be produced by a CVA affecting the right posterior cerebral artery?

170. A 29-year-old woman had an unremarkable pregnancy with her first child. Delivery, however, was long and strenuous. Immediately after delivery, the mother felt tired and very weak, which was thought to be normal for her delivery. Within the next several hours, neurologic problems began to present in the mother, especially when she tried to move from her bed and use her upper limbs. Within 12 hours the woman was evaluated by an attending neurologist and found to have the following deficits: she was quadriplegic, could not speak, had difficulty breathing that required intubation, could not abduct either eye but could look upward and blink on command, and she was alert. By her eye movements, the neurologist recognized that she was fully conscious of the events occurring around her. Which brain-stem lesion would most likely produce this clinical picture?

171. For several months a patient has complained to his family physician of headache and sensations of pressure behind his eyes. The patient and the doctor decided on a thorough neurologic workup. The results were unremarkable except for an apparent paralysis of upward gaze and bilateral pupils that were not reacting normally to light stimuli. A computed tomography study was ordered. The lateral ventricles and the third ventricle were enlarged, and calcification in the region of the pineal gland led to the suspicion of a pinealoma. Which figure most likely explains the neurologic findings as well as the accompanying hydrocephalus in this case?

172. A radiologist's report identifies a patient's neurologic deficits as resulting from occlusion of the posterior inferior cerebellar artery (PICA). Which figure shows the affected area and the distribution of the vessel?

173. Which figure shows the brain-stem level and site of a lesion of a patient who is presenting with signs and symptoms best described as Weber's syndrome?

174. A patient presents with a right-sided paralysis of the tongue. When the patient is asked to stick out his tongue, the tip of the tongue deviates toward the right side. Paralysis of the left side of the body is characterized as weakness and loss of the fine motor control of the left upper extremity. In addition, a Babinski reflex and ankle clonus were elicited. Rigidity to passive movement at the hip and knee on the left was also present. There was sensory loss of two-point touch, vibration on the left. The right side was normal. All other cranial nerve function was normal. Right-sided motor activity was within normal range; and there was no loss of pain and temperature sensation on either side. The initial diagnosis was a lesion in the brain stem and affecting structures. Which figure best illustrates the initial diagnosis?

175. An 85-year-old hypertensive woman is brought to the emergency department after a fall. She describes a progressive weakness in her lower limbs and hands. Neurologic testing shows cranial nerve function normal for a person this age and no major sensory deficits. Bilateral triceps, biceps, wrist, patellar, and Achilles tendon reflexes are brisk to hyperreflexive. A Babinski reflex is present on the left, and present but less obvious on the right. All extremities are weak, and independent finger and toe movement are greatly diminished. The grip in both hands is well below normal strength for a person this age. The patient is generally responsive, alert, and coherent but concerned about what has been happening. Which figure resembles the site and level of the lesion?

176. A 49-year-old construction worker has been hit on the head with a steel beam. He is unconscious when brought to the emergency department, but soon becomes responsive and is aware of the circumstances of his accident. Computed tomography scan shows blood in the posterior cranial fossa. Thorough neurologic testing is done to establish whether the blood was contained or other neurologic structures are in jeopardy. He has left-sided weakness in upper and lower limbs, hyperreflexias at the wrist and elbow, and a Babinski reflex. He also has decreased response to sharp stimuli on the left as compared with the right side. His right eye has a medial strabismus, and he complains of double vision. Paralysis of lateral rectus muscle on the right is found during cardinal eye movement testing. There is a slight right facial asymmetry and puffing outward of the cheek when he speaks. Testing shows that the entire right side of the patient's face is paralyzed and there is no corneal reflex on the right side. Other sensory testing is normal, and the remainder of the cranial nerve testing is within normal range bilaterally. Which figure shows the most likely brain-stem level and site of this infarct or compression?

177. Which figure shows an infarction produced by hemorrhage of penetrating branches of the anterior spinal artery?

Questions 178-180

For each diagram of the eye, compare the illustration with the pretreatment control illustration and select the drug that would produce the depicted ocular effects.

Pretreatment control

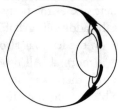

180.

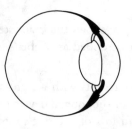

(A) Isoproterenol
(B) Phenylephrine
(C) Propranolol
(D) Atropine
(E) Pilocarpine

178.

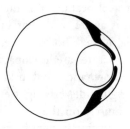

179.

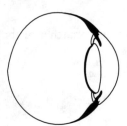

ANSWER KEY

1. B	31. B	61. A	91. C	121. B	151. E
2. B	32. A	62. C	92. A	122. E	152. D
3. D	33. A	63. E	93. A	123. A	153. C
4. C	34. A	64. B	94. C	124. D	154. A
5. C	35. B	65. D	95. B	125. E	155. E
6. C	36. B	66. C	96. C	126. A	156. B
7. C	37. D	67. A	97. D	127. E	157. D
8. D	38. D	68. C	98. B	128. C	158. A
9. C	39. A	69. B	99. C	129. C	159. D
10. C	40. B	70. C	100. D	130. A	160. A
11. A	41. E	71. A	101. D	131. A	161. E
12. C	42. D	72. E	102. A	132. D	162. B
13. D	43. B	73. C	103. C	133. B	163. G
14. A	44. D	74. A	104. B	134. E	164. D
15. B	45. B	75. D	105. B	135. D	165. I
16. D	46. B	76. B	106. E	136. C	166. B
17. B	47. C	77. A	107. B	137. E	167. A
18. C	48. B	78. A	108. C	138. B	168. B
19. E	49. C	79. E	109. E	139. E	169. I
20. B	50. C	80. C	110. D	140. D	170. G
21. B	51. E	81. A	111. E	141. C	171. J
22. D	52. C	82. B	112. B	142. A	172. D
23. A	53. B	83. C	113. E	143. B	173. I
24. A	54. C	84. C	114. B	144. A	174. C
25. B	55. D	85. C	115. C	145. E	175. E
26. E	56. C	86. D	116. E	146. C	176. H
27. D	57. A	87. B	117. C	147. D	177. A
28. E	58. C	88. D	118. B	148. B	178. E
29. C	59. B	89. D	119. D	149. A	179. D
30. C	60. B	90. E	120. A	150. C	180. B

ANSWERS AND EXPLANATIONS

1. The answer is B. *(Anatomy)*
The adductor hiatus is a gap in the inferior portion of the adductor magnus tendon. The femoral artery and femoral vein pass through the adductor canal and then through the hiatus to become continuous with the popliteal artery and vein. Branches of the profunda femoral artery pass through the adductor magnus but not through the adductor hiatus to get from the anterior to the posterior compartment of the thigh. The posterior tibial artery is a branch of the popliteal artery. The saphenous nerve, a branch of the femoral nerve, passes through the adductor canal but does not pass through the adductor hiatus.

2. The answer is B. *(Pathology)*
The figure reveals a round, discolored nodule in the cerebral hemispheres that has shifted the midline structures from the left to the right. The left hemisphere is disproportionately enlarged becuase of the expanding mass and associated edema. Although this is a solitary lesion, the long history of smoking favors the nodule representing metastatic disease from the lung to the brain with cerebral edema leading to uncal herniation. Uncal herniation is characterized by compression of the oculomotor nerve, which produces lid lag, ophthalmoplegia, and mydriasis. Metastasis is the most common cancer in the brain, with the majority coming from the lung in men (small cell cancers in particular) and the breast in women. Malignant melanomas, however, are the most likely of all cancers to metastasize to the brain (more than 50%), though not the overall most common metastasis to the brain. Computerized tomography with contrast and magnetic resonance imaging are the procedures of choice to document metastasis. Any adult patient with new onset seizure activity is suspect for a brain tumor.

A glioblastoma multiforme is the most common primary brain tumor in adults. This tumor commonly occurs in the frontal lobes and characteristically crosses over to the other hemisphere via the corpus callosum. Based on the history of smoking in this patient and the likelihood of uncal rather than cerebellar tonsil herniation into the foreman magnum, metastasis is a better answer. A hemorrhagic infarction of the brain is most commonly associated with embolisms, which are located in the distribution of the middle cerebral artery and are at the periphery of the cerebral cortex. A cerebral abscess from a primary site in the lungs is unlikely because the lesion in the brain is not cystic. A low-grade astrocytoma is unlikely because it is not well circumscribed as with the lesion in this patient.

3. The answer is D. *(Microbiology)*
Conjunctivitis and pneumonia in a newborn best characterize infection caused by *Chlamydia trachomatis*. Chlamydia are obligate intracellular organisms that are passively taken up into phagocytic vacuoles of host cells, where they proliferate and create inclusions (elementary bodies) within the cells that are helpful in their identification on conjunctival scrapings. These organisms are able to inhibit the fusion of lysosomes in phagocytic cells and are protected from attack by oxygen-dependent and independent phagocytic systems. The genus consists of three species that are pathogenic, mainly *Chlamydia psittaci* (ornithosis), *Chlamydia trachomatis*, and *Chlamydia pneumoniae* (TWAR). Serologic tests, direct immunofluorescent tests, and culture techniques are available to secure a diagnosis.

Chlamydia trachomatis produces trachoma, inclusion conjunctivitis, ophthalmia neonatorum, newborn pneumonia, lymphogranuloma venereum, and genitourinary disease. This organism is the most common cause of ophthalmia neonatorum, which occurs in 30%–40% of newborns who pass through a birth canal infected with *Chlamydia*. Topical erythromycin ophthalmic solutions instead of silver nitrate has significantly reduced the incidence of this disease. Approximately one third of all pneumonias that occur in infants between ages 2–6 months are caused by *Chlamydia trachomatis*. Patients present with cough, tachypnea, bilateral inspiratory crackles, scattered expiratory wheezes, hyperinflation, and conjunctivitis (50%). There is a conspicuous absence of fever. The chest radiograph shows hyperinflation and a diffuse interstitial pattern with patchy infiltrates. Peripheral blood eosinophilia is a characteristic laboratory finding. Erythromycin is thought to shorten the clinical illness.

4. The answer is C. *(Pathology)*
Hypersensitive reactions to yeasts may occur in patients who have received recombinant vaccines that use synthetic hepatitis B surface antigen produced in yeast by plasmid gene insertion. Influenza, yellow fever, measles, and mumps are egg-based vaccines and could produce anaphylactic reactions in those patients who are allergic to eggs. Pregnancy or lactation pose no threat for adverse reactions other than the usual local tenderness at the site of injection.

5. The answer is C. *(Microbiology)*
Greenish discoloration of the sputum in a febrile 4-year-old with cystic fibrosis is most likely caused by *Pseudomonas aeruginosa. Pseudomonas* species are motile, thin gram-negative rods that are pigment producers (pyocyanin) and secrete endotoxins and exotoxins. Pathogenic species include *Pseudomonas aeruginosa* (most common), *P. cepacia, P. mallei* (glanders), and *P. pseudomallei* (melioidosis). *Pseudomonas aeruginosa* is the most common cause of malignant external otitis, hot tube folliculitis, osteochondritis associated with nail punctures through rubber-soled sneakers in children, and death caused by burns. This organism is a common cause of pneumonia in patients with cystic fibrosis, urinary tract infections postcystoscopy, external otitis, purulent conjunctivitis, and septic shock in immunocompromised patients. In general, *Pseudomonas* is responsive to aminoglycosides, extended spectrum penicillins, third generation cephalosporins, monobactams, and fluoroquinolones.

   Staphylococcus aureus has a yellow pigment in culture, *Serratia marcescens* has red-pigmented colonies, *Hemophilus influenzae* is not associated with pigment production, and *Bacteroides melanogenicus* has a black pigment in culture.

6. The answer is C. *(Pathology)*
The findings in this patient are consistent with amyotrophic lateral sclerosis (ALS), a motor neuron degeneration disease. ALS appears to be increasing in incidence. In 5%–10% of cases, there is an autosomal-dominant pattern with a strong age-dependent penetrance. Proposed causes include oxidative stress, viral infection, immunologic disease, or some unknown environmental factor. Currently, the oxidative stress theory is favored with the discovery of a defect in the zinc/copper binding superoxide dismutase (SOD1) on chromosome 21. Because SOD1 is an antioxidant that converts the superoxide free radical into peroxide and oxygen, its defective activity may result in apoptosis (individual cell necrosis) of spinal motor neurons. Inhibition of glutamate transport potentiates the toxicity associated with the defective enzyme. ALS most commonly presents with upper motor neuron signs (spastic paralysis) and, eventually, lower motor neuron signs (muscle atrophy, fasciculations). Atrophy of the intrinsic muscles of the hand and forearms with hand weakness and spastic changes in lower legs are early signs. Antioxidant cocktails have been developed, and some symptomatic improvement has been reported.

   A reduction in the synthesis of dopamine is the pathogenesis of Parkinson disease. A defect in the reabsorption of vitamin B_{12} may be associated with subacute combined degeneration, which is a demyelinating disease involving the dorsal columns and lateral corticospinal tract. An HLA-DR2 haplotype is associated with multiple sclerosis. The presence of nucleotide triplet repeats in DNA is seen in Huntington disease.

7. The answer is C. *(Pharmacology)*
Curve C represents the time course of the distribution of thiopental in skeletal muscle and skin. Thiopental is a highly lipid-soluble drug that rapidly diffuses into body tissues at a rate that is proportional to blood flow. The highly perfused tissues (e.g., the brain, heart, liver, kidney) initially receive a high proportion of the total dose. As plasma drug levels fall, thiopental is redistributed from the brain and other highly perfused tissues to those with intermediate blood perfusion such as skeletal muscle and skin. As plasma drug concentrations reach their lowest levels, the drug is redistributed to adipose tissues, which serve as a long-term reservoir for the drug because of its high lipid solubility. Other intravenous anesthetics such as propofol and etomidate have a similar pattern of distribution. It is important to note that the short duration of action of these drugs is a result of their rapid redistribution from the brain to other tissues, including skeletal muscle and adipose tissue.

8. The answer is D. *(Pathology)*
The most common location for a primary brain tumor in adults is the cerebral cortex. Most primary intracranial neoplasms derive from the neuroglia (astrocytes, oligodendrocytes, and ependymal cells). They do not metastasize out of the craniospinal axis. However, metastasis is the overall most common malignancy of the central nervous system (CNS), with lung cancer in men and breast cancer in women representing the primary sites. The majority of adult primary brain tumors are supratentorial (70%). In order of decreasing frequency, the most primary tumors are astrocytoma (glioblastoma multiforme variant), meningioma, and acoustic neuroma.

Astrocytomas are tumors derived from astrocytes. They have been subdivided into these grades: astrocytoma (Grade I and II), anaplastic astrocytoma (Grade III), and glioblastoma multiforme (GBM—Grade IV). Astrocytomas vary in histologic type depending on the age of the patient and the location of the tumor. In children, astrocytomas are more likely to be pilocytic astrocytomas involving the cerebellum, where they have a good prognosis, whereas in adults, they are more likely to be a GBM involving the cerebral cortex. They have a predilection for the frontal lobes and commonly cross the corpus callosum to the other lobe, thus producing a butterfly appearance on computerized tomography (CT) scanning or magnetic resonance imaging (MRI). Prominent histologic features include hemorrhagic necrosis, prominent proliferation of vascular channels in areas of necrosis, and highly pleomorphic astrocytic cells with frequent atypical mitotic figures. They characteristically seed the neuraxis, but rarely metastasize outside the CNS. The five-year survival rate for all astrocytomas, regardless of type, is 25%–40%.

The signs and symptoms of brain tumors relate to their size, location, invasiveness, and rate of growth. A headache is the initial symptom in 50% of patients. Generally, the headache lateralizes to the side of the tumor if it is located in a supratentorial location, or it lateralizes to the orbit or neck if it is located in the posterior fossa. CT scans and MRI are the most useful studies for localizing brain tumors.

9. The answer is C. *(Microbiology)*
The yellow fever virus is an RNA virus in the Togaviridae family. The virus is usually transferred to humans by the bite of the mosquito, *Aedes aegypti*. Humans are the reservoir for the disease. The disease is characterized by fever and jaundice and is associated with midzonal necrosis and Councilman bodies, which are hepatocytes that have died by apoptosis (individual cell death). Mosquito control and vaccination with a live, attenuated strain prevents the disease. The mortality rate is high and no treatment is available.

Tularemia may be transmitted by the bite of a deer fly; plague, by the bite of a flea; African sleeping sickness, by the bite of the tsetse fly; and leishmaniasis, by the bite of the *Phlebotomus* sandfly.

10. The answer is C. *(Pathology)*
In patients who are HIV positive, the two live vaccines that are contraindicated are the oral polio vaccine (Sabin) and the bacille Calmette-Guérin (BCG) vaccine, which contains a live attenuated strain of *Mycobacterium bovis*. The live measles-mumps-rubella (MMR) vaccine is given to HIV-positive patients because the risk for contracting these diseases by the wild viruses, particularly the measles virus, has far worse consequences than the risk for contracting disease associated with the vaccine. Hemophilus influenzae biotype II, diphtheria-pertussis-tetanus (DPT), and the influenza vaccines are not contraindicated in HIV-positive patients.

11. The answer is A. *(Microbiology)*
Nocardia asteroides is an aerobic, gram-positive filamentous bacterium that is also partially acid fast because it contains mycolic acid. Nocardiosis usually occurs in immunocompromised hosts, particularly heart transplant patients. Primary pulmonary disease most commonly occurs with dissemination to the central nervous system and kidney, in descending frequency. Abscess formation with a noncaseous granulomatous reaction is most commonly found in metastatic foci. Sulfadiazine is the treatment of choice. *Nocardia* may also be a pathogen in mycetomas (Madura foot), which are extensive localized skin and subcutaneous infections caused by bacteria (*Actinomyces* or *Nocardia*) or by fungi.

Legionella pneumophila is a gram-negative, motile rod with numerous subspecies. These organisms favor water reservoirs and cooling units. They stain weakly on Gram stain and are best visualized with a Dieterle silver stain or by direct immunofluorescent stains. The laboratory diagnosis is made by culture, direct visualization of organisms in sputum or biopsy specimens, or serologic studies. Erythromycin plus rifampin, which has a synergistic effect, are the drugs of choice. Mortality ranges from 15%–20%.

Infection caused by *Pneumocystis carinii* is considered a fungal disease. This organism is best visualized with silver stains or Giemsa stains and is most commonly contracted in immunosuppressed patients by inhalation. *P. carinii* produces an interstitial pneumonitis with extreme hypoxemia. Pneumocystosis is the most common initial infection in AIDS. Direct immunofluorescent stains are also useful in their identification. The organism cannot be cultured. A gallium scan is strongly positive in the lungs. The treatment of choice is trimethoprim and sulfamethoxazole, and if this has no affect, then pentamidine is used. Prophylaxis against pneumonia is recommended if the CD4 T-helper cell count is less than 200 cells/μl or when the percentage of CD4 lymphocytes is less than 14% of the total lymphocyte count.

Afipia felis, a small pleomorphic gram-negative rod associated with cat scratch disease, is best visualized with a Warthin-Starry silver stain. *Afipia* produces noncaseating, granulomatous microabscesses in lymph nodes draining a cat scratch site. The organism is susceptible to cephalosporins and aminoglycosides.

Chlamydia trachomatis is best visualized with Giemsa stains.

12. The answer is C. *(Pathology)*

A midline, lobulated, mucoid mass occurring in the sphenoccipital or sacrococcygeal region is a chordoma, which is derived from the notochord. A chordoma is a malignant, slow-growing, midline tumor with more than 50% of the cases arising from the sacrococcygeal region and 35% in the sphenoccipital region, with the remainder in the vertebra. These lobulated, firm tumors commonly erode the bone and have a cartilaginous appearance. These masses have cells with droplets of mucus in their cytoplasm that are called physaliphorous (bubble bearer) cells. The only other tumor listed that is located in the sacrococcygeal region is an ependymoma (derived from ependymal cells), involving the filum terminale.

13-19. The answers are: 13-D, 14-A, 15-B, 16-D, 17-B, 18-C, 19-E. *(Anatomy)*

The findings in this case suggest a lesion involving structures located in the lateral aspect of the brain stem medulla. This area is supplied by the posterior inferior cerebellar artery. The superior cerebellar artery supplies the midbrain and cerebellum. The middle cerebral artery, internal carotid artery at the cavernous sinus, and the anterior communicating artery are primarily involved in the vasculature associated with the cerebrum.

Horner's syndrome is a disorder of the sympathetic innervation to structures of the face, specifically glands and smooth muscle. The hypothalamic control of the sympathetic autonomic centers in the spinal cord passes through the lateral aspects of the medulla in the dorsal longitudinal fasciculus. This area is supplied by the posterior inferior cerebellar artery. There is no indication in the case history of parasympathetic dysfunction. Torticollis, conjunctivitis, or hypothalamic cysts may produce specific localized problems, but the case taken as a whole is suggestive of involvement of the descending autonomic system in the medulla.

The anterolateral system (spinothalamic tract) is located in the outer, upper quadrant of the medulla. This pathway carries pain and temperature sensations from the opposite side of the body. This tract also resides in the area of the medulla supplied by the posterior inferior cerebellar artery. The dorsal column–medial lemniscus pathway carries two-point touch, vibration, and conscious proprioception; it lies on the midline of the medulla and out of the territory supplied by the posterior inferior cerebellar artery. The dorsal spinocerebellar tract carries proprioception and the pontocerebellar tract carries motor information from the cerebrum to the cerebellum. The periaqueductal gray pathway is involved in pain modulation; it resides on the midline and out of the territory supplied by the posterior inferior cerebellar artery.

Dysmetria most likely involves some aspect of cerebellum function. In this patient, the most likely cause is ischemia of the inferior cerebellum. The patient is able to move, and does not exhibit any signs or symptoms associated with upper motor palsy (i.e., lesions affecting the pyramidal tract or extrapyramidal motor system). The lateral lemniscus is associated with the auditory system. The dorsal longitudinal fasciculus carries descending autonomic innervation.

The Babinski sign indicates that the pyramidal (corticospinal) tract innervation of the lower limb motor neurons is damaged. Because this patient does not exhibit the Babinski reflex, the physician knows that the descending corticospinal tract is intact through the neuraxis.

Hoarseness and difficulty swallowing indicate a weakness in the muscles of the larynx and pharynx respectively. The motor innervation to these structures is supplied primarily by the vagus nerve from cells of origin in the nucleus ambiguus. The nucleus ambiguus resides in the part of the medulla supplied by the posterior inferior cerebellar artery. The glossopharyngeal nerve is primarily a sensory nerve; its one motor innervation is not enough to influence pharyngeal movement in swallowing. The hypoglossal nerve innervates the tongue. The case does not indicate paralysis of this muscle mass, which is easily tested. The hypoglossal nerve arises and passes through the midline aspects of the medulla, out of the area supplied by the posterior inferior cerebellar artery. The trigeminal nerve may be involved in this syndrome; however, its involvement would be manifested as a loss of pain and temperature sensation in the face. There is no indication that the sternomastoid or trapezius muscles are involved; therefore, the spinal accessory nerve is not the correct answer.

This constellation of neurologic findings and the involvement of the lateral aspect of the medulla suggests Wallenberg's syndrome (lateral medullary syndrome). Occlusion of the vertebral artery or its branch, the posterior inferior cerebellar artery, is the cause of this syndrome. Klüver-Bucy syndrome involves the amygdala and medial temporal lobe. Weber's syndrome involves the midbrain; oculomotor nerve palsy is a key feature. Locked-in syndrome involves the pons. Wernicke's syndrome involves the parietotemporal lobe and is primarily a speech-related disorder.

20. The answer is B. *(Pathology)*
A tumor that might involve the optic nerve, spinal cord, or skull bone and also might be associated with a new onset of seizure activity in an adult is a meningioma, which characteristically has psammoma bodies in tissue sections. Meningiomas are benign tumors arising from arachnoidal cells (not meningeal cells). These masses are the second most common primary brain tumor in adults and are 10 times more frequent

in women than in men. Multiple meningiomas are characteristically seen in von Recklinghausen neurofibromatosis. These tumors are popcorn-shaped, hard neoplasms most commonly located along the parasagittal region, with less common sites in the wing of the sphenoid, olfactory groove, sella turcica, and spinal cord. When located near the skull, these masses often infiltrate into the bone and cause a localized hyperostosis that is seen on a radiograph. Meningiomas do not infiltrate the brain but may compress the brain, thus prompting a new onset of seizure activity. These tumors frequently calcify. Histologically, meningiomas are composed of swirling masses of meningothelial cells, which often encompass psammoma bodies (calcified bodies).

Antoni A and B areas refer to the zebra-like appearance of dark areas (Antoni A) and light areas (Antoni B) in neurilemomas (schwannomas). Physaliphorous cells are notochordal cells filled with lipid in chordomas, a malignant tumor derived from notochordal tissue. Vascular proliferation and necrosis describe a glioblastoma multiforme. Perivascular pseudorosettes are noted in ependymomas.

21. The answer is B. *(Microbiology)*
The patient is a 65-year-old man who recently moved to the Southwest and now has a respiratory condition with a solitary coin lesion in the lung. This presentation is characteristic of coccidioidomycosis (i.e., valley fever, San Joaquin fever). Coccidioidomycosis is caused by the dimorphic fungus, *Coccidiodes immitis*, which is acquired by inhaling arthrospores while in the Southwest or the San Joaquin valley in California. The organism may cause a miliary spread in the lungs and other distant locations. As with histoplasmosis, cryptococcosis, and blastomycosis, coccidioidomycosis is a granulomatous inflammation with both caseating and noncaseating granulomas. The granulomas contain spherules, which harbor endospores. Respiratory precautions are not necessary because the arthrospores in the soil are the primary infective agent. Blacks, Mexicans, and Filipinos are particularly susceptible to severe infections. The diagnosis of coccidioidomycosis is made with culture, direct visualization of the spherules with endospores, skin test, and serologic tests. Amphotericin B is the treatment of choice.

Metastatic disease is an unlikely diagnosis because metastasis is rarely associated with cavitation. Narrow angled septate hyphae with fruiting bodies represent aspergillosis, which is associated with aspergillomas (fungus balls), asthma, and invasive disease, unlike coccidioidomycosis. Budding yeasts with pseudohypha represents candidiasis, which does not produce cavitary lesions in the lungs. A hemorrhagic infarction secondary to a pulmonary embolus may cavitate, but it is usually peripherally located.

22. The answer is D. *(Pathology)*

Bacteremia associated with indwelling urinary catheters is the most common source of gram-negative bacteria in hospitilized patients. Pneumonia, intravenous catheters, right upper quadrant surgery, and septic thrombophlebitis all predispose to septicemia as well, but not as commonly as indwelling urinary catheters. Patient risk factors for bacteremia are immunosuppression (for treatment of cancer), chronic illness (rheumatiod arthritis), diabetes mellitus (glucose is a good culture medium), therapeutic procedures (e.g., ventilators), and some diagnostic procedures (e.g., angiography). Hospital risk factors for bacteremia include venipuncture and any intravenous line in place for over 48 hours.

23. The answer is A. *(Microbiology)*

The findings in this patient are compatible with old histoplasmosis caused by the dimorphic fungus, *Histoplasma capsulatum*. Pulmonary histoplasmosis is acquired by inhaling spores that develop in moist soils, particularly if the soil is enriched with bird or bat droppings. This disorder is the most common systemic fungal disease in patients living in the mid-Atlantic, southeastern, and central states. In tissue, the yeasts are present in macrophages, which is distinctly different than the other systemic fungi but similar to *Mycobacterium tuberculosis* (TB). This fungus has a dormant phase similar to TB and may be reactivated. Old infection sites characteristically contain numerous calcified granulomas. Multiple calcifications in the spleen are almost pathognomonic for histoplasmosis. Another less common association is sclerosing mediastinitis, where excessive fibrous tissue encroaches upon the mediastinal structures resulting in respiratory difficulties. The laboratory diagnosis is made by culture, direct visualization in tissue (organisms in macrophages), skin tests (useful), and serologic tests (useful). Amphotericin B is the mainstay for treatment.

Blastomycosis is caused by the dimorphic systemic fungus, *Blastomyces dermatitidis*. Blastomycosis most commonly occurs in the Midwest and Southeastern parts of the United States. The lung disease is contracted by inhalation of spores. It produces a mixed suppurative and granulomatous inflammatory reaction in the lung parenchyma.

Cyptococcosis is caused by the only encapsulated pathogenic yeast, *Cryptococcus neoformans*, and is commonly found in pigeon excreta. As with *Candida*, *Cryptococcus* is not a dimorphic fungus. Cryptococcosis is primarily an opportunistic infection that most commonly presents in lung (40%). In tissue, it produces a granulomatous reaction, if cellular immunity is intact, but there is no inflammatory reaction if the host is immunocompromised.

Metastatic osteogenic sarcoma is unlikely because the patient is too old for that type of cancer.

Sarcoidosis is a granulomatous disease, but dystrophic calcification is not a common feature.

24. The answer is A. *(Pathology)*

A tumor of the filum terminale in an adult is most likely derived from ependymal cells and represents an ependymoma. Ependymomas are a type of glioma that usually occur in children and are primarily located in the fourth ventricle. Here, they present with an obstructive hydrocephalus, whereas in adults, ependymomas are found in the lumbosacral portion of the spinal cord and filum terminale. The key histologic features of ependymomas are the presence of pseudorosettes (tumor cells arranged around a blood vessel), rosettes (tumor cells arranged around a central space), and blepharoplasts, which are identified with special stains. In the filum terminale, ependymomas are more likely to have a myxopapillary appearance and a tendency for extension into the subarachnoid space. Overall, ependymomas account for slightly less than 60% of all intraspinal gliomas.

A chordoma is a malignant tumor derived from the notochord. Astrocytomas are derived from astrocytes. No tumors are derived from microglial cells. In the past, these cells were implicated as the cell associated with primary lymphomas in the brain, but marker studies indicate that the majority of these tumors are of B-cell origin. Meningiomas derive from the arachnoid granulations.

25. The answer is B. *(Physiology)*
Convergence is a major feature of the retina; there are many more photoreceptors than ganglion cells. The rods outnumber the cones. There is one axon (i.e., the afferent fiber from the ganglion cells) for each ganglion cell. Nerves and blood vessels leave and enter the eye at the optic disk (blind spot); the optic disk does not contain photoreceptors. The refractive index of the cornea exceeds that of the lens.

26. The answer is E. *(Pathology)*
Bacteria are more likely to produce exotoxins or endotoxins as a mechanism for killing host cells than viruses. Exotoxins are secreted by either gram-positive or gram-negative bacteria. Endotoxins are not secreted but are the lipid in the cell wall of most gram-negative organisms. An example of exotoxin-induced damage is the diphtheria toxin. This toxin inhibits protein synthesis by adenosine diphosphate ribosylation of elongation factor 2, which stops protein synthesis. Viral mechanisms for killing include:

- inhibition of host cell DNA, RNA, or protein synthesis.
- lysis of host cells.
- damage host cell membranes.
- alteration of class I antigens on the cell, which leaves these cells susceptible to CD 8 cytotoxic T-cell destruction (e.g., hepatitis B).
- formation of circulating immune complexes (e.g., rubella virus producing arthritis and vasculitis).
- invasion of host cells, which are then killed by cytotoxins that are emitted by natural killer cells.

27. The answer is D. *(Pharmacology)*
Botulinum toxin inhibits the release of acetylcholine (ACh) from cholinergic nerves. When it is injected into ocular muscles, it produces muscle relaxation and relieves spasm. This treatment is now being used for patients with blepharospasm and other types of local muscle spasm, including hemifacial spasm and certain forms of strabismus.

28. The answer is E. *(Pathology)*
The pathogenicity of *Mycobacterium tuberculosis* relates more to its resistance to destruction by nonactivated macrophages than to interference in mucociliary

clearance. Smoking impairs ciliary activity, which allows bacteria to stagnate in the airway and serve as a nidus for infection (e.g., acute chronic bronchitis, pneumonia). In Kartagener's syndrome, the cilia lack the dynein arm, which renders them immotile. Bacterial overgrowth damages the structural integrity of the airways, which predisposes to bronchiectasis. Influenza virus has hemagglutinins to bind to the epithelium and neuraminidase to bore a hole through the mucous layer, which allows the virus to enter into the cells. Damage to the mucosal surface also provides a pathway for bacteria, such as Streptococci and Staphylococcus, to superimpose themselves on the viral inflammation. *Bordetella pertussis* and *Hemophilus influenzae* produce a toxin that paralyzes cilia. *Mycoplasma pneumoniae* produces hydrogen peroxide, which immobilizes the cilia. It then attaches to neuraminic acid receptors on the host cells.

29. The answer is C. *(Physiology)*
The demyelinated axon membrane will either exhibit no change or hyperpolarization (if some potassium channels open). The initial event in an action potential is depolarization caused by opening of the sodium channels; therefore, a membrane that lacks voltage-gated sodium channels cannot generate a normal action potential, much less a larger than normal action potential. Excitatory postsynaptic potentials (EPSPs) and inhibitory postsynaptic potentials (IPSPs) are responses at synapses (not axons) produced by neurotransmitters binding to specific receptors.

30. The answer is C. *(Pathology)*
Asthma, massive hemoptysis, and external otitis are most closely associated with infections caused by *Aspergillus fumigatus*. Aspergillosis produces many different forms of lung disease. An aspergilloma refers to a fungus ball (visible on an radiograph) of matted hyphae and fruiting bodies that develops in a preexisting cavity in the lung, particularly an old tuberculosis cavity. Hemoptysis is the most common sign of this infection. Massive hemoptysis and death may occur in some cases. Another pulmonary manifestation of the disease is allergic bronchopulmonary disease, which involves both type I and type III hypersensitivity reactions. In this disease, immunoglobulin E levels increase, skin tests against *Aspergillus* are positive, and

the serum is positive for precipitin antibodies. Finally, *Aspergillus* produces hemorrhagic infarctions in the lungs caused by direct invasion of vessels by the fungus with subsequent thrombosis. *Aspergillus* is also a common pathogen in external otitis along with *Pseudomonas aeruginosa.*

Pseudomonas aeruginosa is associated with pneumonia and external otitis media but not with asthma. Because this organism is a vessel invader similar to *Aspergillus*, hemorrhagic infarctions and a necrotizing pneumonia may occur.

Candida albicans is often a disseminated disease in the setting of indwelling venous and arterial catheters, immunodeficiency states, diabetes mellitus, mucosal damage, steroid or antibiotic therapy, and the polyendocrinopathy syndromes. This organism produces oropharyngeal disease (thrush) characterized by white patches, which leave raw, bleeding mucosal surfaces when removed.

Steptococcus pneumoniae is the most common cause of community-acquired bacterial pneumonia, which may be associated with rust-colored sputum but not massive hemoptysis. This organism is not a pathogen associated with ashtma or external otitis.

Staphylococcus aureus involving the lung is associated with a severe necrotizing pneumonia and abscess formation. Asthma or massive hemoptysis are not usually present. This organism may be associated with external otitis along with *Pseudomonas aeruginosa* and *Aspergillus.*

31. The answer is B.   *(Anatomy)*

The patient most likely has trigeminal neuralgia. The trigeminal nerve is the somatosensory nerve of the orofacial region, and the tingling and sharp pain follow the distribution of the trigeminal nerve branches. The episodic occurrence of pain is characteristic of aberrant neuronal activity in the nerve or the trigeminal ganglion. Severe pain can induce a seizure-like episode. A meningioma within the tentorium is anatomically distant from the trigeminal nerve and would most likely not produce this type of neurologic phenomenon. Alternating hemiplegia is a motor disorder characterized by paralysis of a cranial nerve on one side and paralysis of the body musculature on the other. Typically, alternating hemiplegia is a lower motor neuron deficit of the cranial nerve distribution and an upper motor neuron deficit of the nerves innervating

the body. Bell's palsy is a lower motor neuron paralysis of the nerves that control facial expression. Aneurysm of the posterior cerebral artery would most likely involve the oculomotor nerve and produce a paralysis affecting positioning of the eye by the extraocular muscles.

32. The answer is A.   *(Pathology)*

Chlamydia pneumoniae would most likely have an interstitial pneumonia rather than a cavitary lesion on a chest radiograph. This organism is transmitted to humans by droplet infection without an avian intermediate and accounts for 10% of all community-acquired pneumonias. The clinical manifestations include acute pharyngitis, sinusitis, bronchitis, and pneumonitis primarily in young adults. These symptoms are similar to those caused by *Mycoplasma pneumoniae* infection, except *Chlamydia pneumoniae* infection is usually preceded by more severe upper respiratory problems and lacks peripheral blood leukocytosis. *Chlamydia pneumoniae* infection qualifies as an atypical pneumonia in that it has a gradual onset, dry nonproductive cough, constitutional symptoms (e.g., headache, sore throat, myalgias, nausea, vomiting), low-grade fever, and a patchy segmental infiltrate on a chest radiograph. Erythromycin or tetracycline are effective in treating the disease.

Reactivation tuberculosis, primary squamous carcinoma of the lung, and histoplasmosis commonly produce cavitary lesions, with a propensity for the upper lobes. A lung abscess is a cavitary lesion usually associated with aspiration of infected oropharyngeal material. In most cases, these abscesses involve the dependent portions of the lung, such as the posterobasal segment of the right lower lobe.

33. The answer is A.   *(Physiology)*

The autonomic nervous system alters heart rate through parasympathetic (vagal) action on muscarinic cholinergic receptors to slow the rate, and sympathetic action on β_1-receptors to increase the heart rate. Atropine, a muscarinic cholinergic blocker, blocks the vagal slowing, thereby increasing the heart rate. Propanolol, a β-adrenergic blocker, would slow the rate. Phenylephrine, an α-adrenergic agonist, has little direct effect on the heart; it has vasoconstrictive activity, which increases the blood pressure and reflexly decreases the heart rate. Curare, a nicotinic cholinergic blocker, acts at the neuromuscular junction.

34. The answer is A. (Pathology)
Both *Mycobacterium tuberculosis* (TB) and sarcoidosis are associated with granulomatous hepatitis. TB is the most common infectious cause of granulomatous hepatitis, and sarcoidosis is the most common noninfectious cause. TB is more likely to produce caseous necrosis in granulomas and constrictive pericarditis caused by a contiguous spread from primary lung disease. Sarcoidosis is more likely to be associated with restrictive lung disease caused by interstitial fibrosis, and a positive Kveim test, which is an intradermal skin test that is positive in 70%–80% of patients with sarcoidosis. Other similarities between the two diseases are that they are granulomatous diseases, involve the skin, utilize cell-mediated immune mechanisms (type IV hypersensitivity), and produce multisystem disease.

35. The answer is B. (Behavioral science)
Positive, or productive, symptoms of schizophrenia include hallucinations, loose associations, strange behavior, and talkativeness. Negative, or deficit, symptoms of schizophrenia include flattening of affect, poverty of speech, thought blocking, poor grooming, lack of motivation, and social withdrawal. Positive symptoms are more responsive to traditional antipsychotic medications and suggest a better prognosis than do negative symptoms.

36. The answer is B. (Pathology)
Hemophilus ducreyi is the cause of the venereal disease called chancroid. Chancroid is characterized by painful genital and perianal ulcers with suppurative inguinal nodes. A Gram stain shows a classic "school-of-fish" orientation of the gram-negative rods. *Hemophilus influenzae* is the most common overall cause of bacterial meningitis and meningitis in children ages 3 months to 6 years and acute epiglottitis, which is characterized by inspiratory stridor with a potential for an acute respiratory arrest. *Hemophilus influenzae* is a common cause of chronic bronchitis in smokers and in patients with cystic fibrosis, otitis media, orbital cellulitis secondary to sinusitis, septicemia, osteomyelitis in children, and bacterial conjunctivitis (pink eye).

37. The answer is D. (Physiology)
β_2-Adrenergic receptors are much less responsive to norepinephrine than other adrenergic receptors. They respond much better to epinephrine than to norepinephrine.

38. The answer is D. (Pathology)
Staphylococcus saprophyticus is a coagulase-negative organism that causes 10%–20% of acute urinary tract infections in young, sexually active females. Unlike *Staphylococcus epidermidis*, the other coagulase-negative Staphylococcus, it is resistant to the antibiotic novobiocin. Trimethoprim and sulfamethoxazole is the treatment of choice.

Staphylococcus aureus is a gram-positive cocci that is coagulase- (virulence factor) and catalase-positive, grows in mannitol salt agar, produces β-lactamase, grows on blood agar (where it exhibits β-hemolysis), and has protein A (antiphagocytic).

Staphylococcus aureus, *S. epidermidis*, and *S. saprophyticus* are the three most important organisms. *Staphylococcus aureus* is the most common cause of:

- osteomyelitis in children
- furuncles (boils)
- carbuncles (more complicated furuncle with multiple sinuses)
- folliculitis (hair follicles)
- acute bacterial endocarditis
- hidradenitis suppurativa (abscess of apocrine glands)
- paronychial infections (nail bed)
- postoperative wound or stitch abscess
- postpartum breast abscesses
- food poisoning (preformed toxin)
- toxic shock syndrome (toxin induced)

Staphylococcus aureus is a common cause of septicemia, acute conjunctivitis, orbital cellulitis, infection in burns, and pneumonia in children with cystic fibrosis, elderly patients, or those with a preexisting viral pneumonia. In children with cystic fibrosis, this organism is associated with tension pneumatocysts, which are air-filled pockets in the pleural lining that rupture and produce a tension pneumothorax.

39. The answer is A. (Anatomy)
Climbing fibers are a major source of input to the cerebellum. The axons from cells in the inferior olivary

nuclei end in terminals described as climbing fibers because of their "ivy-like" relation to the dendrites of the Purkinje cells. The motor cortex does not project directly to the cerebellum. Instead, information is conveyed to the cerebellum from cortical input into the inferior olivary nucleus and the pontine nuclei. Vestibular nuclei send afferent fibers to the cerebellum but end in the granular layer as mossy fibers. Ia muscle afferents do not directly project to the cerebellum. Most likely, information from muscle afferents reaches the cerebellum via the spinocerebellar and cuneocerebellar tracts. The spinocerebellar tract ends in the granule cell layer as mossy fibers.

40. The answer is B. (Pathology)

Progressive degeneration of neurons rather than demyelination is associated with Pick disease, which involves the cerebral cortexas with Alzheimer disease. Pick disease is a rare disease with pronounced cortical atrophy, primarily involving the frontal and temporal regions. There is conspicuous sparing of the posterior two thirds of the first temporal gyrus. The gyri of Pick disease are described as knife edged. Intracytoplasmic silver positive material called Pick's bodies are noted in bizarre, swollen neurons, especially in Ammon's horn. These inclusions represent neurofilaments.

Progressive multifocal leukoencephalopathy is casued by the papovavirus, which infects oligodendrocytes and produces demyelination. Tabes dorsalis is a manifestation of tertiary syphilis and is characterized by demyelination of the posterior columns and dorsal roots. Subacute sclerosing panencephalitis is a demyelinating slow virus disease associated with rubeola. Adrenoleukodystrophy, or Schilder disease, is a sex-linked recessive primary demyelinating disease that differs from multiple sclerosis in that it is a familial disease, occurs earlier in life, has a symmetrical demyelination, and is associated with adrenal insufficiency, thus the term adrenoleukodystrophy. There is a defect in fatty acyl-coenzyme A ligase and an accumulation of long chain fatty acid esters of cholesterol in tissue.

41. The answer is E. (Physiology)

The adrenal medulla is stimulated by preganglionic sympathetic neurons that release acetylcholine (ACh). The adrenal medulla is in effect a specialized group of postganglionic sympathetic neurons.

42. The answer is D. (Pathology)

The skull film exhibits an area of calcification in and around the base of the skull. Because this film is from a child with frontal headaches, growth retardation, and bitemporal hemianopia, the area noted on the film most likely represents a craniopharyngioma, which derives from Rathke's pouch. Craniopharyngiomas are the most common cause of hypopituitarism in children, which is why this child has growth failure. The tumors are located in the suprasellar region and frequently compress the optic chiasm, producing bitemporal hemianopia. These masses might even infiltrate into the hypothalamus or stalk to produce central diabetes insipidus. Craniopharyngiomas are frequently cystic and contain areas of dystrophic calcification that are visible on a radiograph, as in this case. Histologically, these tumors have a squamous component and a component simulating tooth-forming epithelium (adamantinomatous pattern). Surgery is frequently performed, but there is a high rate of recurrence.

43. The answer is B. (Anatomy)

The cerebellum and basal ganglia both project onto neurons of the thalamus and ventral anterior and ventral lateral nuclei. Although the cerebellum and basal ganglia influence the cerebral cortex, brain stem, spinal cord, and contralateral basal ganglia, the convergence that allows for integrated function of the cerebellum and basal ganglia occurs in the thalamus.

44. The answer is D. (Pathology)

Shy-Drager syndrome is associated with extrapyramidal signs and autonomic system failure with severe postural hypotension and urinary incontinence. These patients have many of the same clinical and pathologic findings that are found in idiopathic Parkinson disease and in striatonigral degeneration. The syndrome is characterized by widespread neuronal degeneration in the caudate nucleus, substantia nigra, locus ceruleus, olivary nuclei, and dorsal vagal nuclei. Intracytoplasmic Lewy bodies in the substantia nigra identical to those seen in idiopathic Parkinson disease are also present. The autonomic system is affected bacause of involvement of the cells in the intermediolateral column extending from T1 to T3 in the lateral horn of the thoracic spinal cord. The peripheral autonomic ganglia are involved as well. Most neurologists consider this syndrome to be multisystem degenerative disease that is similar to Parkinsonism but unique in its involvement of the autonomic system.

Wilson disease is associated with toxic damage of the lenticular nucleus by excess copper and extrapyramidal signs, but it does not affect the autonomic system. Wernicke encephalopathy is related to thiamine deficiency and primarily involves the mamillary bodies in the brain. Confusion, ataxia, and nystagmus characterize this syndrome. Huntington disease is associated with destruction of the caudate nucleus and putamen, but it is not associated with autonomic dysfunction.

45. The answer is B. *(Physiology)*
Inhibition of gastrointestinal motility, stimulation of sweat glands, enhancement of cardiac muscle contractility, dilation of the bronchioles, and dilation of the pupil of the eye are all sympathetic actions. However, stimulation of sweat glands, unlike the other sympathetic actions, is produced by sympathetic neurons that release acetylcholine (ACh) to stimulate cholinergic receptors. Therefore, stimultion of sweat glands is the most likely sympathetic action to be blocked by the cholinergic blocker atropine.

46. The answer is B. *(Pathology)*
An alcoholic who develops an acute onset of confusion, ataxia, and nystagmus after the infusion of 5% glucose and isotonic saline has developed acute Wernicke encephalopathy, which results from thiamine deficiency. Thiamine deficiency (B_1) most commonly occurs in malnourished individuals and those with alcoholism. A deficiency of thiamine causes the disease called beriberi. Wet beriberi refers to the congestive (dilated) cardiomyopathy that occurs in these patients, whereas dry beriberi refers to peripheral neuropathy and central nervous system abnormalities related to demyelination and neuronal damage.

In Wernicke encephalopathy, neuronal damage occurs primarily in the mamillary bodies (most common site), tegmentum in the pons, and vestibular nuclei. Initially, edema occurs, followed by the degeneration of neurons in these areas. Astrocytes and microglial cells accumulate around the dying neurons. Capillaries proliferate in the damaged parts of the brain and frequently hemorrhage, producing the characteristic ring hemorrhages with hemosiderin pigmentation of the mamillary bodies. The infusion of glucose into an alcoholic with already borderline thiamine deficiency uses up any remaining thiamine and precipitates acute Wernicke encephalopathy unless thiamine is given intravenously before the glucose is administered. The characteristic triad of Wernicke encephalopathy is confusion, ataxia, and nystagmus (CAN). Korsakoff psychosis is a more advanced stage of Wernicke encephalopathy and is characterized by a memory disorder where the patient cannot form new memories or recall old ones. The peripheral neuropathy of thiamine deficiency usually occurs in the lower extremities, where it produces a sensorimotor neuropathy with burning feet, paresthesias, and muscle atrophy.

Excess copper levels are noted in Wilson disease, which is associated with chronic hepatitis and lenticular degeneration. A direct toxic effect of alcohol occurs in the cerebellum with the drop out of Purkinje cells, leading to cerebellar atrophy. Niacin deficiency is associated with dementia. Vitamin B_{12} deficiency results in subacute combined degeneration in the spinal cord.

47. The answer is C. *(Anatomy)*
The lentiform nuclei comprise the putamen and globus pallidus. On cross-section, these nuclei together have a lens-like appearance, hence the name. The subthalamic nucleus and substantia nigra are midbrain and diencephalic components of the basal ganglia. The caudate nucleus and the putamen together are referred to as the striatum. The caudate nucleus, putamen, and globus pallidus comprise the nuclei of the basal ganglia. The ventral anterior and ventral lateral thalami are the thalamic-specific nuclei related to the motor system. Cerebellar and basal ganglion projections converge here before being relayed to cerebral cortex.

48. The answer is B. *(Pathology)*
The site in the brain that is a favored location for ischemic damage, rabies virus infestation, and toxic damage resulting from alcohol is the Purkinje cells in the cerebellum. In chronic ischemia, the Purkinje cells undergo apoptosis (individual cell necrosis) and assume a shrunken, deeply eosinophilic cytoplasm with fading out of the nucleus (red neuron). The eosinophilic Negri inclusion body of rabies is located in the cytoplasm of the Purkinje cells. Alcohol has a direct toxic effect on Purkinje cells, resulting in cerebellar atrophy.

The nucleus basalis of Meynert is associated with neuronal loss in Alzheimer disease. The third, fifth, and sixth cortical layers of neurons in the cerebral hemispheric gray matter, the neurons in Ammon's horn of the hippocampal gyrus, and the watershed zones between overlapping blood supplies are susceptible to ischemic damage.

49. The answer is C. *(Physiology)*
A concave lens is a diverging lens. In myopia, the eyeball is too long for the refractive power of the eye's lens at rest; therefore, the image comes into focus in front of the retina and appears blurred on the retina. A diverging lens moves the image further back onto the retina where it can be seen clearly. In presbyopia (lengthening of the near point of vision with age) and hyperopia, the image tends to come into focus beyond the retina and a converging (convex) lens is needed. Astigmatism is caused by greater curvature in some planes of vision than in others; it requires a cylindrical lens. Emmetropia is normal vision.

50. The answer is C. *(Pathology)*
This patient has tabes dorsalis, which is a form of neurosyphilis where the spirochete attacks the posterior columns and the dorsal roots of the spinal cord. This attack produces:

1. impaired joint position sense (proprioception), leading to a broad-based ataxia and a positive Romberg test
2. loss of pain and vibration sensation
3. joint damage (Charcot joints) caused by loss of pain sensation
4. sensory disturbances manifesting as "lightening pains"
5. absent deep tendon reflexes
6. an Argyll Robertson pupil

Demyelinization first begins in the middle portion of the dorsal root zone close to the posterior horns and then extends into the dorsal columns. Laboratory findings in the spinal fluid include a positive VDRL (25-50%), a positive FTA-ABS (80-95%), a mild pleocytosis consisting of lymphocytes and mononuclear cells (not neutrophils), an increased protein with oligoclonal bands on high-resolution electrophoresis, and a normal glucose. An elevated protein and cell count

is an indicator of disease activity. The treatment is aqueous penicillin G, 12 million to 24 million units daily given intravenously for 10–14 days.

The history is not compatible with cryptococcosis (encapsulated yeast cells), Toxoplasmosis, or leptomeningeal spread of malignant cells.

51. The answer is E. *(Behavioral science)*
Infantile autism is a pervasive developmental disorder of childhood. Males are more likely to be affected with infantile autism than females, and onset is before 6 years of age. In autism, while there is no family history of schizophrenia, there is evidence of neurologic abnormalities; seizures and perinatal complications are often seen in children with infantile autism.

52. The answer is C. *(Pathology)*
This patient has a bacterial meningitis, which would most likely be the gram-negative coccobacillus, *Hemophilus influenza*, in her age bracket. Leptomeningitis, or inflammation of the meninges, is the most common type of central nervous system infection and is transmitted primarily by the hematogenous route.

Group B streptococcus infection occurs during the first week after birth (early onset) or less than 7–10 days after birth (late onset). Early onset infections are contracted from the maternal genital tract usually in association with premature rupture of the membranes and the spread of infection from the vagina. The source of the organism for the late onset type is paradoxical because the vagina is frequently not colonizes by the streptococcus when cultures are taken. *Hemophilus influenza* meningitis is the most common overall bacterial meningitis regardless of age. Hopefully, the incidence will decrease in the future because of immunization with the type b vaccine.

Symptoms and signs associated with bacterial meningitis include:

• fever in more than 90% of cases
• generalized headache (80%–90%)
• nuchal rigidity (more than 80%)
• an altered sensorium (more than 80%)
• positive Kernig sign, where a patient in the supine position and hips flexed 90 degrees cannot fully extend the knees because of traction on inflamed meninges

- a positive Brudzinski neck sign, where passive flexion of the neck causes flexion of both legs and thighs because of traction on the inflamed meninges
- cranial nerve palsies (IV, VI and VII) in 10%–20% of cases

The spinal fluid findings in bacterial meningitis include an increased total white blood cell count with predominantly neutrophils, an increased protein resulting from increased vessel permeability, a low glucose resulting from use of glucose by the cellular elements, and a positive Gram stain in approximately 75% of cases. Direct antigen detection of specific organisms is more sensitive and specific than counter-immunoelectrophoresis techniques. Direct antigen detection is performed by utilizing latex agglutinations or coagglutination techniques. Methods are available for the detection of most of the pathogenic bacteria including *Escherichia coli, Hemophilus influenza,* Group B streptococcus, *Neisseria meningitidis, Streptococcus pneumoniae,* and the most common opportunistic encapsulated yeast, *Cryptococcus neoformans.*

53. The answer is B. *(Physiology)*
Light activates both "on" centers and "off" centers through hyperpolarization of the photoreceptors. What distinguishes "on" centers from "off" centers is the response of the bipolar cells to the hyperpolarization of the photoreceptors. In the "on" centers, light on the photoreceptor leads to a depolarization of the ganglion cells, which initiates an increase in action potentials (hence the name, "on" center). The ganglion cells of "off" centers are hyperpolarized, decreasing the rate of action potential production.

54. The answer is C. *(Pathology)*
This patient most likely has cerebral toxoplasmosis. *Toxoplasma gondii* is a protozoan parasite that is contracted usually through contact with cat litter, eating contaminated meat, blood transfusion, or organ transplantation. This organism is part of the TORCH complex in congenital infections in newborns. Acute toxoplasmosis in the immunocompetent host usually presents as a mononucleosis-like syndrome with cervical lymphadenopathy. However, in immunocompromised patients (e.g., patients with AIDS), the central nervous system is the most common site. Cerebral toxoplasmosis in AIDS is thought to be a reactivation of a previous infection.

Toxoplasma encephalitis develops when the CD4 T-helper cell count is less than 100 cells/μl. Clinical manifestations include encephalitis, meningoencephalitis, or focal dysfunction caused by mass lesions. Altered mental status is the most common finding, with the most common involved areas being the brainstem, basal ganglia, pituitary gland, and corticomedullary junction. A double dose contrast computerized tomography (CT) scan and magnetic resonance imaging are highly sensitive techniques, which are useful in making a presumptive diagnosis, along with the proper history. Serologic studies and, in cases that are resistant to therapy, brain biopsies with tissue examination for the parasite may be necessary. A combination of pyrimethamine and clindamycin has been tried for treatment with varying success.

The other choices are all lesions that frequently involve the central nervous system in patients with AIDS, but they are not the most common cause of space-occupying lesion. The radiologic findings and clinical presentation are often enough to make a presumptive diagnosis and to begin treatment.

55. The answer is D. *(Anatomy)*
This patient most likely has a lower motor neuron lesion of the left hypoglossal nerve. Atrophy of the muscle is characteristic of this type of motor neuron disorder. The deviation of the tongue is caused by the unopposed contraction of the normally innervated genioglossus muscle. The vector of contraction of this muscle is from the lateral toward the midline. With two normal genioglossus muscles contracting, the vectors cancel each other at the midline, causing the tip of the tongue to protrude forward. If one side is not contracting, the tip of the tongue continues to point past the midline and to the opposite side. Therefore, a lower motor neuron lesion of the tongue causes the tongue to point toward the side of the lesion. A lesion of the corticobulbar fibers in the internal capsule produces an upper motor neuron lesion that does not cause atrophy to the muscles of the tongue. The paralysis is a spastic paralysis with movement, especially of the affected intrinsic skeletal muscle fibers. Articulation is most affected, resulting in poor speech. The patient's paralysis is on the left side. If the right hypoglossal nerve had been affected, this case scenario

would be reversed. The motor cranial nerves innervate skeletal muscles on the same side that the nerve exits the brain stem. The exception to this is the trochlear nerve, which is the only nerve to cross to the opposite side in the brain stem. The left nucleus ambiguus is the origin of motor axons in the glossopharyngeal and vagus nerves. The distribution of these fibers is to the skeletal muscles of the palate, pharynx, and larynx.

56. The answer is C.   *(Pathology)*
The cause of this complication is most commonly a cytomegalovirus (CMV). Ophthalmologic abnormalities occur in more than 50% of patients with AIDS. The most common abnormal finding is the presence of cotton-wool exudates in the retina, which represents areas of ischemia secondary to microvascular disease. However, this finding is not associated with visual loss. The second most common manifestation is CMV retinitis. This disorder is usually a late manifestation of the disease and often correlates with a CD4 T-helper cell count that is less than 100 cells/μl. It produces a necrotizing retinitis with cotton-wool exudates and perivascular hemorrhages.

Oxygen-free radical damage is more commonly seen in neonates on 100% oxygen for management of the respiratory distress syndrome. Optic neuritis secondary to demyelinating disease produces inflammation around the optic nerve, but it is not associated with exudates. Cerebral edema secondary to encephalitis would have papilledema and hemorrhage but not the presence of cotton-wool exudates. Retinitis caused by *Candida albicans* may occur in AIDS, but it is not more common than CMV.

57. The answer is A.   *(Anatomy)*
The talus articulates with the tibia and fibula to form the talocrural joint. This joint permits dorsiflexion and plantar flexion. The talus also articulates with the calcaneus and the navicular to form the subtalar joint. The subtalar joint permits inversion and eversion.

58. The answer is C.   *(Pathology)*
This 25-year-old woman most likely has acute maxillary sinusitis. The maxillary and ethmoid sinuses are present at birth, and the frontal and sphenoid sinuses develop much later in childhood, with the sphenoid sinus developing last. Obstruction of the ostia draining the sinuses is the most common cause of sinusitis. Viral infections, allergic rhinitis, nasal polyps, intranasal catheters in a hospital, and barotrauma are predisposing causes for these infections. The maxillary sinus is most frequently infected, followed by the ethmoids, frontal, and sphenoid sinuses. Maxillary sinusitis has malar pain and pain in the upper teeth because the infraorbital nerve supplying the first two molars runs through the sinus. Anterior ethmoiditis has pain in the upper nose or retro-orbital or temporal area. Posterior ethmoiditis produces pain over the mastoid area. Sphenoid inflammation produces pain over the retro-orbital, frontal, or facial area. The most common organisms are *Streptococcus pneumoniae* and *Hemophilus influenza*. Sinus films, including laterals or computerized tomography scans, are ordered sometimes depending on which sinuses are involved. Complications include orbital cellulitis, epidural, subdural, or cerebral abscesses, and cavernous sinus thrombosis, with involvement of cranial nerves II through VI.

Orbital cellulitis is associated with periorbital edema and proptosis of the eyes, but eye movement is still present. Erysipelas refers to a cellulitis caused by group A streptococcus and is associated with a raised, red confluent rash. A frontal lobe abscess would present with localizing signs.

59. The answer is B.   *(Anatomy)*
Wernicke's aphasia is characterized as a fluent aphasia because the patient has no difficulty in forming and speaking words. The speech, however, is often filled with nonsense and inappropriate words to describe objects and events. The abnormal brain activity is related to gyri that include the Wernicke's speech center. There is no specific aphasia related to Jacksonian motor disorders, but the patient may have slow and deliberate speech with perseveration. Speech usually is understandable and coherent. Parkinsonism is not associated with a specific aphasia, but the speech may be deliberate and halting, with quivering detected in the speech pattern. It is normally coherent. Speech in Alzheimer's disease is confused as a result of the dementia, but no specific aphasia is involved. Broca's aphasia, or motor aphasia, is characterized by the inability to form words. The patients usually know what they want to say, and what they do say is appropriate and meaningful. This disorder occurs from a cortical

lesion involving the opercular area of the left frontal lobe.

60. The answer is B.   *(Pathology)*
The photomicrograph reveals necrotic tissue that are ribbons of nonseptate hyphae consistent with mucormycosis. Diabetics in ketoacidosis can have invasion of the frontal lobes by this fungus, usually originating from a preexisting frontal sinusitis (rhinocerebral abscess). The organisms are from the genera *Mucor, Rhizopus,* or *Absidia.* Patients present with periorbital swelling, pain, and bloody nasal discharge. Cavernous sinus thrombosis and internal jugular vein and dural sinus thromboses can occur. Surgery and amphotericin B are required for treatment. *Aspergillus, Candida, Cryptococcus,* and *Histoplasma* do not have an increased incidence in patients with diabetic ketoacidosis, particularly those patients who have invasion into the frontal lobe.

61. The answer is A.   *(Behavioral science)*
Episodes of major depression tend to increase in both length and frequency with age. When treated, episodes of major depression last for about 3 months. If untreated, depression lasts from 6 to 12 months. Episodes of major depression often have a gradual onset and occur an average of 5 to 6 times over a 20-year period.

62. The answer is C.   *(Pathology)*
Strabismus refers to a malalignment of the eyes so that only one eye at a time is able to view an object. This disorder occurs in 2%–3% of children and has a strong familial tendency. In descending order of frequency, the eyes may deviate inward (esotropia), outward (exotropia), upward (hypertropia), or downward (hypotropia). The child may unconsciously suppress vision in the affected eye. Diplopia is a common finding. The corneal light reflex is useful in identifying inequality between the pupils. The unaffected eye is usually patched, which forces the affected eye to be used by the visual cortex. Failure to correct strabismus before 6 years of age may result in amblyopia, which is reduced vision in the eye that is uncorrectable with lenses.

Cataracts refer to the opacification of the lens and are most commonly the result of aging. Glaucoma refer to the elevation of the intraocular pressure (greater than 21 mm Hg). These disorders are caused by a defect in the Schlemm canal, which drains the aqueous humor in the anterior chamber, or acquired conditions that obstruct the outflow of aqueous humor in the angle between the cornea and iris. Macular degeneration is the leading cause of visual loss and legal blindness in old age. Otosclerosis refers to sclerosis and fixation of the middle ear ossicles associated with a conductive type of hearing loss and possible deafness. It is the most common cause of conductive hearing loss in adults.

63. The answer is E.   *(Anatomy)*
The alpha motor neurons in lamina IX innervate skeletal muscle associated with the axial and appendicular skeleton. The neurons of the nucleus ambiguus innervate the skeletal muscle in the pharynx, larynx, and palate. Like the alpha motor neurons in lamina IX, the neurons in the nucleus ambiguus use acetylcholine (ACh) as their neurotransmitter and are susceptible to diseases that affect alpha motor neurons, such as amyotrophic lateral sclerosis (Lou Gehrig's disease). The neurons in the dorsal root ganglia are sensory and would be similar to neurons found in the superior and inferior ganglia of the vagus nerve located in the jugular foramen. The dorsal motor nucleus of the vagus consists of preganglionic parasympathetic neurons. Similar cells would be found in the sacral spinal cord, which innervates the lower gastrointestinal and pelvic viscera. The sympathetic chain ganglia are postganglionic sympathetic neurons. The otic ganglion consists of postganglionic parasympathetic neurons.

64. The answer is B.   *(Pathology)*
This 32-year-old woman most likely has myasthenia gravis (MG) with either thymic hyperplasia or a thymoma in the anterior mediastinum. Myasthenia gravis is a predominantly female autoimmune disease characterized by autoantibodies directed against acetylcholine receptors, thus, blocking the uptake of acetylcholine. This disorder qualifies as type II hypersensitivity reaction. Thymomas are associated with myasthenia gravis in approximately 15% of cases, whereas thymic hyperplasia is noted in 65%–75% of cases. Thymectomy often improves the symptoms of myasthenia gravis. Patients with MG present with muscle

weakness that becomes more prominent with repeated contraction. Weakness of the ocular muscles and ptosis is the most common initial presentation. These symptoms are followed by progressive weakness of the facial muscles, limb girdle muscles, and respiratory muscles, which will result in death of the patient if left untreated. Patients should avoid aminoglycosides, which also block acetylcholine release. The Tensilon (edrophonium) stimulation test shows improvement of muscle weakness because the drug has a short-acting anticholinesterase activity. Anti-acetylcholine receptor antibodies and antistriated muscle antibodies are present in the serum.

Antismooth muscle antibodies are seen in autoimmune hepatitis. MG is not a sex-linked recessive disease or a lower motor neuron disease. Toxin blockade of acetylcholine release is the mechanism of paralysis in botulism caused by *Clostridium botulinum.*

65. The answer is D.   *(Anatomy)*
The large, flask-shaped Purkinje cells of the cerebellum separate the molecular layer on the outside and the granular layer on the inside. The Purkinje cell has a single axon, which is an outflow source of the cerebellum. They possess several dendrites that arborize in the molecular layer. Few neurons are present in the molecular layer, so it stains diffusely. In contrast, many cell bodies of small neurons are seen in the granular layer. Satellite cells are not found in the cerebellum. Glial cells perform the supporting function of satellite cells in the central nervous system. Pyramidal cells or neurons are present in the cerebrum, which has six layers of cells. The white matter of the cerebellum stains diffusely in the midst of the granular layer. A silver stain is necessary to resolve the contrast in fiber presence between the white matter and gray matter.

66. The answer is C.   *(Pathology)*
Malignant melanomas, squamous cell carcinomas (SCC), and basal cell carcinomas (BCC) are associated with sun-damaged skin. BCC is the most common of the three, but malignant melanoma is the most rapidly increasing in incidence in the United States.

BCCs are not associated with metastasis. SCCs and melanomas are present in many other areas in the body other than the skin. SCC is the most common primary cancer in the oral pharynx, esophagus, and larynx. Not all malignant melanomas and SCCs are nodular tumors. None of the three cancers need to be pigmented tumors.

67. The answer is A.   *(Behavioral science)*
The area of the brain most closely associated with memory is the temporal lobe, particularly the hippocampus.

68. The answer is C.   *(Pathology)*
Immunosuppression is most likely associated with a squamous cell carcinoma of the skin. There is an increased incidence of cervical squamous cancer in the United States. Lymphoma cutis refers to a malignant lymphoma involving skin. A Merkel tumor is a malignancy of neural crest-derived Merkel cells, which are normally thought to have a tactile function in skin.

69. The answer is B.   *(Anatomy)*
The tibialis anterior is the major dorsiflexor of the ankle. Its segmental innervation primarily is from spinal nerve L_4. A patient with a lesion to spinal nerve L_4 (e.g., herniation of the L_3/L_4 intervertebral disk) may present with difficulty in dorsiflexing at the ankle.

70. The answer is C.   *(Pathology)*
Exposure to excessive sunlight is the single most important predisposing cause of malignant melanoma. Other risk factors include the following:

1. a history of severe sunburn
2. fair skin, blue eyes, blond or red hair
3. the dysplastic nevus syndrome
4. freckling on exposure to the sun (melanoma syndrome)
5. history of a melanoma in a first- or second-degree relative
6. xeroderma pigmentosum (autosomal recessive disease with a lack of DNA repair enzymes)

Although uncommon, certain nevi (modified melanocyte) can evolve into a malignant melanoma, particularly those that are congenital and those that are referred to as dysplastic nevi.

The basal cell nevus syndrome is an autosomal dominant disorder characterized by the development of basal cell carcinomas early in life, with associated abnormalities of bone, skin, nervous system, eyes, and the ovaries. Young age is not a risk factor because of the need for long-term exposure to the sun. A family history of breast cancer offers no increased risk, but a history of malignant melanoma in a first or second degree relative does pose an increased risk. Blacks rarely have malignant melanomas, except for the acral lentiginous variety.

71. The answer is A.   *(Behavioral science)*
Reduced motivation and depression are most likely to reflect damage to the frontal lobes. Damage to the temporal lobes is associated primarily with memory problems, while damage to the parietal lobes is associated primarily with difficulty processing sensory information. Damage to the occipital lobes and basal ganglia results in visual problems and movement disorders respectively.

72. The answer is E.   *(Pathology)*
The patient most likely has acute intermittent porphyria. Her urine would turn a port-wine color after sitting on a window sill for a short time because light oxidizes the colorless porphobilinogen into the colored porphobilin.

The two most common porphyrias in the United States are acute intermittent porphyria (AIP) and porphyria cutanea tarda (PCT). Porphyrins are involved in oxidative or oxygen-transferring functions and in heme synthesis. Enzyme defects in the heme synthesis pathway account for the clinical porphyrias (see figure).

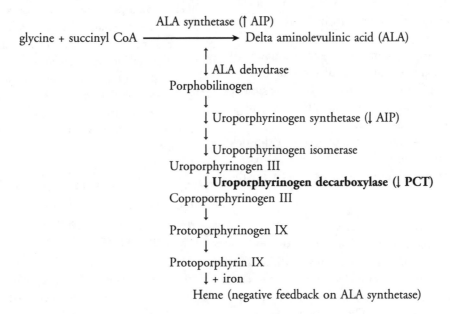

$$\text{glycine + succinyl CoA} \xrightarrow{\text{ALA synthetase (}\uparrow\text{ AIP)}} \text{Delta aminolevulinic acid (ALA)}$$

↑
↓ ALA dehydrase
Porphobilinogen
↓
↓ Uroporphyrinogen synthetase (↓ AIP)
↓
↓ Uroporphyrinogen isomerase
Uroporphyrinogen III
↓ **Uroporphyrinogen decarboxylase (↓ PCT)**
Coproporphyrinogen III
↓
Protoporphyrinogen IX
↓
Protoporphyrin IX
↓ + iron
Heme (negative feedback on ALA synthetase)

ALA synthetase is the rate-limiting enzyme in heme synthesis and has a negative feedback with its end product, heme. Heme is used up when drugs (e.g., alcohol, phenobarbital) are being metabolized in the liver by the cytochrome P-450 system. When the heme levels drop, ALA synthetase activity increases, which may precipitate an acute porphyria attack if enzymes along the pathway are deficient. Porphyrinogen compounds are colorless and nonfluorescent in the reduced state. However, when "oxidized" in voided urine upon exposure to light, they become "porphyrins," which have a red wine color. Oxidized porphyrins under ultraviolet (UV) light have an intense red–orange fluorescence.

Acute intermittent porphyria (AIP) has two basic defects, an increased activity of ALA synthetase and a decreased activity of uroporphyrinogen synthetase. The net effect of the two defects in AIP is an excessive quantity of δ-aminolevulinic acid (ALA) and porphobilinogen (PBG) in the urine. This autosomal dominant disease is characterized by intermittent exacerbations of neurologic dysfunction, including psychosis, neuropathy, and severe colicky abdominal pain, with the last often mistaken for a surgical emergency requiring surgery. Many patients with AIP presenting with abdominal pain often have the classic "bellyful of scars" from previous surgeries. Similar to PCT, AIP is often precipitated by drugs, which induce hepatic ALA synthetase activity by the mechanisms previously discussed. Laboratory findings in AIP include (1) a colorless fresh-voided urine, which when left standing in light turns a red wine color (windowsill test), (2) low red blood cell uroporphyrinogen synthetase activity even when the patient is asymptomatic, and (3) increased amounts of porphobilinogen in the urine, as well as increased amounts of ALA. Intravenous infusion of heme is considered the treatment of choice for acute attacks, rather than intravenous infusion of glucose.

The urine does not contain an increase in uroporphyrin or coproporphyrin. However, both are increased in the urine in porphyria cutanea tarda.

The urine does not contain an excess amount of urobilinogen. Increased amounts of urobilinogen are seen in the jaundice states, particularly those disease associated with increased extravascular hemolysis (e.g., sickle cell disease) and hepatitis.

The urine would not be positive with a dipstick for blood because porphobilinogen is not related to hemoglobin or myoglobin, which do react with the dipstick.

73. The answer is C.   *(Anatomy)*
The substantia nigra is the most likely site of this lesion. A persistent, or resting, tremor that diminishes with intention of movement is characteristic of disease in this location. This patient has classic akinetic, tardive akinesia, or dyskinesia. The pause and the apparent resistance to movement are caused by a delay in motor processing of information through the basal ganglia associated with a neurotransmitter deficiency (dopamine). These findings are consistent with parkinsonism. The patient apparently clearly understands the request, and there is no hearing deficit or apparent dementia described. The auditory cortex does not play any immediate role in motor activity. It could only be determined if the dentate nucleus of the cerebellum was involved by asking the patient to do this activity simultaneously with both extremities. A lesion in the dentate nucleus would result in a lack of coordination

and the tremor would differ in that it would worsen as the patient tried to perform the requested task (intention tremor). Lesions of the red nucleus would cause manifestations similar to those caused by a lesion in the dentate nucleus. The red nucleus is primarily involved in motor control of proximal axial and appendicular muscle groups. Through the rubrospinal tract, the red nucleus affects postural muscles involved in voluntary motor activity. It is coordinated with corticospinal innervation of the distal limb musculature. The post-central gyrus is the somatosensory cortex. A lesion in this area would not produce the findings observed in the patient.

74. The answer is A.   *(Pathology)*
A 45-year-old African-American man who has widespread metastatic malignant melanoma would most likely have a primary lesion located in the subungual area (under the nails). Black skin has a decreased incidence of malignant melanoma because of the protective effect of increased melanin pigmentation on damaging the DNA in the squamous cells. Acral lentiginous melanoma is the least common type of melanoma in the white population. The lesions are commonly found on the palms, soles, or subungual regions.

75. The answer is D.   *(Behavioral science)*
Inhalation of carbon dioxide or infusion of sodium lactate will induce a panic attack in individuals who have panic disorder.

76. The answer is B.   *(Pathology)*
The figure shows a hyperkeratotic-appearing, irregularly bordered scaly patch on the upper lip consistent with an actinic keratosis. These lesions are caused by chronic sun exposure. They commonly appear on older patients, primarily on the face and arms, and are usually multiple rather than solitary lesions. They may predispose the patient to a squamous cell carcinoma.

There is no evidence of melanin hyperpigmentation around the lips to suspect Peutz-Jegher's syndrome, which is the second most common hereditary polyposis syndrome. It is autosomal dominant and is also associated with hamartomatous polyps in the small intestine.

Pemphigus vulgaris is an autoimmune disease that may involve the lips and oral pharynx, but it is a bullous disease, rather than one associated with a scaly lesion.

There are no vesicles suggesting a herpes infection of the upper lip.

Inflammation of the minor salivary glands is associated with Sjögren syndrome, which involve autoimmune destruction of the minor salivary glands and the lacrimal ducts. This condition produces xerostomia (dry mouth) and keratoconjunctivitis (dry eyes). Rheumatoid arthritis rounds out the clinical picture.

77. The answer is A. *(Anatomy)*
All input to the cortex of the cerebellum collateralizes and sends axon branches to both the cortex and the deep cerebellar nuclei. The activity of the deep cerebellar nuclei depends on the integrated response of the direct excitatory input from the collaterals and the inhibitory influence of the Purkinje cells of the cerebellar cortex.

78. The answer is A. *(Pathology)*
The figure shows flat lesions that are stated to be erythematous and pruritic. They are sharply bordered, raised lesions, some having a circular appearance. Leading edge is darker than the more central portions of the lesion. The patient has tinea corporis (ringworm), which is due to a superficial dermatophytic infection by *Trichophyton rubrum* in this particular case. Scrapings should be taken from the leading edge of the lesion and examined under the microscope after digestion by a few drops of potassium hydroxide on a slide. The morphology of the lesion is against a contact dermatitis, which is usually the result of sensitization to an antigen (cellular immunity). Often they are weeping lesions and do not have the dry, scaly appearance noted in this case. There is no autoimmune disease of skin that is associated with this type of lesion. Erysipelas, a group A β-hemolytic streptococcal infection would have a raised, hot erythematous cellulitis involving the skin. Atopic dermatitis, representing an IgE-mediated type I hypersensitivity reaction, is not usually located on the buttocks but is more likely to be seen in the flexor creases of the arms and legs, or on the face of infants.

79. The answer is E. *(Behavioral science)*
Although dissociative fugue and dissociative amnesia both involve a failure to remember important information about oneself, dissociative fugue is further characterized by the wandering away from home. Depersonalization disorder is characterized by feelings of detachment from one's own body or social situation. In dissociative identity disorder, an individual possesses at least two distinct personalities. Individuals with anterograde amnesia cannot put down new memories following a traumatic event. Anterograde amnesia may occur following head trauma.

80. The answer is C. *(Pathology)*
The figure shows thick, crusty-appearing lesions on the chin and cheek with a few blisters located along the edge of the lesion, which is consistent with impetigo, most commonly due to group A streptococcus and/or *Staphlococcus aureus*. In either case, the bacteria are gram-positive cocci, the former often in chains and the latter in clusters. They must be treated with antibiotics.

Gram-negative rods involved with skin infections would most likely involve *Pseudomonas aeruginosa*, which is associated with ecthyma gangrenosum and malignant external otitis.

Gram-positive diplococci are most likely *Streptococcus pneumoniae*, which is not associated with skin infections.

Gram-negative diplococci are most likely *Neisseria* species, none of which produce this type of skin lesion.

Gram-positive filamentous bacteria represent Actinomyces and Nocardia, neither of which produces superficial skin infections.

81. The answer is A. *(Physiology)*
Atropine blocks muscarinic cholinergic receptors, which mediate parasympathetic activity in the eye. Therefore, the nerves that mediate constriction of the pupil and contraction of the ciliary muscles are affected. Ciliary muscle contraction decreases the near point to allow accommodation for near vision. Atropine blockage will reverse these actions, increasing both pupil size and the near point.

82. The answer is B. *(Pathology)*
The photograph shows papular lesions on the upper arm of a 25-year-old homosexual who has a positive

antibody test for the human immunodeficiency virus. The lesions are stated to be pearl-colored and nonpruritic. Some of the lesions are beginning to show central umbilication, characteristic of molluscum contagiosum, which is due to a poxvirus. The craters frequently fill up with a sandy-like material, which contains the viral inclusions. They may spread with close physical contact. When disseminated as in this patient, they indicate that the person is immunocompromised.

83. The answer is C.   *(Anatomy)*
The substantia nigra has a direct input to the caudate nucleus, using dopamine as its primary neurotransmitter. Research also shows projections to other basal ganglia and the thalamus by collaterals, but the primary effect of the dopaminergic input seems to be on caudate nucleus neurons. The globus pallidus receives input from the caudate nucleus and cerebral cortex and projects to the thalamus.

84. The answer is C.   *(Pathology)*
The Gram stain reveals neutrophils with diplococci. Since they are pustular lesions on the wrist of a febrile 25-year-old woman who has a swollen right knee, the bacteria are most likely gram-negative diplococci representing *Neisseria gonorrhoeae* associated with disseminated gonococcemia. *N. gonorrhoeae* is the most common cause of septic arthritis, particularly in the urban population. Many of the strains are resistant to complement-mediated bactericidal activity in serum, particularly in patients who have C5 through C8 complement deficiencies. The disease is more common in young women and presents with (1) septic arthritis, most commonly in the joints of the hands, feet, and knee; (2) a dermatitis consisting of macules, papules, or pustules, as in this case; and (3) a tenosynovitis, typically in the wrist, fingers, toes, and ankles. The organism is recovered in synovial fluid in 50% of patients.

85. The answer is C.   *(Pharmacology)*
Meperidine is a full opiate agonist and may produce considerable drug dependence. Buprenophine, pentazocine, nalbuphine, and butorphanol are partial agonists or mixed agonists/antagonists at the opiate receptors. These agents do not fully activate μ receptors and have less tendency to cause euphoria and drug

dependence than the full agonists. Mixed or partial agonists also have less capacity to produce severe respiratory depression because of their reduced ability to activate μ receptors.

86. The answer is D.   *(Pathology)*
The photograph shows multiple, flat, and raised pigmented areas of varying coloration, with a lighter area noted in the center of the lesion. The borders of the lesions are irregular. With a history of non-tender inguinal adenopathy on the same side as the lesion, a malignant melanoma with metastasis to the nodes is the most likely diagnosis. An excisional biopsy of this lesion reported it as an invasive superficial spreading melanoma.

Malignant melanomas derive from melanocytes. The incidence is increasing in the United States, which may in part be explained by an increase in outdoor recreational activities. It affects both sexes equally, is more common in whites than blacks, and has a predilection for fair-skinned, blue-eyed persons with red or blond hair. Exposure to excessive sunlight is the single most important predisposing cause of malignant melanomas. They may arise de novo, from a preexisting lesion (e.g., congenital nevus, dysplastic nevus), or from a lentigo maligna. Most variants have an initial radical growth phase that lasts for a few years to a decade or longer. During this phase, the malignant melanocytes proliferate laterally within the epidermis, dermoepidermal junction, or the papillary dermis. Metastasis does not occur while a malignant melanoma is in this phase. After a variable amount of time, they may enter a vertical growth phase, where the malignant melanocytes penetrate into the underlying reticular dermis. The appearance of a nodule along the lateral margin of the radial growth phase is a marker for the vertical phase. Superficial spreading melanoma is the most common type of melanoma. It primarily effects women over 50 years of age. The lower extremities and back are the favored locations. Lentigo maligna melanoma is an extension of a lentigo maligna. It primarily occurs on the sun-exposed face in elderly people. They have an irregular, mottled pigmentation. The radial growth phase continues for 10 to 15 years before entering a vertical growth phase. A nodular melanoma is a particularly agressive type that is more common in elderly men than women. It lacks a radial growth phase and invades into the dermis very early in its natural history. Acral lentiginous melanomas are the least common type of melanoma in the white population. However, it has an increased incidence in the Affrican-American population, who, as a rule, are not predisposed to melanomas by virtue of the protective effect of melanin against ultraviolet light. They primarily occur on the palms, soles, or subungual regions. Excisional biopsy is the recommendation for all suspicious lesions. The stage of the disease is the single most important prognostic factor. The Breslow system measures the depth of invasion from the outermost granular layer to the deepest margin of the tumor. In general, lesions with less than 0.76 mm of invasion do not metastasize, whereas those with more than 1.7 mm of invasion have lymph node metastasis. The Clark system uses levels of invasion from I to V. Level I is limited to the epidermis (in situ); level II is invasion into the papillary dermis; level III is where tumor impinges on the reticular dermis, which is a marker for the vertical growth phase; level IV refers to invasion of the reticular dermis without invasion of subcutaneous tissue; and level V is invasion of the subcutaneous fat. The overall 5-year survival rate is 81%. Nodular melanomas and acral lentiginous melanomas have the worst prognosis. Other factors influencing prognosis are (1) the mitotic rate, with decreased survival associated with increased mitoses; (2) the degree of lymphocytic response around the tumor, with less response indicating a poorer prognosis; (3) the location of the tumor, with melanomas on the extremities in general having a better prognosis than those on the head, neck or trunk; and (4) evidence of depigmentation in a previously pigmented area, which is a poor prognostic sign (present in this patient).

87. The answer is B.   *(Anatomy)*
At the wrist, the ulnar artery lies along the lateral border of the flexor carpi ulnaris tendon. The radial artery lies along the lateral border of the flexor carpi radialis tendon. The median nerve lies lateral to the flexor digitorum superficialis tendon and the palmaris longus tendon and medial to the flexor carpi radialis tendon.

88. The answer is D.   *(Pharmacology)*
Bronchodilation can be produced by both β_2-adrenoceptor agonists such as isoproterenol and muscarinic

antagonists such as atropine. Several organs have dual and opposing innervation from the parasympathetic and sympathetic nervous systems. In these organs, the effects of adrenoceptor agonists are the same as those of muscarinic antagonists (and muscarinic agonists have the same effects as adrenoceptor antagonists). Examples of such opposing innervation and corresponding drug effects can be observed in the iris, sinoatrial node, and bronchial smooth muscle. Clinically, bronchodilation is usually achieved with the use of selective β_2-agonists such as albuterol. Ipratropium, the isopropyl derivative of atropine, can be administered by aerosol and is a valuable agent for use in patients with chronic obstructive pulmonary disease.

89. The answer is D.   *(Anatomy)*
Among the proximal row of carpal bones, the scaphoid and the lunate articulate with the radius. The triquetrum articulate with the articular disk of the ulna. The pisiform is a sesamoid bone within the tendon of the flexor carpi ulnaris; it articulates with the triquetrum. The distal row of carpal bones (trapezium, trapezoid, capitate, and hamate) does not articulate with the bones of the forearm.

90. The answer is E.   *(Anatomy)*
Neither the cerebellum nor the basal ganglia (which includes the neostriatum, the substantia nigra, and the globus pallidus) gives rise to tracts that descend directly to the spinal cord. These areas modulate motor activity through feedback loops to the motor cortex. The reticular formation, on the other hand, does give rise to a descending tract that influences motor control (the reticulospinal tract).

91. The answer is C.   *(Anatomy)*
The radial nerve lies medial to the humerus as it leaves the axilla. At this point it may be damaged by a dislocation of the head of the humerus. The nerve then enters the musculospiral groove of the humerus. Here it may be damaged by a midshaft fracture of the humerus. The radial nerve crosses the elbow on the anterolateral surface in the interspace between the brachialis and the brachioradialis muscles. The radial nerve provides motor innervation to the extensor muscles of the arm and forearm and provides sensory innervation to the dorsal surface of the lateral portion

of the hand and the lateral $3\frac{1}{2}$ digits, except for the distal phalanx.

92. The answer is A.   *(Physiology)*
Normal physiologic control of motor function requires dopaminergic stimulation of the receptors on cells whose axons give rise to both pathways. Although the indirect pathway has D_2 receptors that are inhibited by dopamine, it requires a dopamine agonist to accomplish this. A D_1 agonist would not "stimulate" the indirect pathway, so this is not the best choice. Similarly, administration of a D_2 antagonist or a combination of a D_1 agonist and a D_2 antagonist would not be the best course of action. Both dopamine and L-dopa could stimulate both types of dopaminergic receptors. However, dopamine cannot cross the blood–brain barrier. Therefore, administration of an L-dopa precursor would be the best therapy for a patient with Parkinson's disease.

93. The answer is A.   *(Anatomy)*
The muscles responsible for keeping the pelvis level while standing on one foot are the gluteus medius and gluteus minimus muscles of the supporting side. These muscles are innervated by the superior gluteal nerve. In the Trendelenberg test, the patient stands on one foot. If the unsupported side of the pelvis drops, this indicates that the gluteus medius and gluteus minimus muscles of the supporting side are weak.

94. The answer is C.   *(Anatomy)*
Neurons from the temporal portions of the eyes do not cross at the optic chiasm, but neurons from the nasal portions do. The optic tract is beyond the optic chiasm. Therefore, the optic tract on the right side carries impulses on the uncrossed neurons coming from the temporal portion of the right eye plus impulses on the crossed neurons coming from the nasal portion of the left eye.

95. The answer is B.   *(Anatomy)*
The iliofemoral ligament (Y ligament of Bigelow) is an especially strong ligament that reinforces the anterior surface of the hip joint capsule. This ligament resists extension of the hip joint and can maintain the stability of the hip joint during erect posture without the action

of any of the muscles that cross the hip. The pubofemoral ligament is a less important ligament of the hip joint capsule that resists abduction of the hip. The ligament of the head of the femur serves as a pathway for the artery of the head of the femur to reach the head of the femur and has little, if any, mechanical effect on the hip joint. The sacrospinous and sacrotuberous ligaments are not part of the hip joint. They help to maintain the stability of the sacroiliac joint and form part of the boundary of the sciatic foramina.

96. The answer is C.   *(Pharmacology)*
All nonsteroidal antiinflammatory drugs and acetaminophen have antipyretic activity and may be used to counteract fever. Only aspirin inhibits platelet aggregation, exerts a significant antiinflammatory effect, and has been associated with Reye's syndrome. Only acetaminophen typically causes fatal hepatic necrosis after overdose.

97. The answer is D.   *(Anatomy)*
The medial meniscus of the knee is fused to the medial collateral ligament of the knee. In contrast, the lateral collateral ligament is not attached to the lateral meniscus. This attachment makes the medial meniscus less mobile than the lateral meniscus and more likely to be injured. The attachment of the medial meniscus to the medial collateral ligament accounts for the frequency with which these two structures are injured together. The common triad of knee injuries are tears of the medial meniscus, medial collateral ligament and anterior cruciate ligament.

98. The answer is B.   *(Pathology)*
A Wood's lamp generates 360 nm ultraviolet light, or black light, that causes certain types of skin lesions to fluoresce.

Pityriasis rosea is not an infectious disease and does not fluoresce with a Wood's lamp evaluation. This disorder is characterized by an initial "herald patch" on the trunk, followed days or weeks later by an eruption of rose-colored papules scattered along the lines of skin cleavage.

Tinea veriscolor produces hypopigmented or hyperpigmented skin lesions. *Malassezia furfur* is responsible for the disease and is located in the stratum corneum. The lesions fluoresce yellow, and potassium hydroxide scrapings reveal a "spaghetti-and-meatball" appearance of the hyphae and yeast, respectively. Topical selenium sulfide or clotrimazole are useful in therapy.

Corynebacterium minutissimum causes erythrasma, which is a patchy erythematous rash that has a red fluorescence with Wood's light. The bacteria are located in the stratum corneum. Erythromycin is the treatment of choice.

Tinea capitis refers to infection of the hair and scalp and is most common in children. The infection is caused by *Microsporum* or *Trichophyton* species but not *Epidermophyton* species, which are restricted to the skin. These infections are characterized by circular or ring-shaped patches of alopecia with erythema and scaling. Tinea capitis, caused by both *Microsporum canis* (most common overall cause) and *Microsporum audouinii*, is associated with yellow fluorescence with the Wood's lamp. The organisms infect the outer portion of the hair shaft (ectothrix) causing damage to the hair with breaking off of the hair at the level of the skin surface ("ink-dot" appearance). Micronized griseofulvin is the treatment of choice.

99. The answer is C. *(Anatomy)*
The posterior cruciate ligament attaches to the anterior portion of the medial femoral condyle and descends posteriorly and laterally to attach to the tibia. This ligament resists posterior displacement of the tibia and anterior displacement of the femur. The posterior "drawer sign" is an indication of a tear of the posterior cruciate ligament. The cruciate ligaments are within the fibrous capsule of the knee joint but are outside of the synovial cavity.

100. The answer is D. *(Microbiology)*
Staphylococcus epidermidis is a gram-positive, coagulase-negative, catalase-negative, novobiocin-sensitive bacterium. It is the most common infection involving prosthetic devices. Other infections include infective endocarditis in intravenous drug users, infection of intravenous peritoneal dialysis catheters and intracranial shunts, and urinary tract infections. Vancomycin is the drug of choice for *Staphylococcus epidermidis* infections. *Escherichia coli, Pseudomonas aeruginosa, Actinomyces israelii*, and *Streptococcus pyogenes* are not associated with any of the above infections.

101. The answer is D. *(Anatomy)*
The popliteus muscle arises from the lateral condyle of the femur and passes between the lateral collateral ligament and the lateral meniscus to insert on the posterior surface of the tibia. The muscle is innervated by the tibial nerve and assists in flexion of the knee. During the early phase of extension, the popliteus rotates the femur laterally, "unlocking" the knee.

102. The answer is A. *(Pathology)*
An enhanced computerized tomography (CT) scan of the brain in this patient shows hematogenous spread of infection from the heart to the brain with the formation of multiple cerebral abscesses. A spinal tap is unlikely in this case. However, if a spinal tap could be performed safely, it would reveal a normal glucose, a variable increase in white blood cells, an elevated protein, a normal chloride, and the absence of organisms on a Gram stain of the spun down sediment because the infection is not leptomeningeal. A cerebral abscess develops from an adjacent focus of infection (40%), most commonly nasal, mastoid sinus of middle ear in location or from a hematogenous spread from a patient with cyanotic congenital heart disease, infective endocarditis, or infection in the lung. Most cerebral abscesses are located in the frontal and parietal lobes. On a CT scan, these abscesses have characteristic ring-enhancing lesions, as described in this patient.

103. The answer is C. *(Anatomy)*
The median nerve does not innervate any muscles in the arm. The muscles responsible for flexion of the forearm at the elbow include the brachialis and biceps brachii (innervated by the musculocutaneous nerve) and the brachioradialis (innervated by the radial nerve). The median nerve provides sensory innervation to the palmar surface of the lateral $3\frac{1}{2}$ digits and the lateral portion of the palm. The major pronators (pronator teres and pronator quadratus), the thumb flexors (flexor pollicis longus and flexor pollicis brevis), and the opponens pollicis are innervated by the median nerve.

104. The answer is B. *(Pathology)*
A vegan diet is not detrimental to any of the host defenses in the gastrointestinal tract. In fact, the types of bacteria that develop in individuals with a pure

vegetable diet have considerable metabolic potential in breaking down possibly harmful metabolites that are present in food.

The alimentary tract has a number of protective mechanisms against microorganisms, which have to be overcome for the pathogen to gain access into the mucosa. Saliva has a flushing action in the mouth that mechanically removes bacteria from the mouth and a bactericidal property associated with lysozyme activity. Xerostomia (dry mouth), which is seen in Sjögren syndrome, predisposes to dental caries and periodontal disease. The acidity of gastric secretions impedes the transit of many organisms through the stomach. Most bacteria are acid sensitive and enjoy slightly alkaline conditions. Glycoproteins on the intestinal mucosal surface prevent bacterial adhesion. *Vibrio cholerae* produce a mucinase that helps them propel themselves through the mucus and attach to specific receptors on the intestinal epithelium. Hydrochloric acid in the stomach kills enveloped viruses. Acid-fast bacteria, such as *Mycobacterium tuberculosis*, are resistant to acid because of their high lipid content. The cysts of *Entameba histolytica* are also resistant to acid injury and excyst in the alkaline environment of the cecum, where they emit powerful necrotoxins that aid them in gaining entrance into the bowel wall.

Achlorhydria predisposes to infections caused by salmonella organisms and *Vibrio cholerae*. Antibiotic therapy often changes the flora of the bowel and favors the overgrowth of *Clostridium difficile*, which elaborates a powerful exotoxin responsible for pseudomembranous enterocolitis. Reduced motility of the small intestine predisposes to bacterial overgrowth. Secretory immunoglobulin A protects the gastrointestinal mucosa from viral, bacteria, and parasitic infections.

105. The answer is B.   (Pharmacology)
Although the precise mechanism by which gold compounds exert their antiarthritic effect is unknown, it is suspected that their suppression of leukocyte activity, including lysosomal enzymes, phagocytosis, and mediator release, is likely responsible for their therapeutic effects. Unlike nonsteroidal antiinflammatory drugs (NSAIDs), gold compounds do not inhibit cylooxygenase and prostaglandin synthesis.

106. The answer is E.   (Pathology)
Central nervous system (CNS) disease in AIDS is not associated with primary brain tumors of astrocyte origin, such as glioblastoma multiforme. These tumors are most commonly secondary B-cell malignant lymphomas of the non-Hodgkin's type that metastasize to the brain or, in 20% of cases, AIDS-associated primary CNS lymphomas. AIDS is considered the most common risk factor for primary malignant lymphomas of the brain. Primary lymphomas are frequently multifocal and usually involve the cerebral cortex, whereas metastatic lymphomas most commonly involve the leptomeninges.

Four syndromes in the central/peripheral nervous system have been ascribed to HIV. These include aseptic meningitis (resembling viral meningitis), subacute encephalitis associated with dementia (develops in 60% of patients), vacuolar myelopathy (20%–30%) within the spinal cord resembling the subacute combined degeneration of vitamin B_{12} deficiency, and peripheral neuropathy (95%) with demyelination resembling Guillain-Barré syndrome.

107. The answer is B.   (Behavioral science)
This patient probably has panic disorder. Panic attacks commonly occur twice per week with each attack lasting about 30 minutes. Patients with panic disorder are more likely to be female than male and most commonly are young adults. Mitral valve prolapse is found in up to 50% of panic disorder patients. For diagnostic purposes, panic attacks can be precipitated in the physician's office by carbon dioxide inhalation effected by breathing in and out of a paper bag or by infusion of sodium lactate.

108. The answer is C.   (Pathology)
The most likely diagnosis of this patient is Alzheimer disease (AD). AD is responsible for 55% of dementia cases that develop in either the presenile age bracket (less than 65) or the senile age bracket (greater than 65 years of age). AD is characterized by cerebral atrophy preferentially involving the frontal lobes with associated neuronal loss leading to dementia. Although the cause of AD is unknown, the following relationships have been implicated:

- neuronal toxicity of amyloid β-protein, which is derived from amyloid precursor protein coded for on chromosome 21

- reduced levels of choline acetyltransferase, an important catalyst for the synthesis of acetylcholine, an important learning agent
- high aluminum levels in the brain tissue
- inheritance of the APOEε4 allele, which is involved in lipid transport in the brain
- an autosomal-dominant inheritance pattern, particularly in those who present with disease in the fourth or fifth decade

The pathology of AD is not specific for the disease but includes:

- neurofibrillary tangles (silver stain positive tangles of neurofilaments containing an abnormal phosphorylated form of the microtubule protein tau and ubiquitin)
- senile plaques, which consist of a core of amyloid β-protein polymerized into fibrils that are surrounded by dystrophic neurites
- Hirano bodies, representing glassy eosinophilic inclusions found in neurons in the hippocampus
- granulovacuolar degeneration consisting of small, clear, intraneuronal cytoplasmic vacuoles with a silver positive inclusion
- decreased number of neurons in the nucleus basalis of Meynert cell (not the locus ceruleus)

The usual clinical course for AD is progressive dementia over the ensuing 5–10 years with total incapacitation and eventual death. Clinically, the disease is characterized by general impairment of higher intellectual functions in the absence of focal neurologic deficits. Loss of recent memory is one of the first signs of the disease. Similar to other types of dementia, AD is associated with behavioral disturbances [psychosis (30%), agitation (85%), and depression (10%–30%)—PAD].

109. The answer is E.   *(Pharmacology)*
Prednisone is a steroidal antiinflammatory agent with a rapid onset of action that has a limited role in the treatment of arthritis because chronic use of prednisone produces intolerable side effects. A number of slow-acting drugs have been used in patients with severe arthritis, with varying degrees of success. The considerable toxicity of these agents usually limits their use to those patients with severe and progressive illness.

The exact mechanism by which these drugs work remains uncertain. This class of drugs includes the gold compounds (auranofin), antimalarials (hydroxychloroquine), chelating agents (penicillamine), and the immunostimulant, levamisole.

110. The answer is D.   *(Pathology)*
The Sturge-Weber syndrome is a congenital abnormality characterized by:

1. benign cutaneous angiomas of the face ("port wine stain"), usually in the distribution of the trigeminal nerve
2. ipsilateral venous angiomatous masses involving the leptomeninges, with a potential for subarachnoid bleeds
3. mental retardation
4. epileptic seizures
5. calcific deposits in the leptomeninges with peculiar "railroad" calcifications visible on skull radiographs

Cerebellar hemangioblastoma and secondary polycythemia are associated with von Hippel-Lindau disease, which is an autosomal-dominant disease.

The Dandy-Walker syndrome consists of failure of development of the cerebellar vermis and obstruction of the fourth ventricle with subsequent development of the noncommunicating hydrocephalus.

Anencephaly is a defect in closure of the upper part of the neural tube associated with the elevation of α-fetoprotein (AFP). This disorder is the worst form of open neural tube defects and is usually associated with absence of the brain and fetal adrenal cortex, a frog-like appearance, and polyhydramnios (excess fluid in the amniotic sac) caused by leakage of spinal fluid into the amniotic fluid. Folic acid taken before pregnancy protects against the development of open neural tube defects.

Spina bifida refers to failure of the posterior vertebral arches to properly close, leaving an open defect for the meninges and spinal cord to protrude through the opening. In its mildest form, spina bifida occulta (10% of population), the defect is very small and marked by the presence of a dimple or tuck of hair in the overlying skin. A meningocele refers to spina bifida with associated protrusion of the meninges through the defect. A meningomyelocele refers to a spina bifida where the spinal cord is present in the defect, which results in severe neurologic deficits in the lower extremity, bladder, and rectum.

The Arnold-Chiari malformation is characterized by elongation of the medulla oblongata and cerebellar tonsils through the foremen magnum, a communicating hydrocephalus (50% of cases), flattening of the base of the skull (platybasia), an increased incidence of syringomyelia, and a meningomyelocele.

111. The answer is E. *(Anatomy)*
The tibial nerve is one of the components of the sciatic nerve. The other component is the common peroneal nerve. The tibial nerve innervates all of the muscles of the posterior compartment of the thigh except for the short head of the biceps femoris, which is innervated by the common peroneal nerve.

112. The answer is B. *(Pathology)*
Pityriasis rosea differs from tinea versicolor because it is not a fungal disease, whereas tinea versicolor is a superficial dermatophyte infection. Pityriasis rosea is an eruption that develops in children and young adults in the spring and fall. This disorder first presents a single, scaly, pink plaque on the trunk called a herald patch. Days to weeks later, there is an eruption of rose-colored papules that follow the lines of cleavage in a christmas-tree distribution.

Tinea versicolor is caused by infestation of the stratum corneum by *Malassezia furfur*, a superficial dermatophyte. Skin lesions may be hypo- or hyperpigmented. The lesions fluoresce yellow with Wood's light. Potassium hydroxide preparations of scrapings of superficial skin reveals the classic "spaghetti (hyphae)-and-meatball (yeast)" morphology. Topical antifungal therapy is curative.

113. The answer is E. *(Pharmacology)*
The earliest acid–base disturbance observed in patients following aspirin overdose is respiratory alkalosis secondary to centrally mediated hyperventilation. Respiratory alkalosis is gradually replaced by metabolic acidosis as serum salicylate levels increase. Higher levels are associated with coma, vasomotor collapse, and, finally, respiratory failure and death. Tinnitus and dizziness are early signs of aspirin toxicity and may even occur at the upper end of therapeutic serum levels. Aspirin toxicity is more likely, especially in the

elderly, because salicylate elimination processes are saturated at higher serum levels (zero-order kinetics).

114. The answer is B. *(Pathology)*
The skin cancer that is least likely to metastasize is a basal cell carcinoma (epithelioma). Skin cancers associated with ultraviolet light damage include basal call carcinoma (most common), squamous cell carcinoma, and malignant melanoma. A basal cell carcinoma (BCC) occurs primarily on sun-exposed, hair-bearing surfaces, located on the inner aspect of the nose, around the orbit, or on the upper lip. These locally aggressive, infiltrating cancers arise from the basal cell layer of the epidermis and infiltrate the underlying superficial dermis. BCCs rarely, if ever, metastasize. They appear as crateriform lesions, with the skin surface displaying numerous vascular channels. Microscopically, BCCs have cords of basophilic-staining cells infiltrating the dermis. Because they are multifocal, BCCs commonly recur if they are not totally excised. Basal cell nevus syndrome is an autosomal dominant disorder characterized by the development of BCCs early in life with associated abnormalities of bone, skin, nervous system, eyes, and ovaries.

Squamous cell carcinomas (SCC) of the skin are commonly located on the face and favor areas such as the ears, nose, and lower lip. Unlike BCCs, SCCs can develop on both exposed and nonexposed areas of the body, and they do have a small potential for metastasis, particularly if located on a mucosal surface. Predisposing conditions other than sunlight include arsenic poisoning, chronic ulcers or sinus tracts, chewing tobacco, radiation, burn scars, and patients who are immunocompromised. SCCs commonly present as a shallow ulcer with a raised edge that may resemble a BCC. The majority of SCCs are well-differentiated tumors.

Malignant melanomas derive from melanocytes, and all of them, regardless of type, have the potential to metastasize.

115. The answer is C. *(Behavioral science)*
Female children are less at risk than male children for alcoholism. Alcoholism is more common in the

children of alcoholics than in the children of nonalcoholics, and has a higher concordance rate in monozygotic than in dizygotic twins. Both genetic and envrionmental factors are involved in the etiology of alcoholism.

116. The answer is E.   (Pathology)

If not contraindicated, estrogen is the gold standard for the prevention of osteoporosis and should be given to all postmenopausal women. Other benefits include (1) a 35% to 50% reduction in the risk for death due to coronary artery disease, (2) a 25% reduction on risk for developing osteoporosis-related fractures (vertebral followed by Colles' fracture), (3) a reduction in vasomotor symptoms (flushing) related to menopause, and (4) decreased urinary urgency, incontinence, and frequency. Adding progestin protects against developing endometrial carcinoma; however, recent research suggests that it may increase the risk for breast carcinoma (1.25–2.0). Contraindications for estrogen include (1) pregnancy, (2) breast cancer (use of tamoxifen, a weak estrogen, in estrogen-positive cancers), (3) undiagnosed vaginal bleeding, (4) active thrombophlebitis, and (5) thromboembolic disorders previously associated with estrogens. Preventive measures that are prescribed along with estrogen are calcium supplementation, vitamin D, and weight-bearing exercise.

117. The answer is C.   (Anatomy)

Autonomic, or motor, ganglia contain multipolar neurons. Sensory ganglia, such as the dorsal root ganglion, contain unipolar neurons. Satellite cells are present in autonomic ganglia although they are not as plentiful as in the sensory ganglia, where they completely surround the neuron. Schwann, or sheath, cells enwrap the axon of the multipolar neurons, which conduct impulses to smooth and cardiac muscle and glands. Lipofuscin pigment is an age pigment that is seen frequently in ganglion neurons, especially motor ganglion neurons. Synaptic connections are made upon the motor ganglion cell body by preganglionic cell fibers. The reduction is satellite cells allows for passage of these potential synapses.

118. The answer is B.   (Behavioral science)

Use of heroin is not associated with increased aggressiveness. In contrast, cocaine, amphetamines, PCP,

and high doses of marijuana are associated with increased levels of aggressiveness.

119. The answer is D.   (Anatomy)

The extensor expansion is formed by the tendons of the extensor digitorum, the lumbricals, and the interosseous muscles. Lumbricals I through IV insert into the expansions of digits II through V respectively. The first dorsal interosseous muscle inserts into the expansion of digit II, the second and third insert into the expansion of digit III, and the fourth inserts into the expansion of digit IV. The three palmar interosseous muscles insert into the expansion of digits II, IV, and V. There is no palmar interosseous insertion into digit III.

120. The answer is A.   (Behavioral science)

Alcoholism is more common in European Americans than in Asian Americans, and it is more common in the Northeastern states. Of the children of alcoholics, sons are more vulnerable than daughters. The life expectancy of alcoholics is reduced by about 10 years.

121. The answer is B.   (Anatomy)

The popliteal fossa is a diamond-shaped area behind the knee. It is bounded inferiorly by the two heads of the gastrocnemius and superiorly by the biceps femoris and the semimembranosus. The floor of the fossa consists of the popliteal surface of the femur, the posterior surface of the knee joint capsule, and the popliteus muscle. The neurovascular contents of the fossa include the popliteal artery and vein and the tibial nerve.

122. The answer is E.   (Anatomy)

The genu of the internal capsule contains neuronal axons that distribute to the orofacial area. The question asks for localization of cells and fibers innervating the distal upper limb. This area is located in the posterior limb of the internal capsule. The crus cerebri contains all the descending motor axons innervating the brain stem and spinal cord motor centers (the corticobulbar and corticospinal tracts, respectively). The lateral hemispheres of the cerebellum are involved in coordination of the distal muscle groups of the limbs, including muscles in the hands. The cervical enlargement of the spinal cord contains the lower motor neurons that directly innervate the skeletal muscle of the distal upper extremity. The ventral anterior and ventral lateral nuclei of the thalamus are the site of convergence of the cerebellum and basal ganglion influence over motor systems to both the proximal and distal muscles of the limbs.

123. The answer is A.   *(Anatomy)*
The tendon of the flexor digitorum superficialis inserts on the middle phalanx immediately distal to the proximal interphalangeal joint. The tendon does not cross the distal interphalangeal joint and therefore cannot cause movement at this joint. The flexor digitorum profundus is responsible for flexion and the distal interphalangeal joint. The tendons of both the flexor digitorum superficialis and the flexor digitorum profundus cross the metacarpophalangeal joint, the midcarpal joint, and the radiocarpal joint; therefore, both muscles can cause flexion at these joints.

124. The answer is D.   *(Pharmacology)*
Opiates, such as morphine, do not act peripherally to block activation of pain receptors on primary afferent neurons or to inhibit the transmission of pain impulses to the spinal cord. Morphine is believed to act at supraspinal structures and in the spinal cord to inhibit transmission of pain impulses. The opiates activate receptors in the periaquaductal gray matter to activate descending inhibitory pathways. The descending inhibitory pathways lead to the release of enkephalins and serotonin at the spinal cord. These substances are inhibitory transmitters that block ascending pain impulses. The opiates also directly activate these spinal cord opiate receptors; this may be their most important mechanism of action. In the spinal cord, opiates act pre- and postsynaptically to block ascending pain impulses, possibly by inhibiting the release of substance P and other pain mediators.

125. The answer is E.   *(Gross anatomy)*
Many of the muscles of the gluteal region are external rotators of the hip. These muscles include the gluteus maximus, piriformis, obturator internus, obturator externus, quadratus femoris, superior gemellus, and inferior gemellus. The sartorius is a flexor and external

rotator of the hip. The gluteus minimus is an abductor and internal rotator of the hip.

126. The answer is A.   *(Behavioral science)*
Hypothermia is not a sign of acute opiate withdrawal. Signs of acute opiate withdrawal include fever and sweating, insomnia, piloerection, mydriasis, yawning, nausea, and diarrhea. The syndrome is said to resemble severe influenza. The symptoms are most severe approximately 2 days after discontinuation of the opiates and persist for up to 10 days, with some residual effects lasting several weeks. During the withdrawal period, addicts have an intense craving for opiates.

127. The answer is E.   *(Anatomy)*
The major extensors of the hip are the hamstring muscles. The hamstring muscles arise from the ischial tuberosity and occupy the posterior compartment of the thigh; they include the semimembranosus, semitendinosus, and the long head of the biceps femoris. The gluteus maximus muscle is used as an additional extensor of the hip when additional force is required, such as when climbing steps or rising from a chair. The short head of the biceps femoris arises from the femur and does not cross the hip. Therefore, it cannot extend the hip.

128. The answer is C.   *(Pharmacology)*
Pure opiate antagonists (e.g., naltrexone) and mixed agonist/antagonists (e.g., nalbuphine) can precipitate a withdrawal syndrome in opiate addicts. Naltrexone and naloxone are antagonists at mu, kappa, and delta opioid receptors, whereas nalbuphine and pentazocine are weak antagonists at mu receptors and agonists or partial agonists at delta and kappa receptors. The abstinence syndrome may be suppressed by administration of any full agonist such as morphine, methadone, or heroin. Clonidine, an α_2-adrenoceptor agonist, can suppress the syndrome, apparently by inhibiting activation of noradrenergic fibers in the locus ceruleus, a brain stem nucleus whose activity is suppressed by opiates and increased during the withdrawal syndrome.

129. The answer is C.   *(Anatomy)*
The trigeminal, or semilunar, ganglion is a sensory ganglion. Autonomic fibers distribute with the three

divisions of the trigeminal but are not truly parts of the nerve. The otic ganglion is found in the infratemporal fossa near the exit of the mandibular division of the trigeminal from the foramen ovale. It contains postganglionic neurons that stimulate the parotid gland. The small ciliary ganglion is found in the orbit between the optic nerve and the lateral rectus muscle. Parasympathetic fibers arise from neurons in this ganglion to control the sphincter pupillae muscle of the iris and the ciliary muscle of accommodation. The submandibular ganglion contains cell bodies for the secretory control of the submandibular and sublingual glands. The pterygopalatine ganglion lies in the pterygopalatine fossa and contains cell bodies that control glands in the nose and palate.

130. The answer is A. *(Physiology)*
In general, the parasympathetic nervous system causes contraction of smooth muscles, except the vascular smooth muscle and sphincters of the intestines and bladder. Atropine blocks parasympathetic activity to cause relaxation of most smooth muscles. The lower esophageal sphincter behaves physiologically as a sphincter but is anatomically composed of smooth muscle similar to that found in the body of the stomach and intestinal walls; therefore, administration of atropine causes the sphincter to relax and should be used with caution in patients with reflux esophagitis. Muscarinic agonists such as bethanechol cause contraction of this sphincter and are used in treating reflux esophagitis. Bronchial, intestinal, ciliary, and bladder smooth muscles are all contracted by parasympathetic stimulation and relaxed by atropine.

131. The answer is A. *(Anatomy)*
Age is associated with a decrease, not an increase, in the curvature of the lens. This decrease in curvature causes presbyopia and the need for reading glasses as people approach 45 years of age. In individuals older than 65 years of age, the lens usually develops some degree of opacity. The lens is suspended by zonule fibers attached to the ciliary body and is avascular. Contraction of the ciliary muscles increases its refractory power.

132. The answer is D. *(Physiology)*
There are no Renshaw cells at the neuromuscular junction. Renshaw cells inhibit motor neurons in the anterior gray horn of the spinal cord. Action potentials

on the alpha motor neuron release acetylcholine (ACh) from the axon terminal. The ACh diffuses across the synaptic cleft and stimulates nicotinic receptors on the muscle endplate, generating an action potential that causes contraction of the muscle fiber. Cholinergic receptors on the muscle endplate are cation channels.

133. The answer is B. *(Anatomy)*
All of the muscles of the anterior compartment of the leg are innervated by the deep peroneal neve. These include the tibialis anterior, peronus tertius, extensor hallucis longus, and extensor digitorum longus. The muscles of the lateral compartment of the leg, which include the peroneus longus and peroneus brevis, are innervated by the superficial peroneal nerve. The muscles of the anterior compartment are primarily dorsiflexors of the ankle. Therefore, a lesion of the deep peroneal nerve results in foot drop.

134. The answer is E. *(Pathology)*
A child living with a mother who has chronic hepatitis B (HBV) and who is negative for both HBe antigen (HBeAg) and HBV-DNA is not at great risk for developing hepatitis B because HBeAg and HBV-DNA are associated with infectivity. The mother is an example of a "healthy" carrier. However, the child is still a candidate for active immunization. People who are at high risk for developing HBV infections include prostitutes, health care workers who are exposed to blood and blood products, sexually active homosexuals or bisexuals, intravenous drug abusers who share dirty needles, any patient in a long-term facility, and heterosexuals who recently had a sexually transmitted disease.

135-138. The answers are: 135-D, 136-C, 137-E, 138-B. *(Pharmacology)*
Drugs can lower intraocular pressure either by reducing the formation of aqueous humor or increasing the outflow of aqueous humor.

Atropine and other muscarinic blockers can cause acute angle-closure glaucoma by relaxing the iris sphincter muscle (site B) so as to cause mydriasis. As the sphincter relaxes, it occludes the trabecular meshwork in patients with a narrow angle between the iris and cornea, leading to a precipitous rise in intraocular pressure.

Pilocarpine can be used to reduce intraocular pressure in patients with chronic open-angle glaucoma. Pilocarpine contracts the meridianal fibers of the ciliary muscle (site C), thereby increasing tension on the trabecular meshwork at the angle of the iris and cornea and opening the spaces through which aqueous humor drains into Schlemm's canal. Epinephrine reduces the intraocular pressure in patients with open-angle glaucoma, primarily by causing vasoconstriction and "decongestion" in the trabecular area so that aqueous humor drains out more easily. The end result is much the same as that obtained with pilocarpine.

Timolol, a β-adrenoceptor blocker, acts on the ciliary process (site A) to inhibit the production of aqueous humor, thereby lowering intraocular pressure.

Carbonic anhydrase inhibitors, such as acetazolamide, act to block the formation of bicarbonate required for aqueous humor secretion by the ciliary body (site A), thereby lowering intraocular pressure.

139-143. The answers are: 139-E, 140-D, 141-C, 142-A, 143-B. *(Anatomy)*
Dyscalculia, a problem with simple calculation, is associated with dysfunction of the dominant parietal lobe. Broca's aphasia, associated with damage to the dominant frontal lobe, is characterized by inability to speak, although understanding is intact. Patients suffering from Wernicke's aphasia cannot understand language. Wernicke's aphasia is associated with damage to the dominant temporal lobe. Damage to the nondominant parietal lobe would result in an inability to copy a simple drawing. Alexia, which is characterized by the inability to read what one has written, is associated with damage to the occipital lobe.

144-147. The answers are: 144-A, 145-E, 146-C, 147-D. *(Pharmacology)*
Uricosurics are drugs that increase uric acid excretion in the urine, thereby reducing serum uric acid levels. Sulfinpyrazone and probenecid, the currently available uricosuric drugs, are used in the chronic prevention of gout.

Today, the most frequently used drugs for acute gout are the potent nonsteroidal antiinflammatory drugs such as indomethacin. Indomethacin inhibits prostaglandin synthesis.

Allopurinol acts by inhibiting xanthine oxidase and uric acid synthesis. It also reduces serum uric acid levels and prevents gout.

Drugs for the treatment of acute gouty arthritis are directed at inhibition of the marked inflammatory reaction to uric acid deposition in the joints. Colchicine is the time-honored treatment, but produces considerable gastrointestinal toxicity and other adverse effects. Colchicine inhibits leukocyte migration and phagocytosis secondary to inhibition of tubulin polymerization.

148-152. The answers are: 148-B, 149-A, 150-C, 151-E, 152-D. *(Behavioral science)*
Schizotypal personality disorder is characterized by peculiar appearance and odd thought patterns and behavior. Schizoid personality disorder is characterized by a lifetime of social withdrawal and isolation. Paranoid personality disorder is characterized by suspiciousness and attribution of problems to others. Sensitivity to rejection and feelings of inferiority characterize avoidant personality disorder. Patients suffering from antisocial personality disorder display criminality and an inability to conform to social norms.

153-156. The answers are: 153-C, 154-A, 155-E, 156-B. *(Pharmacology)*
Chronic, high-dose therapy with glucocorticoids such as dexamethasone is associated with a number of adverse metabolic effects, including protein catabolism and muscle wasting as well as the redistribution of fat to the face and trunk.

β₂-Adrenoceptor agonists such as albuterol often cause skeletal muscle tremor as a result of activation of β₂ receptors in skeletal muscle.

Thioridazine can cause the neuroleptic malignant syndrome, characterized by muscle rigidity, fever, involuntary movements, and cardiovascular instability. The neuroleptic malignant syndrome is quite similar to malignant hyperthermia and is occasionally observed in patients receiving chronic medication for psychiatric disorders.

Genetically susceptible patients may experience a rare malignant hyperthermia when they are exposed to inhalational anesthetics such as halothane. This potentially lethal syndrome can be treated with dantrolene and other agents. Although ketamine may increase muscle tone, it has not been associated with malignant hyperthermia.

157-158. The answers are: 157-D, 158-A. *(Physiology)*
Micturition is initiated by relaxation of the external urethral sphincter and contraction of the detrusor muscle. Urinary retention may be caused by inadequate parasympathetic activity or excessive sympathetic activity. The sympathetic nervous system tends to promote urinary retention, partly by contracting the internal sphincter of the bladder. α_1-Adrenergic blockers such as terazosin may be used to increase bladder emptying in patients with incomplete voiding due to excessive sympathetic tone at the internal sphincter (site B). α_1-Receptors also mediate increased prostate gland tone that may contribute to urethral obstruction in patients with benign prostatic hypertrophy.

In patients with neurogenic urinary retention or urinary retention caused by anesthetics, bethanechol may be used to increased urination by activating muscarinic receptors and contracting the detrusor muscle (site A).

159-162. The answers are: 159-D, 160-A, 161-E, 162-B. *(Pharmacology)*
Cocaine inhibits the neuronal membrane transporter for catecholamines and prevents reuptake of norepinephrine, thereby increasing the synaptic concentration of norepinephrine and producing a sympathomimetic effect.

Guanethidine inhibits norepinephrine release, reducing the synaptic concentration of norepinephrine and producing a sympatholytic effect.

Methyltyrosine inhibits norepinephrine synthesis and has a sympatholytic effect.

Reserpine inhibits norepinephrine storage, producing a sympatholytic effect.

163-177. The answers are: 163-G, 164-D, 165-I, 166-B, 167-A, 168-B, 169-I, 170-G, 171-J, 172-D, 173-I, 174-C, 175-E, 176-H, 177-A. *(Anatomy)*
The basilar artery runs along the ventral surface of the pons and sends penetrating branches into the substance of the brain stem. A hemorrhage of this vessel

or its branches often produces bilateral neurologic deficits. The multiple crossing fibers of the pontine nuclei and the trapezoid body provide naturel planes for blood to follow across the midline, destroying structures bilaterally.

The indications from the history of the 42-year-old athletic man point to a lesion of the lateral medulla. The cluster of neurologic findings should always be noted and an attempt made to identify where neural structures might be clustered and lesioned, with a relatively small focal lesion destroying these anatomically juxtaposed structures:

Ataxia	Posterior Spinocerebellar tract
Loss of pain and temperature on left side of body	Spinothalamic tract (anterolateral system)
Numbness and paresthesia on right face	Spinal tract and nucleus of trigeminal
Horner's syndrome	Descending hypothalamic–sympathetic fibers in dorsal longitudinal fasciculus
Dizziness	Vestibular nuclei
Nausea	Dorsal motor nucleus of vagus; emetic centers

All of the structures provided in the table are clustered in the upper outer quadrant of the medulla; with a relatively small lesion, they could all be destroyed, producing specific neurologic deficits. Normal findings are important as well. The major ascending and descending systems found near the midline are functioning normally and are therefore out of the lesioned site.

It it important to find a link between findings affecting the body (motor and sensory) and deficits associated with cranial nerves. The cranial nerves can be the most helpful indicator of the level of the lesion. In the case of the 56-year-old woman who lost consciousness while swimming, the cranial nerve testing isolated a problem with the oculomotor nerve. The external strabismus was caused by the unopposed pull of the normally innervated lateral rectus muscle (abducens nerve) and the superior oblique muscle (trochlear nerve). These muscles acting in isolation from the oculomotor innervated muscles pull the eye downward and outward. Therefore, the diagnosis can be localized to the level of the midbrain where oculomotor nerve nuclei are located. The upper motor neuron paralysis is a result of a lesion of the corticospinal and corticobulbar tracts. Where are the oculomotor nerve and the descending motor system juxtaposed so that a focal lesion could affect both? The ventral aspect of the midbrain is the site of exit of oculomotor nerve fibers and the cerebral peduncles. In fact, the axons of both these nerve fiber systems interweave to travel to their designated targets. The extraocular muscle paralysis is on the opposite side from the upper motor neuron paralysis of the extremities because the exiting right oculomotor nerve innervates muscles on the same side as its origin. The corticospinal tract is not crossed at the midbrain, but crosses at the pyramidal decussation in the medulla, therefore if these fibers are lesioned in the midbrain on the right, their ultimate effect is going to be on neurons in the left side of the spinal cord innervating skeletal muscles on the left side. This is one example of an alternating hemiplegia. In the eye, the dilated pupil results from a loss of preganglionic parasympathetic innervation by the Edinger-Westphal nucleus component of the oculomotor nerve to the sphincter pupillae muscle.

The lesion in the 14-year-old patient involves the dorsal column nuclei and the spinal nucleus and tract of the trigeminal nerve. Both nuclei are innervated by sensory neurons coming from the same (ipsilateral) side of the body. The nucleus gracilis and nucleus cuneatus receive synapses from the dorsal root ganglion neurons ascending in the dorsal columns of the spinal cord (fasciculus gracilis and fasciculus cuneatus). This system carries the modalities of two-point touch discrimination, vibration, and conscious proprioception. The spinal nucleus and tract of the trigeminal nerve are the pain and temperature pathways from the face. The spinal nucleus of the trigeminal nerve receives input from cells in the trigeminal ganglion. Each nucleus represents the second neuron in the somatosensory pathway. The axons of the second neurons cross to the opposite side. If these nuclei are damaged, the symptoms would be on the same side as that of the nucleus that was damaged.

Another factor in determining the site of lesions is to think about where the ascending and descending systems decussate. If the decussation is at a specific site (in the case of the man who sought treatment because of difficulty using his hands is was the low medulla), a focal lesion at this site produces bilateral deficits. In this case, note that the medial lemniscus is lesioned and consists of the dorsal column–medial lemniscal fibers that have already crossed and the internal arcuate fibers, which are ipsilateral fibers crossing to the opposite side to form the medial lemniscus on the opposite side, are also lesioned. The result is a bilateral loss of two-point touch discrimination, vibration sensation, and conscious proprioception. The lesion in this case has also affected the right pyramids. The resulting upper motor neuron deficit is observed on the left side since this system crosses lower in the medulla to form the lateral corticospinal tract. Upper motor neuron paralysis is tested in the upper limb by rapid independent finger movements (pulp-to-pulp opposition of individual digits in rapid succession), which are exclusively corticospinal movements. The Babinski reflex is an abnormal dorsiflexion that occurs when the sole of the foot is stroked. A normal response in humans over the age of 2 is planter flexion. Clonus is alternating flexion and extension of muscle groups, in this case, around the ankle, and is usually elicited by the examiner.

The posterior spinal arteries are paired and run along the dorsal surface of the low medulla and spinal cord. They arise from the vertebral arteries. Before reaching the spinal cord proper, where their distribution is augmented by radicular branches of the aorta, they supply the dorsal portion of the medulla. An occlusion of one of these posterior spinal arteries could produce the lesioned area shown in figure B.

The posterior cerebral arteries are paired and are the terminal branches of the vertebro-basilar system. The posterior cerebral vessel branches from the basilar artery at the level of the midbrain and travels along the lateral surface of the cerebral peduncles to reach the inferior and lateral surfaces of the temporal and occipital lobes of the cerebrum. In passing around the midbrain, the posterior cerebral arteries send penetrating branches into the midbrain. Here, penetrating branches from the right posterior cerebral artery either hemorrhaged or were occluded, producing the lesion shown and affecting the exiting fibers of the oculomotor nerve and the descending motor fibers in the cerebral peduncles.

The severe brain-stem lesion in the woman who had the very difficult delivery is referred to as the locked-in syndrome. Note that the patient is completely alert and aware of her surroundings. This lesion in the ventral pons spares all areas of the ascending reticular activating systems in the pons and midbrain. The quadriplegia results from a loss of all descending fibers in the ventral pons headed for spinal cord motor centers via the corticospinal pathway. Breathing is often difficult due to paralysis of laryngeal muscles that maintain the airway. The nucleus ambiguous loses its descending input. The patient is unable to talk (form words) because both hypoglossal nuclei have been denervated from their descending corticobulbar input. Upward movement of the eyes is retained because the oculomotor nucleus and nerve are above the level of this lesion. However, lateral gaze is paralyzed because the abducens nerve and nuclei are denervated.

Finding the pinealoma is a major hint in finding the cause of the impairment in the man who had headaches and eye pressure because the pineal gland is a formation of the epithalamus and overhangs the midbrain and superior colliculus. Enlargement of the gland compresses the superior colliculi, affecting the processing of visual input to the colliculus and affecting certain visual reflex mechanisms. Specifically, upward gaze when following an object and appropriate response to light stimuli are affected. Physical compression of the colliculi is translated into compression of the cerebral aqueduct (Sylvian), which affects the normal flow of cerebrospinal fluid through the ventricles. The third ventricle and the lateral ventricles enlarge due to this restricted flow—an example of a noncommunicating hydrocephalus.

The upper outer quadrant of the medulla, if lesioned, produces a constellation of neurologic deficits called either the lateral medullary syndrome or Wallenberg's syndrome. The posterior inferior cerebellar artery (PICA) supplies this area of the medulla with penetrating branches as the PICA travels to the cerebellum. The organization of the vascular supply essentially defines this area. Long circumferential branches specifically of the posterior inferior cerebellar artery supply the territory outlined by this lesion. Occlusion of this vessel, or sometimes occlusion of the vertebral artery, produces the most obvious neurologic findings due to compromise of the distribution of this vessel. The constellation of neurologic deficits includes nausea, vertigo, ataxia, Horner's syndrome, dysphagia, anesthesia of face ipsilaterally, and loss of pain and temperature sensations from areas of the body contralateral to the lesion.

Weber's syndrome is an alternating hemiplegia affecting the oculomotor nerve on one side and causing upper motor neuron paralysis of the extremities on the opposite side. The combination of the cranial nerve and the descending motor system suggests the level of the lesion. Oculomotor nerve fibers exit the ventral midbrain by passing through the cerebral peduncles and into the interpeduncular fossa. The cranial nerve lesion affects the structures on the ipsilateral side, whereas the descending motor fibers cross to the opposite side at lower brain-stem levels and therefore have their ultimate effect on skeletal muscle innervation on the opposite side.

The patient with paralysis of the tongue has an alternating hemiplegia that involves the cranial nerve. The hypoglossal nerve exits the ventral surface of the medulla to innervate the ipsilateral half of the tongue; that is, the right hypoglossal nerve innervates the right half of the tongue. The genioglossus muscles are attached on the midline, and the left and right genioglossus muscles normally function as a unit. In protruding the tongue, both genioglossus muscles have vectors that point toward the opposite side. If both muscles are functioning normally, the vectors cancel and the tip of the tongue protrudes on the midline. With paralysis of one half, the vectors do not cancel, and the tongue continues to point toward the opposite side. The rule is that the tongue points toward the side of the lesion in cases of hypoglossal nerve lesions. The upper motor neuron deficits result from lesions of the pyramids and are found on the opposite side to the hypoglossal nerve paralysis. When lesions include the midline above the pyramids, the medial lemniscus is affected. The dorsal column–medial lemniscus system has already decussated in the low medulla, and these fibers are carrying sensory modalities from the opposite side of the body. Note that negative findings are carried in systems that reside in the lateral aspects of the brain stem and also help to narrow the selection of lesion sites.

The 85-year-old woman with hypertension has findings that are classical upper motor neuron deficits and they are present bilaterally. Cranial nerve testing was normal. The choice in real life is either spinal cord or low medulla. The only choice here is that both pyramids are affected in lesion E. Note that the corticospinal tracts are closest together on the midline in the low medulla and through the decussation at the transition from medulla to spinal cord. This decussation of the corticospinal tract occurs within about 2-3 cm longitudinally. A focal lesion here can produce widespread bilateral upper motor neuron effects. In the spinal cord the lateral corticospinal tracts are in the lateral funiculi and distant from each other. The likelihood of only those paths being lesioned in the spinal cord is remote.

The presentation and examination of the construction worker who was hit on the head with a steel beam indicate that the sixth and seventh cranial nerves are involved. The medial strabismus is due to the paralyzed lateral rectus muscle as a result of the abducens nerve lesion. The muscle asymmetry is due to a lower motor neuron deficit of the muscles of facial expression. Note that the whole side of the face is affected, indicating a seventh nerve lower motor neuron lesion as opposed to an upper motor neuron lesion, which would affect only the lower muscles of the face. Both the sixth and seventh cranial nerves are located in the pons. Pain and temperature are affected because of the spinothalamic tract coursing through the outer half of the pons. This pathway is crossed; therefore, the sensory loss would be opposite the cranial nerve involvement. The upper motor neuron paralysis is on the opposite side because this lesion affects the descending pyramidal system in the pons before the decussation in the medulla. The Millard-Gubler syndrome is characterized by an alternating hemiplegia affecting the ipsilateral sixth and seventh cranial nerves. An upper motor neuron syndrome affects skeletal muscles on the contralateral side of the lesion. In reviewing these cases and syndromes, note that each is a template of brain-stem lesions and associated syndromes. Patients may fit these templates very closely, or they may show only some of the deficits. For example, some patients may have a paralysis

of the sixth and seventh cranial nerves, but the upper motor neuron paralysis—although on the opposite side—may affect only the upper limb. In such a case, the lesion (e.g., infarct from ischemia, tumor, abscess) has not completely infiltrated the ventral pons, and some of the descending fibers are spared. However, the lesion is still located in the outer lower quadrant of the pons and is a variant of the Millard-Gubler syndrome. By the nature of the central nervous system, no two patients will ever present with identical tumor, vascular, or demyelination disease affecting the cranial nerves and the ascending and descending systems. However, localization is critical, especially to monitor the progression of a neurologically related disease or to evaluate the permanency of a particular deficit for assistance in planning the appropriate lifestyle alternatives.

The blood supply to the medulla is derived from penetrating branches of the anterior spinal artery. The anterior spinal artery, which is formed by branches from the vertebral arteries. The inferior and midline zones of the medulla, up to the ponto-medullary junction, are supplied by these vessels. In this review, therefore, infarctions represented in figures C and E would be produced by occlusion of these vessels.

178-180. The answers are: 178-E, 179-D, 180-B. *(Pharmacology)*
Activation of the parasympathetic division of the third cranial (oculomotor) nerve serves to contract the iris sphincter and ciliary muscles, thereby causing miosis and accommodation for near vision. Pilocarpine activates muscarinic receptors in these tissues to cause miosis and accommodation, whereas atropine blocks both of these effects, leading to mydriasis and cycloplegia.

The sympathetic nervous system activates the dilator muscle of the iris, leading to mydriasis, but the sympathetic nervous system has little effect on accommodation (there is a slight relaxation of the ciliary muscle mediated by β_2 receptors). Phenylephrine activates α_1 receptors in the dilator muscle to cause mydriasis without cycloplegia.

Test 4

QUESTIONS

DIRECTIONS:

Each of the numbered items or incomplete statements in this section is followed by answers or by completions of the statement. Select the ONE lettered answer or completion that is BEST in each case.

1. An 88-year-old man has developed progressive weakness in and loss of sensation from both lower extremities. The resulting generalized loss of bladder and rectal control has caused him to become socially debilitated. Cranial nerve and upper limb innervation are within normal range for an individual of this age. The neurological workup shows impairment below the T1 to T3 spinal cord segments. Previous tests have ruled out lesions in the cerebral cortex and brain stem, and no mass or space-occupying lesions were found in the vertebral canal. Noted in the history and physical exam was hypertension and progressive atherosclerosis (producing vascular occlusion). The most likely explanation for this patient's findings is

(A) occlusion of the posterior spinal arteries
(B) breakdown in the tenuous radicular artery distribution at this level
(C) absence of anterior spinal arteries from vertebral arteries
(D) vertebro-basilar insufficiency
(E) drug toxicity

2. Which of the following is more likely to be associated with osteomalacia than with osteoporosis?

(A) Aluminum in dialysate solutions
(B) Chronic metabolic acidosis
(C) Space travel
(D) Long-term corticosteroid therapy
(E) Heparin

3. Both physostigmine and bethanechol

(A) increase acetylcholine concentration at cholinergic synapses
(B) increase skeletal muscle tone
(C) produce miosis
(D) relax the detrusor muscle
(E) activate nicotinic receptors at the autonomic ganglia

4. The best test to evaluate a patient for osteoporosis is

(A) routine bone radiographs
(B) dual photon absorptiometry
(C) serum calcium and phosphorus
(D) a bone marrow biopsy
(E) radionuclide bone scans

5. Which one of the following retinal cells undergoes an action potential when stimulated?

(A) Ganglion cell
(B) Bipolar cell
(C) Horizontal cell
(D) Photoreceptor cell
(E) Postganglion cell

6. A 45-year-old man with bilateral palmar erythema has contraction of the fourth and fifth fingers associated with a thick band of tissue that is palpable on drawing the examining finger across the right palm. The latter finding is most closely associated with

(A) rheumatoid arthritis
(B) a fibromatosis
(C) hyperestrinism
(D) a neoplasm involving fibroblasts
(E) Gardner syndrome

7. A patient presents to the clinic with eyelid ptosis and low hand grip strength. A test dose of edrophonium produces further loss of facial muscle tone and increased muscle weakness. The most probable conclusion is that

(A) the patient does not have myasthenia gravis
(B) the patient most likely has muscular dystrophy
(C) the patient is in "cholinergic crisis"
(D) the muscle weakness can be reversed with larger doses of neostigmine
(E) atropine should be given to reverse the muscle weakness

8.   A 32-year-old woman is pregnant with her fourth child. She notes a mass in the anterior portion of her abdominal wall. A biopsy reveals a nonencapsulated, infiltrating, fibroblastic process with no evidence of atypical mitotic spindles. It appears to have its origin from the musculoaponeurotic wall. The pathogenesis of this lesion is in the same category of disease as

(A) malignant fibrous histiocytoma
(B) fibromatosis colli
(C) fibrosarcoma
(D) a leiomyoma
(E) a keloid

9.   An infection in the synovial sheath of the flexor pollicis longus is most likely to spread to the

(A) flexor synovial sheath the of second digit
(B) flexor synovial sheath of the third digit
(C) flexor synovial sheath of the fourth digit
(D) flexor synovial sheath of the fifth digit
(E) synovial sheath of the flexor carpi radialis

10. The most common benign tumor in women is also the most common benign tumor in the gastrointestinal tract. This tumor most likely originates from

(A) adipose tissue
(B) bone
(C) smooth muscle
(D) endothelium
(E) Schwann cells

11. Acetylcysteine is used in the treatment of acetaminophen toxicity because acetylcysteine

(A) reduces the viscosity of pulmonary secretions
(B) increases the renal excretion of acetaminophen
(C) accelerates conversion of acetaminophen to its acetylated metabolite
(D) promotes catabolism of the toxic metabolite of acetaminophen
(E) exerts a cytoprotective effect on tissues which might be damaged by acetaminophen

12. Angiomyolipomas are frequently associated with an autosomal dominant disease, which is also associated with a neoplasm in the

(A) stomach
(B) heart
(C) peripheral nerve
(D) frontal lobe
(E) eighth cranial nerve

13. Presbycusis results from degenerative changes and loss of supportive cells, hair cells, and ganglion cells in the base of the cochlea. Which of the following is the MOST LIKELY to occur in this condition?

(A) Loss of sensitivity to high-frequency sounds
(B) Loss of sensitivity to low-frequency sounds
(C) Loss of sensitivity to angular acceleration
(D) Loss of sensitivity to linear acceleration
(E) Nystagmus

14. Nail infections and an association with polyendocrinopathy syndromes characterize infection due to

(A) *Trichophyton* species
(B) *Microsporum* species
(C) *Candida albicans*
(D) *Staphylococcus aureus*
(E) *Herpes simplex*

Questions 15-19

For each of the numbered descriptions of poisoning, select the causative substance from column I and the appropriate antidote or treatment from column II.

	I		II
A.	Amitriptyline	I.	Ethanol, hemodialysis
B.	Heroin	J.	Activated charcoal, sodium bicarbonate
C.	Acetaminophen	K.	Atropine, pralidoxime
D.	Ethylene glycol	L.	Naltrexone
E.	Parathion	M.	Diazepam, bicarbonate
F.	Aspirin	N.	Deferoxamine
G.	Ferrous sulfate	O.	Acetylcysteine
H.	Methanol		

15. Paramedics were called to attend a comatose and cyanotic young man who was found in the streets with a respiratory rate of 4/min, 3-mm pupils, and needle marks on his forearms.

(A) A-M
(B) H-O
(C) B-L
(D) E-K
(E) B-O

16. A 36-year-old man was brought by coworkers to the emergency room, where he was found to be restless, confused, and cyanotic with labored breathing. He had 2-mm pupils and was markedly salivating and lacrimating. He subsequently exhibited urinary incontinence and defecated.

(A) G-N
(B) F-M
(C) D-L
(D) A-K
(E) E-K

17. A young woman came to the emergency room complaining of nausea, vomiting, abdominal pain, and tinnitus. She was diaphoretic and displayed tachypnea. A urine ferric chloride test was positive, and blood gas studies showed a mixed respiratory alkalosis and metabolic acidosis.

(A) F-J
(B) H-K
(C) B-M
(D) A-O
(E) C-L

18. A young man presents to the emergency room with nausea, vomiting, malaise, and diaphoresis. He has been treating himself for 3 days to relieve severe discomfort from a neck injury. His physical exam is otherwise normal, but laboratory studies reveal markedly elevated serum transaminases.

(A) F-J
(B) B-L
(C) A-K
(D) C-O
(E) G-N

19. A man is brought to the emergency room after ingesting an unknown substance in an attempt to kill himself. He was mildly agitated, but the physical exam was unremarkable. Laboratory studies revealed a severe metabolic acidosis with an anion gap of 37 mEq/L and an osmolar gap of 28 mosm/L. His urine was brightly fluorescent and contained oxalate crystals.

(A) F-M
(B) C-M
(C) D-I
(D) E-K
(E) H-I

20. Which of the following pathogens is more likely to produce fever, rash, and neurologic abnormalities rather than bone or joint diseases?

(A) *Treponema pallidum*
(B) *Salmonella* species
(C) Parvovirus
(D) Rubella
(E) *Borrelia recurrentis*

21. In which of the following subtypes of schizophrenia are delusions of persecution most characteristic?

(A) Disorganized
(B) Catatonic
(C) Paranoid
(D) Undifferentiated
(E) Residual

22. A 32-year-old woman who recently moved from the Northeast to the Midwest presents with fever, headache, myalgias, and arthralgias. Physical exam reveals an erythematous rash arranged in concentric circles on her right leg. Which of the following questions would most likely shed light on the etiology of this patient's disease?

(A) Have you had any recent exposure to ticks?
(B) Have you had a sore throat recently?
(C) Have you ever had infectious mononucleosis?
(D) Is there any history of rheumatoid arthritis in your family?
(E) Have you ever had rheumatic fever?

23. On equilibrium receptor cells in the ear, the bending of the sterocilia and kinocilium toward the side of the cell having the kinocilium causes

(A) hyperpolarization and an increase in the release of neurotransmitter
(B) hyperpolarization and a decrease in the release of neurotransmitter
(C) hyperpolarization and no change in the release of neurotransmitter
(D) depolarization and an increase in the release of neurotransmitter
(E) depolarization and a decrease in the release of neurotransmitter

24. Which one of the following statements best distinguishes type I from type II muscle fibers?

(A) Type I muscle fibers are rich in glycogen
(B) Type I muscle fibers are rich in mitochondria
(C) Type I muscle fibers function best in anaerobic exercise conditions
(D) Type I muscle fibers are the dominant fiber in the biceps muscle
(E) Type I muscle fibers hypertrophy with exercise

25. The anterior recess of the ischiorectal fossa is between the

(A) superior and inferior fascia of the pelvic diaphragm
(B) inferior fascia of the pelvic diaphragm and the superior fascia of the urogenital diaphragm
(C) superior and inferior fascia of the urogenital diaphragm
(D) inferior fascia of the urogenital diaphragm and Colles fascia
(E) inferior fascia of the pelvic diaphragm and the obturator internus fascia

26. A 42-year-old man with frontal balding and wasting of the facial muscles is noted to have difficulty in releasing his grip after a handshake. An additional finding to expect is

(A) improvement in muscle function after a Tensilon test
(B) autoantibodies against acetylcholine receptors
(C) testicular atrophy
(D) an autosomal recessive pattern of inheritance
(E) a dislocated lens

27. Spasticity is

(A) another name for rigidity
(B) a common symptom of Parkinson's disease
(C) a condition exhibiting hypotonus
(D) a velocity-dependent resistance to passive movement of antigravity muscles
(E) a condition produced by lesions in the medial lemniscus

28. A peripheral neuropathy associated with demyelination rather than axonal degeneration is most likely associated with

(A) lead poisoning
(B) ethanol
(C) diphtheria toxin
(D) organophosphate esters
(E) vincristine

29. A 70-year-old woman who has had a stroke cannot identify a camouflaged object in a picture. The part of her brain that is injured is most likely to be the

(A) temporal lobe
(B) frontal lobe
(C) parietal lobe
(D) occipital lobe
(E) cerebellum

30. A 26-year-old man, who recently had an acute influenza-like illness, presents with ascending muscle weakness that began in the lower extremities. The deep-tendon reflexes in the lower extremities are absent. A spinal tap would be expected to reveal

(A) an increased cell count composed primarily of neutrophils
(B) low glucose
(C) increased protein with oligoclonal bands on high-resolution electrophoresis
(D) increased pressure
(E) positive syphilis serology

31. Which one of the following statements about gamma motor neurons is true?

(A) They are stimulated by 1a afferents
(B) They are inhibited by 1a afferents
(C) They are inhibited by descending motor tracts
(D) They are inhibited by afferents by Golgi tendon organs
(E) They are located in the posterior horn of the spinal cord

32. A 33-year-old man with neurofibromatosis complains of tinnitus and some hearing loss in his right ear. There is no history of vertigo or trauma to the ear. His Weber test lateralizes to the left ear, and the Rinne test exhibits air conduction longer than bone conduction in both ears. The patient probably has

(A) an acoustic neuroma involving the eighth nerve on his right side
(B) Meniere disease involving his right ear
(C) otosclerosis involving the right ear
(D) a glomus jugulare tumor beneath the floor of the right middle ear
(E) early development of prebycusis involving the right ear

33. Which structure includes the inguinal ligament?

(A) Anterior rectus sheath
(B) External oblique aponeurosis
(C) Transversus abdominis aponeurosis
(D) Iliacus tendon
(E) Internal oblique aponeurosis

34. Sequestrum and involucrum describe a disease in children that is primarily located in the

(A) joint space
(B) epiphysis of bone
(C) metaphysis of bone
(D) diaphysis of bone
(E) cortical surface of bone

35. What would be the effect on the smooth muscle of the airways in an asthmatic given a drug that inhibits the enzyme phosphodiesterase?

(A) Relaxation due to an increase in cyclic adenosine monophosphate (cAMP)
(B) Constriction due to an increase in cAMP
(C) Relaxation due to a decrease in cAMP
(D) Constriction due to a decrease in cAMP
(E) Constriction but no change in cAMP

36. Which of the following histologic findings matches the associated description?

(A) Langerhans cells—has an immune function in the skin
(B) Rete ridge hyperplasia—classic feature of lichen sclerosis et atrophicus
(C) Acanthosis—most commonly secondary to spongiosis
(D) Acantholysis—associated with ichthyosis vulgaris
(E) Macule—raised, colored lesion on the epidermis

37. Manic patients commonly show

(A) good judgment
(B) grandiosity
(C) psychomotor retardation
(D) lack of energy
(E) excessively sleepiness

38. In the differential list for a malignant small round cell tumor involving bone, which of the following small round cell malignancies is also associated with hypertension?

(A) Ewing sarcoma
(B) Burkitt lymphoma
(C) Small cell carcinoma of lung
(D) Neuroblastoma
(E) Acute lymphoblastic leukemia

39. Which of the following is MOST LIKELY to be found in the muscles of a patient with spasticity caused by an upper motor neuron lesion, such as damage to descending motor tracts?

(A) Atrophy
(B) Increased muscle tone
(C) Paresthesia
(D) Less active stretch reflexes
(E) Fasciculations

40. Which one of the following descriptions about bone is true?

(A) Bone is composed of type III collagen
(B) Osteoclasts operate independently of osteoblasts
(C) Osteoblasts differentiate into osteoclasts
(D) Osteoblasts primarily have receptors for hormones and cytokines
(E) Woven rather than lamellar bone is the normal, structurally stronger bone

41. During an examination of a patient, the physician notices that the patient's right knee is fully extended and locked during the right midstance phase of gait. This locking suggests a lesion of the

(A) right sciatic nerve
(B) right tibial nerve
(C) right obturator nerve
(D) right deep peroneal nerve
(E) right femoral nerve

42. Osteoblasts play a dominant role in

(A) osteopetrosis
(B) the early phase of Paget disease
(C) bone lesions in multiple myeloma
(D) bone disease in primary hyperparathyroidism
(E) bone lesions in prostate cancer

43. Damage to the basal ganglia can produce a variety of motor disturbances. Some, such as Parkinson's disease, produce hypokinesia; others, such as Huntington's chorea, produce hyperkinesia. Which one of the following BEST describes the effects of a drug on these conditions?

(A) Cholinergic agonists exacerbate hyperkinetic disorders and alleviate hypokinetic disorders
(B) Dopaminergic agonists exacerbate hyperkinetic disorders and alleviate hypokinetic disorders
(C) Cholinergic agonists exacerbate hyperkinetic disorders, and dopaminergic agonists exacerbate hypokinetic disorders
(D) Dopaminergic agonists alleviate hyperkinetic disorders, and cholinergic agonists alleviate hypokinetic disorders
(E) Dopaminergic agonists alleviate hyperkinetic disorders, and cholinergic agonists exacerbate hyperkinetic disorders

44. Which of the following lesions most closely resembles the clinical and microscopic features of Kaposi sarcoma?

(A) Molluscum contagiosum
(B) Bacillary angiomatosis
(C) Seborrheic dermatitits
(D) Dermatofibrosarcoma protuberans
(E) Dermatofibroma

45. During an examination of a patient, the physician notices that the patient enters the right stance phase of gait with a toe strike. This action suggests a lesion of the

(A) right superficial peroneal nerve
(B) right deep peroneal nerve
(C) right tibial nerve
(D) right femoral nerve
(E) right obturator nerve

46. A 1-year-old boy has a scaly eruption on the trunk and scalp, hepatosplenomegaly, generalized lymphadenopathy, and osteolytic lesions in the skull. A biopsy of skin reveals a dermal infiltrate composed of large cells with indented nuclei and foamy cytoplasm. The cells are CD1 antigen-positive. The cells most likely represent

(A) neutrophils
(B) lymphocytes
(C) natural killer cells
(D) histiocytes
(E) melanocytes

47. Which of the following adrenergic receptors produce(s) its effect by increasing intracellular levels of cyclic adenosine monophosphate (cAMP)?

(A) α_1, α_2, β_1 and β_2 receptors
(B) α_2, β_1 and β_2 receptors
(C) β_1 and β_2 receptors
(D) Only β_1 receptors
(E) α_1 and α_2 receptors

48. A 58-year-old man has numerous, raised, erythematous plaques and nodules with focal areas of necrosis. A biopsy reveals a band-like infiltrate of atypical, irregularly contoured lymphocytes, some of which are located in small pockets within the epidermis. Marker studies of these cells would identify them as

(A) CD4 helper T cells
(B) CD8 suppressor/cytotoxic T cells
(C) natural killer cells
(D) histiocytes
(E) melanocytes

49. During an examination of a patient, the physician notices that the patient displaces his shoulders posteriorly at right heel strike. This displacement suggests a paralysis or paresis of the

(A) right gluteus maximus muscle
(B) right gluteus medius muscle
(C) right quadriceps femoris muscle
(D) right tibialis anterior muscle
(E) right gastrocnemius muscle

50. A 23-year-old man has pruritic dermatitis in the intertriginous areas of his second and third left fingers. The pathogen responsible for this finding is most likely

(A) a mite
(B) a louse
(C) a *Leishmania* species
(D) *Trichinella spiralis*
(E) an *Ancylostoma* species

51. Changing the focus of the eye from far to near vision involves which of the following?

(A) Dilation of the pupil
(B) Contraction of the ciliary muscles
(C) Divergence of the eyeballs
(D) All of the above
(E) None of the above

52. Which of the following statements concerning poisonous reptiles is correct?

(A) Pit vipers include the coral snake and the Gila monster
(B) Pit vipers envenomate into the wound whenever they strike an individual
(C) Pit vipers have an acute sense of hearing, which helps localize their prey
(D) "Red and yellow kill a fellow, red and black, friend of Jack" is the mnemonic that separates a coral snake from a scarlet kingsnake, respectively
(E) The treatment of pit viper bites is enhanced by applying a tight tourniquet above the envenomation site and putting ice on the envenomation site

53. The spinal nerve that provides cutaneous branches to the skin around the umbilicus is

(A) T_8
(B) T_{10}
(C) T_{12}
(D) L_2
(E) L_4

54. Which of the following disorders would most likely explain blurry vision in a child with a recent onset of polyuria, polydipsia, and weight loss?

(A) Cataracts
(B) Retinoblastoma
(C) Refractive error
(D) Amblyopia
(E) Retinal hemorrhages

55. Most of the levator ani muscle has its origin on the arcus tendineus. The arcus tendineus is a thickening of the fascia covering the

(A) psoas major
(B) iliacus
(C) coccygeus
(D) piriformis
(E) obturator internus

56. Most patients over 40 years of age with Down syndrome develop neuropathologic changes characteristic of

(A) lower motor neuron disease
(B) upper motor neuron disease
(C) stroke, secondary to essential hypertension
(D) Alzheimer disease
(E) ischemic encephalopathy

57. The skeletal muscle innervated by the glossopharyngeal nerve is the

(A) styloglossus
(B) stylohyoid
(C) stylopharyngeus
(D) posterior belly of the digastric
(E) palatoglossus

58. A 22-year-old military recruit has fever, nuchal rigidity, and generalized palpable petechial lesions. A spinal tap reveals increased protein, decreased glucose, and an increased white blood cell count, predominantly with neutrophils. The Gram stain would most likely reveal

(A) thin gram-negative coccobacilli
(B) gram-positive diplococci
(C) fat gram-negative rods
(D) gram-negative diplococci
(E) gram-positive cocci in chains

59. Which spinal cord tract receives the cells in the dorsal nucleus of Clarke?

(A) Anterolateral tract
(B) Dorsal column–medial lemniscal tract
(C) Posterior spinocerebellar tract
(D) Reticulospinal tract
(E) Spino-olivary tract

60. A 48-year-old man who is a nonsmoker presents with frontal headaches. In the course of the work-up, a computerized tomography (CT) scan locates a necrotic mass in the frontal lobe that crosses over the corpus callosum into the other hemisphere. The mass is most likely derived from

(A) astrocytes
(B) oligodendrocytes
(C) microglial cells
(D) ependymal cells
(E) choroid plexus

61. A 35-year-old patient with a head injury has problems with sleep and arousal. Which area of his brain is most likely to be damaged?

(A) Cerebellum
(B) Basal ganglia
(C) Thalamus
(D) Reticular system
(E) Amygdala

Questions 62-63

A 22-year-old man is brought to the emergency room by his wife. According to his wife, her husband was raking leaves in the back yard when he suddenly lost consciousness, became rigid, and fell to the ground. His respiration temporarily ceased. This situation lasted for about 45 seconds and was followed by jerking of all four limbs that lasted for about 2 or 3 minutes; then the patient was unconscious for 3 to 4 minutes. On examination, the patient is drowsy. He has a large laceration on his lip. The neurologic examination is otherwise unremarkable. The vital signs are normal.

62. The patient most likely had a

(A) simple partial seizure

(B) complex partial seizure

(C) absence seizure

(D) grand mal (tonic–clonic) seizure

(E) myoclonic seizure

63. Which of the following tests would be most useful in the workup of this patient?

(A) Electroencephalogram

(B) Computerized tomography scan

(C) Serum electrolytes

(D) Serum glucose

(E) Skull radiograph

64. The ligament of the vertebral column that resists its extension is the

(A) ligamentum flavum

(B) supraspinous ligament

(C) posterior longitudinal ligament

(D) anterior longitudinal ligament

(E) interspinous ligament

65. Which of the following descriptions characterizes a schwannoma (neurilemoma) rather than a neurofibroma? They

(A) are more likely to undergo malignant transformation

(B) are typically solitary encapsulated tumors

(C) are typically difficult to remove at surgery

(D) often involve large nerve trunks

(E) are pigmented, pedunculated lesions on the skin

66. Huntington disease is most closely associated with damage to the

(A) cerebellum

(B) basal ganglia

(C) thalamus

(D) reticular system

(E) amygdala

67. In general, the spinal fluid findings in both bacterial meningitis and viral meningitis exhibit

(A) low glucose

(B) neutrophil-dominant cell count

(C) elevated protein

(D) elevated C-reactive protein

(E) normal pressure

68. Which bony landmark is used to locate the appropriate site for a lumbar puncture?

(A) Ischial tuberosity

(B) Ischial spine

(C) Top of iliac crest

(D) Anterior superior iliac spine

(E) Anterior inferior iliac spine

69. In a series of interviews, a physician determines that a 65-year-old man shows progressive memory loss and progressive reduction in good judgment but no evidence of depression. Which statement about this patient is most likely to be true?

(A) His condition is reversible
(B) His level of consciousness is normal
(C) His symptoms are owing to normal aging
(D) Pharmacotherapy is an effective way to reverse his memory loss
(E) He most likely has a nutritional deficiency

70. The bony landmark that is used to perform a pudendal nerve block is the

(A) ischial tuberosity
(B) ischial spine
(C) sacral promontory
(D) pubic tubercle
(E) posterior superior iliac spine

71. The neurotransmitter most closely associated with the development of anxiety is

(A) dopamine
(B) neurotensin
(C) vasopressin
(D) γ-aminobutyric acid (GABA)
(E) somatostatin

72. Which muscle may be paralyzed by a superficial knife wound to the posterior triangle of the neck?

(A) Trapezius
(B) Sternocleidomastoid
(C) Anterior scalene
(D) Splenius capitis
(E) Posterior scalene

73. Which of the following statements about attention deficit hyperactivity disorder (ADHD) is a common misconception?

(A) Genetic factors are implicated in its etiology
(B) Emotional lability is commonly seen
(C) Stimulants are the treatment drugs of choice
(D) Irritability is commonly seen
(E) It is associated with a very low intelligence quotient (IQ)

74. A 52-year-old woman has been referred to your service. Her radiographic report indicates a brain tumor located in the falx cerebri of the longitudinal fissure in the vicinity of the precentral and postcentral gyri. In following the growth of this tumor, which of the following indications might be expected first?

(A) Decreasing pain and temperature in shoulder area
(B) Diminishing strength in forearm flexors
(C) Tremor in lower extremities
(D) Diminishing sensation and strength in leg and foot
(E) Diminishing affect in response to social situations

75. The electroencephalogram (EEG) of a 29-year-old man is dominated by theta waves. Which stage of sleep is this patient most likely in?

(A) Stage 1
(B) Stage 2
(C) Stage 3
(D) Stage 4
(E) REM

76. Which of the following neuroactive substance belongs to the largest group of putative (proposed) neurotransmitters?

(A) Glutamate
(B) Acetylcholine
(C) Serotonin
(D) Enkephalin
(E) Norepinephrine

77. A couple married for 10 years tells their primary care physician that they are having sexual problems. When the physician questions the wife, she reveals that she was raped by her father throughout her childhood and has never had a satisfactory sexual experience. The most correct response would be to

(A) refer the couple to a professional therapist

(B) tell the wife to relax

(C) advise her to masturbate to demonstrate that she has a normal sexual response

(D) describe to both of them the physiological changes of the normal sexual response cycle

(E) provide them with sensate focus exercises

78. Alzheimer disease is characterized by disruption of the tubule and filament organelles of selected cerebral cortex neurons. Which of the following statements describes the cellular physiology most affected?

(A) Golgi complex does not package enzymes for transmitter synthesis

(B) Inclusion bodies increase significantly during treatment

(C) Axonal transport systems may be disrupted

(D) RNA transcription is blocked

(E) Nuclear pores are closed, blocking nuclear and cytoplasmic interaction

79. Which cells form the scar tissue of the brain or spinal cord?

(A) Microglia

(B) Fibrocytes

(C) Astrocytes

(D) Ependymal

(E) Oligodendroglia

80. Mrs. Smith presented with a sudden onset of facial asymmetry. Seven days later, neurological evaluation showed flattening of the lower half of her face on the right side but retention of full activity in muscles of her forehead on both sides. Which one of the following is most likely responsible for this neurological deficit?

(A) Parotid tumor

(B) Cerebrovascular accident (CVA) affecting the internal capsule

(C) CVA affecting tegmentum of medulla

(D) Acoustic neuroma

(E) CVA of anterior cerebral artery

81. Which of the following best describes the vision in a typical patient with hyperopia?

(A) Objects at a distance (>20′) are not seen as clearly as they are by a person with emmetropia

(B) Objects close to the eye (3′ to 20′) are not seen as clearly as they are by a person with emmetropia

(C) Objects close to the eye (3′ to 20′) and objects at a distance (>20′) are not seen as clearly as they are by a person with emmetropia

(D) Objects at a distance (>20′), as well as those close to the eye (3′ to 20′), are seen clearly

(E) Objects in different planes of vision are not seen as clearly as they are by a person with emmetropia

82. The computed tomography (CT) scan shows an area of severe hemorrhage in the region of the calcarine fissure. To determine the most likely neurologic deficit produced by this space-occupying lesion, which capability should be tested?

(A) Rapid independent finger movements

(B) Visual fields

(C) Cognitive functions in word definition

(D) Tongue movements

(E) Muscle tone and coordination

83. The effects of therapeutic doses of dobutamine could be most effectively opposed by the administration of

(A) atropine
(B) phentolamine
(C) labetalol
(D) trimethaphan
(E) prazosin

84. A muscle that opens the jaw is the

(A) masseter
(B) temporalis
(C) buccinator
(D) medial pterygoid
(E) lateral pterygoid

85. The following image is of a special preparation on cerebrospinal fluid (CSF) taken from a patient with nuchal rigidity. Spinal fluid glucose is low and protein is increased. A few scattered mononuclear cells are noted in the white blood cell count. This patient is most likely a/an

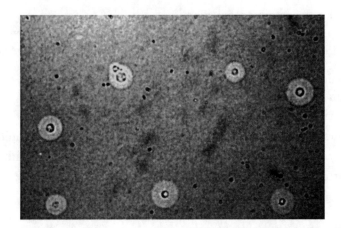

(A) newborn, with a mother who experienced premature rupture of the membranes
(B) immunocompromised adult
(C) previously healthy 3-year-old child
(D) previously healthy 20-year-old military recruit
(E) adult with infective endocarditis

DIRECTIONS:

Each of the numbered items or incomplete statements in this section is negatively phrased, as indicated by a capitalized word such as NOT, LEAST, or EXCEPT. Select the ONE lettered answer or completion that is BEST in each case.

86. Experimental evidence indicates that serotonin is involved in all of the following factors EXCEPT

(A) mood
(B) sexuality
(C) learning
(D) anxiety
(E) sleep

87. Which of the following statements concerning HIV in the central nervous system (CNS) is NOT correct?

(A) Autoimmune destruction of neurons is secondary to crossreactivity with proteins in the virus
(B) Macrophages carry the virus to the CNS
(C) Apoptosis of astrocytes is cytokine induced
(D) Astrocytes are directly infected by the virus
(E) Multinucleated giant cells are derived from infected astrocytes

88. The potential adverse effects of propranolol include all of the following EXCEPT

(A) hyperglycemia
(B) bradycardia
(C) atrioventricular (AV) block
(D) sleep disturbances
(E) bronchoconstriction

89. A 28-year-old man with AIDS has clinical evidence of tremor, ataxia, memory loss, and confusion. Which of the following cells is LEAST likely to be involved in the progression of this complication?

(A) Microglial cells
(B) Astrocytes
(C) Oligodendrocytes
(D) Multinucleated giant cells
(E) CD4 T-helper cells

90. In the eye, the physiological reflex of pupillary constriction during accommodation involves all of the following structures EXCEPT

(A) the optic nerve
(B) the medial geniculate body
(C) the cerebral cortex
(D) the Edinger Westphal nucleus
(E) the ciliary ganglion

91. Primary malignant lymphomas of the brain differ from malignant lymphomas that secondarily involve the brain in that they are

(A) more common
(B) more likely to be of T-cell origin
(C) more likely to be multifocal
(D) always associated with the AIDS
(E) less likely to involve the brain parenchyma

92. A patient is brought to the emergency room after ingesting a bottle of atropine (hyoscyamine) tablets. All of the following would be expected findings EXCEPT

(A) blurred vision
(B) delirium
(C) mydriasis
(D) absence of bowel sounds
(E) hypothermia

93. All of the following muscles are attached to the scapula EXCEPT

(A) deltoid
(B) trapezius
(C) pectoralis major
(D) pectoralis minor
(E) biceps brachii

94. Administration of trimethaphan would be expected to cause all of the following effects EXCEPT

(A) mydriasis
(B) decreased heart rate
(C) decreased blood pressure
(D) urinary retention
(E) dry mouth

95. Which one of the following tracts or systems does NOT synapse in the thalamus, a relay station for most sensory pathways?

(A) The spinocerebellar tract
(B) The lateral spinothalamic tract
(C) The dorsal column medial lemniscal system
(D) The central tract of the auditory nerve
(E) The optic tract

96. The following effects of atropine are correctly matched with a corresponding receptor type EXCEPT

(A) decreased heart rate—stimulation of vagal nucleus in the brain stem
(B) increased heart rate—blockade of M_2 receptors in the heart
(C) bronchodilation—blockade of M_1 receptors in the lung
(D) mydriasis—blockade of M_3 receptors in the iris
(E) urinary retention—blockade of M_3 receptors in the bladder

97. Functions of the right hemisphere of the brain are commonly thought to include all of the following EXCEPT

(A) perception of social cues
(B) musical ability
(C) spatial relations capability
(D) language skills
(E) perceptual ability

98. Hemodialysis is an appropriate treatment for poisoning by all of the following substances EXCEPT

(A) methanol
(B) ethylene glycol
(C) aspirin
(D) paraquat
(E) theophylline

99. Stretch of a muscle, as in the knee jerk, produces all of the following changes EXCEPT

(A) elongation of the intrafusal fiber in the muscle spindles
(B) excitation of the annulospiral (primary) endings in the spindles
(C) excitation of the flower spray (secondary) endings in the spindles
(D) increased frequency of action potentials over Ia afferents from the muscle
(E) inhibition of the alpha motor neurons returning to that muscle

100. The early signs of acute nicotine poisoning include all of the following EXCEPT

(A) hypertension
(B) salivation
(C) nausea
(D) constipation
(E) diaphoresis

101. Muscles that can flex the hip joint include all of the following EXCEPT

(A) psoas major
(B) vastus intermedius
(C) sartorius
(D) rectus femoris
(E) iliacus

102. All of the following drugs are useful in the treatment of acne vulgaris EXCEPT

(A) triamcinolone
(B) ethinyl estradiol
(C) tretinoin (retinoic acid)
(D) benzoyl peroxide
(E) minocycline

103. All of the following nerves pass through the greater sciatic foramen EXCEPT

(A) superior gluteal nerve
(B) inferior gluteal nerve
(C) pudendal nerve
(D) sciatic nerve
(E) lateral femoral cutaneous nerve

104. All of the following substances may cause or contribute to the development of acneiform skin lesions EXCEPT

(A) beclomethasone
(B) doxycycline
(C) methyltestosterone
(D) lithium
(E) cooking oils

105. All of the following bones have one or more air-filled cavities EXCEPT

(A) frontal
(B) sphenoid
(C) parietal
(D) temporal
(E) ethmoid

106. All of the following dermatologic agents are correctly matched with a clinical indication EXCEPT

(A) mupirocin—treatment of impetigo due to staphylococci or streptococci
(B) haloprogin—treatment of dermatophyte infections such as tinea corporis
(C) benzoyl peroxide—a sunscreen for the prevention of sunburn
(D) trioxsalen—repigmentation of skin in patients with vitiligo
(E) malathion—treatment of pediculosis

107. Specific evidence of child abuse in a 6-year-old includes all of the following EXCEPT

(A) old healed fractures
(B) bruised buttocks
(C) rupture of the liver
(D) bruised knees
(E) subdural hematoma

108. Isotretinoin may cause all of the following adverse effects EXCEPT

(A) hypertriglyceridemia
(B) birth defects
(C) pruritus
(D) muscle and joint pain
(E) hirsutism

109. A peripheral nerve includes all of the following EXCEPT

(A) fibrocytes
(B) perineurium
(C) afferent fibers
(D) efferent fibers
(E) oligodendroglia

110. All of the following dermatologic agents are correctly paired with a descriptive characteristic EXCEPT

(A) fluorinated corticosteroids—better absorbed from scalp than the forearm
(B) podophyllum resin—inhibits DNA synthesis in Condyloma acuminatum
(C) minoxidil—topical application may reverse hair loss in androgenic alopecia
(D) coal tar preparations—useful in treating psoriasis
(E) salicylic acid—acts as a keratolytic agent when applied topically

111. The benzodiazepines are effective in treating all of the following conditions EXCEPT

(A) alcohol withdrawal
(B) panic attacks
(C) psychotic agitation
(D) musculoskeletal problems
(E) passive–aggressive personality disorder

112. All of the following cranial nerves arise from or enter the brain stem EXCEPT

(A) vagus nerves
(B) hypoglossal nerves
(C) olfactory nerves
(D) optic nerves
(E) oculomotor nerves

113. Stimulation of photoreceptors in the retina does all of the following EXCEPT

(A) hyperpolarizes the cell
(B) decreases the level of cyclic guanosine monophosphate (cGMP)
(C) reduces sodium influx through sodium channels
(D) produces photopigment breakdown
(E) increases the rate of neurotransmitter release

114. All of the following statements about electroconvulsive therapy (ECT) are true EXCEPT

(A) it is a relatively safe treatment
(B) it involves induction of a generalized seizure
(C) its most common indication is schizophrenia
(D) it is an effective treatment for major depression
(E) maximum response is usually seen after 5 to 10 treatments

115. All of the following adrenergic receptor antagonists are correctly identified EXCEPT

(A) acebutolol—selectively antagonizes β_2 receptors
(B) prazosin—selectively antagonizes α_1 receptors
(C) propranolol—equally antagonizes β_1 and β_2 receptors
(D) labetalol—antagonizes α_1, β_1 and β_2 receptors
(E) atenolol—selectively antagonizes β_1 receptors

116. A muscle biopsy exhibits atrophy that is primarily limited to type II muscle fibers. This finding is LEAST likely associated with

(A) poliomyelitis
(B) Parkinson disease
(C) Charcot-Marie-Tooth disease
(D) Werdnig-Hoffmann disease
(E) amyotrophic lateral sclerosis (ALS)

DIRECTIONS:

Each set of matching questions in this section consists of a list of four to twenty-six lettered options (some of which may be in figures) followed by several numbered items. For each numbered item, select the ONE lettered option that is most closely associated with it. To avoid spending too much time on matching sets with a large number of options, it is generally advisable to begin each set by reading the list of options. Then for each item in the set, try to generate the correct answer and locate it in the option list, rather than evaluating each option individually. Each lettered option may be selected once, more than once, or not at all.

Questions 117-120

The effects of four procedures (designated Q, R, S, and T) on heart rate and blood pressure following pretreatment with saline, phentolamine, propranolol, atropine, or a combination of atropine and propranolol are illustrated in the figure below. The illustrations show the effects of the procedures but not the effects of the pretreatments.

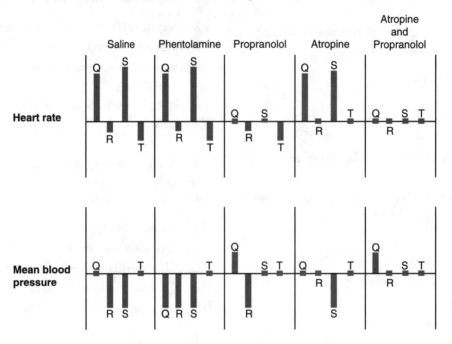

(A) Epinephrine administration
(B) Isoproterenol administration
(C) Phenylephrine administration
(D) Acetylcholine administration
(E) Sympathetic nerve stimulation
(F) Parasympathetic nerve stimulation

117. Procedure Q is most likely

118. Procedure R is most likely

119. Procedure S is most likely

120. Procedure T is most likely

Questions 121-123

Match each clinical description with the appropriate seizure disorder.

(A) Simple partial seizure, jacksonian type
(B) Complex partial seizure
(C) Absence seizure
(D) Grand mal (tonic–clonic) seizure
(E) Myoclonic seizure
(F) Temporal lobe epilepsy

121. A mother brings her 12-year-old daughter to a physician. The mother states that, for the past 6 months, she and her daughter's teacher have noticed the child staring into space. The child's lack of concentration usually lasts 5 to 10 seconds. Sometimes her limbs briefly twitch during this staring episode. The child's neurologic exam is normal. An electroencephalogram is performed on an outpatient basis and reveals a 3-Hz spike-and-wave pattern.

122. A 38-year-old woman has a history of seizure characterized by an aura of either a foul smell or a taste sensation. This aura is followed by isolated, rhythmic jerking of the face or extremities, sometimes involving a sequential movement around the body without any loss of consciousness.

123. A 39-year-old woman complains of experiencing "loss of contact" with her surroundings. She has had these experiences over the last 14 months. Her first episode was brought to her attention by a close friend who said that she had a vague look in her eyes and started smacking her lips and rubbing her right thumb against her other hand for about 30 to 60 seconds. Since that time, the patient has noticed a foul smell and taste in her mouth and a rising feeling in her stomach before havng one of these episodes. Lately, she is aware of people during these episodes, but they seem to be in the distance.

Questions 124-126

Identify the pharmacologic effects that are mediated by the numbered receptors in the diagram below.

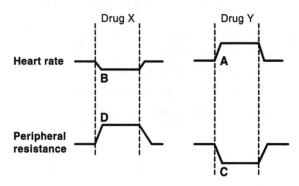

124. Beta$_2$ receptors

125. Alpha$_1$ receptors

126. Beta$_1$ receptors

Questions 127-130

Match the following types of *Mycobacteria* species with the most appropriate clinical description.

(A) *Mycobacterium tuberculosis*
(B) *Mycobacterium scrofulaceum*
(C) *Mycobacterium kansasii*
(D) *Mycobacterium avium-intracellulare*
(E) *Mycobacterium bovis*
(F) *Mycobacterium ulcerans*
(G) *Mycobacterium marinum*
(H) *Mycobacterium leprae* (tuberculoid)
(I) *Mycobacterium leprae* (lepromatous)

127. Grentz zone on skin biopsies, beneath which are macrophages filled with numerous organisms

128. Nonphotochromogen associated with Whipple-like syndrome in a patient with AIDS

129. Scotochromogen associated with painless cervical adenopathy in children

130. Positive lepromin skin reaction in a patient with autoamputation of the digits of the hands

Questions 131-135

Select the most appropriate treatment for poisoning by each of the numbered compounds.

(A) Methylene blue
(B) Hyperbaric oxygen
(C) Diazepam and phentolamine
(D) Nitrite, thiosulfate, hydroxocobolamin
(E) Airway and respiratory support

131. Carbon monoxide

132. Cyanide

133. Aniline dyes; nitrites

134. Barbiturates; ethchlorvynol

135. Methamphetamine

Questions 136-143

For each patient or situation, identify the approximate location of the cerebral infarction.

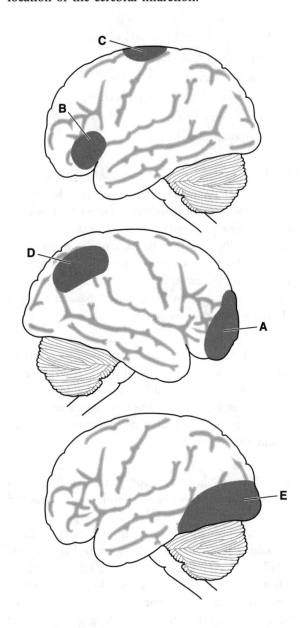

136. A 74-year-old man suffered a stroke that has affected his speech. The attending neurologist suggests that the accompanying aphasia in this gentleman is of a Broca's type.

137. A young women has discussed with you her father's decreasing ability to take care of himself. When she is questioned, you discover there have been episodes of mood changes, confusion, and that he "just has not been himself." Your examination of her father results in a poor performance in a routine mental status examination.

138. A 20-year-old college student was found unconscious in his dorm room. The student was taken to the hospital, where he regained consciousness with no assistance but complained of a funny feeling in his head. When questioned, he did remember experiencing a severe pain in his head before "the lights went out." He has no other complaints. Cranial nerve testing was complete, and except for some weakness in the right lower limb, the neurologic examination was unremarkable. During the day, this student had another episode of headache and difficulty with motor activity on the right side of the body. Continuing from this episode, there was an upper motor neuron paralysis of the right lower extremity, including a Babinski reflex and clonus. Angiography showed an AVM (arteriovenous malformation) in the left cerebral hemisphere.

139. A 45-year-old truck mechanic blacked out on the job. CT scan showed that an area of the brain supplied by the posterior cerebral artery was infarcted.

140. A neurologist was consulted on a rather unusual case observed in the clinic of a local geriatric care unit. A 70-year-old resident was being examined during a routine visit by a PA. The PA noted that he was essentially ignoring the left side of his body, including dressing and hygiene habits. The neurologist concluded that this man was demonstrating sensory neglect due to multiple strokes within a part of the cerebral cortex.

141. Location of a lesion resulting from an occlusion of branches of the middle cerebral artery

142. Area of the brain affected by ischemia in the watershed zone between the middle cerebral and anterior cerebral arteries

143. Area of the cerebral cortex infarcted by an embolism that travelled into the vertebral artery

Questions 144-148
Select the most appropriate drug for the treatment of each disease or disorder.

(A) Ipratropium
(B) Propranolol
(C) Bethanechol
(D) Terazosin
(E) Epinephrine

144. Urticaria, laryngeal edema, severe wheezing, and hypotension in a patient who was stung by a wasp.

145. Urinary retention in a post-surgical patient without outflow obstruction.

146. Increasing dyspnea in an older woman with emphysema.

147. Dysuria due to benign prostatic hypertrophy in an older male.

148. Prophylaxis of migraine headache in a young woman who has had frequent attacks during the past several months.

Questions 149-158

For each phrase or term, select the one lettered heading below that best describes or is most closely associated with the statement. Lettered headings may be used more than once or not at all.

(A) Lower motor neuron syndrome
(B) Upper motor neuron syndrome
(C) Dorsal column-medial lemniscal system
(D) Spinothalamic (anterolateral system)
(E) Extrapyramidal system

149. Spasticity and hyperreflexia

150. Romberg's sign

151. Vibratory, two-point touch discrimination

152. Associated with abnormal movement disorders including dystonia, difficulty in postural maintenance, and dyskinesia

153. Associated with pain and temperature stimuli

154. Atrophy of skeletal muscle

155. Flaccidity

156. Paresthesias

157. Decussation of pyramids in medulla

158. Nucleus and fasciculus cuneatus

Questions 159-161

For each of the numbered descriptions of heavy metal poisoning, select the appropriate antidote(s) for treatment of acute poisoning from the list below.

(A) Penicillamine
(B) Dimercaprol (BAL)
(C) Disodium EDTA
(D) Deferoxamine
(E) Trientine

159. A child with seizures is brought to the emergency room with a history of irritability, apathy, and anorexia. He has also had headaches and other diffuse aches and pains. After controlling seizures, the physical exam revealed a blue line at the base of the gums, and the neurologic exam revealed depressed deep tendon reflexes.

160. After swallowing a half a bottle of tablets, a patient vomits blood and complains of abdominal distress. Endoscopic examination reveals diffuse hemorrhagic gastritis with extensive necrosis. The neurologic exam was normal.

161. A young man presents to the emergency room after intentionally ingesting several teaspoons of a compound from his chemistry set. He repeatedly vomited blood-tinged material and showed graying discoloration of buccal mucosa. The physical exam was unremarkable except for abdominal tenderness. Urinalysis was consistent with acute tubular necrosis.

Questions 162-163

Match the following pathogens with the correct clinical description.

(A) Rubeola
(B) Papovavirus
(C) *Herpes zoster*
(D) Adenovirus
(E) Mumps virus
(F) *Herpes simplex*
(G) Arborvirus
(H) *Naegleria fowleri*
(I) *Acanthamoeba* species
(J) *Taenia solium*

162. Painful vesicular lesions on the right side of the forehead, dorsum of the nose, upper eyelid, and cornea, producing a keratitis in an immunocompromised patient

163. Meningoencephalitis after swimming in fresh water

Questions 164-167

Match each disorder with the drug of choice.

(A) Benzene hydrochloride
(B) Metronidazole
(C) Chloroquine
(D) Mefloquine
(E) Primaquine
(F) Suramin
(G) Nifurtimox
(H) Stibogluconate sodium
(I) Pyrantel pamoate
(J) Mebendazole
(K) Thiabendazole
(L) Ivermectin
(M) Diethylcarbamazine
(N) Praziquantel
(O) Albendazole

164. The following urine sediment finding, from a 3-year-old girl with a urinary tract infection

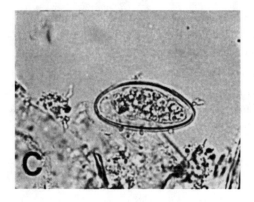

165. Hematuria in an Egyptian man whose bladder biopsy reveals squamous metaplasia

166. Chronic diarrhea in a patient who has a genetic deficiency of immunoglobulin A (IgA)

167. Gram-positive protozoan associated with the gay bowel syndrome

Questions 168-180

Match each clinical description with the most likely causative organism.

(A) *Brucella* species

(B) *Erysipelothrix*

(C) *Yersinia* species

(D) *Staphylococcus aureus*

(E) Anaerobic streptococcus

(F) *Neisseria gonorrhoeae*

(G) *Streptococcus pneumoniac*

(H) *Branhamella catarrhalis*

(I) *Bacillus* species

(J) *Clostridium* species

(K) *Neisseria meningitidis*

(L) *Nocardia*

(M) *Actinomyces*

(N) *Listeria monocytogenes*

(O) *Francisella* species

(P) *Streptococcus agalactiae*

(Q) *Escherichia coli*

(R) *Pseudomonas aeruginosa*

168. Large, red areas of denuded skin and generalized bulla in an infant

169. Bilateral adrenal hemorrhage, disseminated intravascular coagulation (DIC), and hemorrhagic vasculitis in a 6-year-old girl

170. Bilateral ophthalmia neonatorum in a 4-day-old infant

171. A neonate develops septicemia, maculopapular lesions on the legs and trunk, pneumonia, diarrhea, and seizures within a few hours of birth and dies a short time later

172. Chronic otitis media in a 9-year-old boy

173. A pruritic, creeping violaceous rash on the hands of a fish-packing plant employee

174. Examination of exudate in a woman fitted for an intrauterine device reveals yellow granules

175. Associated with granulomatous microabscesses in mesenteric lymph nodes

176. An infant develops ophthalmoplegia, hypotonia, and constipation after drinking milk sweetened with honey

177. A weaver who cards her own wool develops insect bite–like lesions on her hands that eventually swell and form black scabs with central areas of necrosis

178. A veterinarian experiences undulant fever

179. A swollen tongue and difficulty in breathing in a 32-year-old man

180. Granulomatous inflammation in the lymph nodes of a rabbit hunter

ANSWER KEY

1. B	31. C	61. D	91. C	121. C	151. C
2. A	32. A	62. D	92. E	122. A	152. E
3. C	33. B	63. A	93. C	123. F	153. D
4. B	34. C	64. D	94. B	124. C	154. A
5. A	35. A	65. B	95. A	125. D	155. A
6. B	36. A	66. B	96. C	126. A	156. D
7. C	37. B	67. C	97. D	127. I	157. B
8. B	38. D	68. C	98. D	128. D	158. C
9. D	39. B	69. B	99. E	129. B	159. A, B, C
10. C	40. D	70. B	100. D	130. H	160. D
11. D	41. E	71. D	101. B	131. B	161. A
12. B	42. E	72. A	102. A	132. D	162. C
13. A	43. B	73. E	103. E	133. A	163. H
14. C	44. B	74. D	104. B	134. E	164. I
15. C	45. B	75. A	105. C	135. C	165. N
16. E	46. D	76. D	106. C	136. B	166. B
17. A	47. C	77. A	107. D	137. A	167. O
18. D	48. A	78. C	108. E	138. C	168. D
19. C	49. A	79. C	109. E	139. E	169. K
20. E	50. A	80. B	110. B	140. D	170. F
21. C	51. B	81. D	111. E	141. B	171. N
22. A	52. D	82. B	112. C	142. A	172. H
23. D	53. B	83. C	113. A	143. E	173. B
24. B	54. C	84. E	114. C	144. E	174. M
25. B	55. E	85. B	115. A	145. C	175. C
26. C	56. D	86. C	116. B	146. A	176. J
27. D	57. C	87. E	117. A	147. D	177. I
28. C	58. D	88. A	118. D	148. B	178. A
29. D	59. C	89. E	119. B	149. B	179. E
30. C	60. A	90. B	120. F	150. C	180. O

ANSWERS AND EXPLANATIONS

1. The answer is B. *(Anatomy)*
The anterior spinal artery requires augmentation by segmental radicular arteries to adequately supply the spinal cord with arterial blood. Without other indicators, and given the fact that segments T1 through T3 are susceptible to a deficiency in this radicular arterial supply, the best selection is a deficiency in this blood supply.

2. The answer is A. *(Pathology)*
Aluminum in dialysate solutions is deposited in the area of mineralization of bone and inhibits the deposition of calcium hydroxyapatite crystals in the osteoid, which produces osteomalacia. Osteoporosis is a decrease in bone mass. The most common cause is estrogen deficiency in a postmenopausal woman. Other causes include primary hyperparathyroidism; hypercortisolism (Cushing syndrome); chronic metabolic acidosis, in which bone is being used up as a buffer for excess hydrogen ions (e.g., in chronic renal failure); heparin therapy; the lack of gravity in space; lithium; multiple myeloma; and hyperthyroidism, which involves an increase in bone turnover.

3. The answer is C. *(Pharmacology)*
Physostigmine is a reversible cholinesterase inhibitor that increases acetylcholine concentrations at all cholinergic synapses, including the central nervous system. Neostigmine, a quaternary amine, does not cross the blood–brain barrier and lacks central effects. Only physostigmine leads to activation of nicotinic receptors in skeletal muscle, thereby increasing muscle tone in patients with myasthenia gravis. Physostigmine also activates nicotinic receptors in autonomic ganglia at high doses and can augment sympathetic and parasympathetic tone. Both drugs cause activation of muscarinic receptors, leading to contraction of the iris sphincter muscle and miosis. Neither drug relaxes the detrusor muscle, which is an effect of the muscarinic antagonist, atropine.

4. The answer is B. *(Pathology)*
The best test to evaluate a patient for osteoporosis is dual photon absorptiometry. This noninvasive study measures bone density. It is considered the gold standard test. Densitometry is analogous to a static photograph of bone. Tests that evaluate bone turnover provide an evaluation of bone dynamics. These tests include an increase in the urinary concentration of (1) hydroxyproline, (2) osteocalcin, and (3) pyridinoline. The serum calcium and phosphorus are usually normal in most cases of osteoporosis. A bone marrow biopsy is an expensive and subjective test for osteoporosis. Radionuclide bone scans do not evaluate bone density. Routine bone radiographs show only osteopenia, which may be a feature of osteomalacia as well.

5. The answer is A. *(Physiology)*
Only a ganglion cell undergoes an action potential. Bipolar, horizontal, and receptor cells undergo fluctuations in membrane potential, such as depolarizations or hyperpolarizations.

6. The answer is B. *(Pathology)*
The patient has a Dupuytren's contracture, which is the most common type of fibromatosis. It refers to a group of non-neoplastic, proliferative connective tissue lesions that commonly infiltrate tissue and recur after surgical excision. Dupuytren's contractures are commonly bilateral and are often associated with alcoholism. Palmar erythema in this patient is probably due to hyperestrinism from alcoholic cirrhosis and inability to degrade estrogens and 17 ketosteroids (e.g., androstenedione), the latter aromatized in fat into estrogen.

Rheumatoid arthritis is not associated with the fibromatoses. Abnormalities in the hand in rheumatoid arthritis include trigger finger, swan-neck deformity, and boutonnière deformity, but these are problems with the muscles and tendons in the fingers rather than a proliferative phenomenon involving fibroconnective tissue.

Hyperestrinism is not the cause of Dupuytren's contracture, but is responsible for the palmar erythema, as previously discussed.

Gardner syndrome is an autosomal dominant polyposis syndrome associated with desmoid tumors. This type of fibromatosis involves the abdominal wall, not the hand.

7. The answer is C.   *(Pharmacology)*
Edrophonium is short-acting cholinesterase inhibitor that is administered intravenously in order to distinguish myasthenic crisis from cholinergic crisis in patients with myasthenia gravis. If the patient improves after administration of edrophonium, then the patient probably has myasthenia gravis and would benefit from longer-acting cholinesterase inhibitors. If the patient's muscle strength decreases after giving edrophonium, it suggests that the patient is in "cholinergic crisis" resulting from excessive doses of a cholinesterase inhibitor and the resulting depolarization blockade of skeletal muscle similar to that produced by succinylcholine. The treatment for cholinergic crisis is to withhold further cholinesterase inhibitor treatment until the patient improves. Atropine has no direct effect on skeletal muscle tone affected by cholinesterase inhibitors, but it is used on conjunction with these drugs to block the muscarinic side effects resulting from increased acetylcholine concentrations at parasympathetic neuroeffector junctions.

8. The answer is B.   *(Pathology)*
This patient has a desmoid tumor, which is a type of fibromatosis. The fibromatoses are a group of nonneoplastic, proliferative connective-tissue lesions that commonly infiltrate tissue and recur after surgical excision. A desmoid tumor is a fibromatosis of the anterior abdominal wall in women. These tumors are associated with previous trauma, multiple pregnancies, and Gardner syndrome. The tumors originate from the musculoaponeurotic wall.

The pathogenesis of this lesion is in the same category of disease as a fibromatosis colli (torticollis), which produces severe contractures of the neck muscles. Other examples include Peyronie disease, which is a fibromatosis of Buck's fascia that causes painful contracture of the penis, and retroperitoneal fibrosis, which frequently obstructs the ureters and leads to renal failure. The latter condition may be associated with methysergide, an ergot derivative, and other diseases associated with dense fibrosis including sclerosing cholangitis, Reidel fibrosing thyroiditis, and sclerosing mediastinitis.

A malignant fibrous histiocytoma or a fibrosarcoma may be confused with a fibromatosis, except mitotic activity would be increased and often atypical. A leiomyoma is a benign tumor of smooth muscle. A keloid is abnormal scar tissue formation commonly seen in the African American population. The scar tissue consists of thick bands of type III collagen.

9. The answer is D.   *(Anatomy)*
The synovial sheath of the flexor pollicis longus extends proximally through the carpal tunnel and is known as the radial bursa. The common synovial sheath around the tendons of the flexor digitorum superficialis and flexor digitorum profundus in the palm of the hand is known as the ulnar bursa. The ulnar bursa is continuous with the digital tendon sheath of the fifth digit. The digital synovial tendon sheaths of the second, third, and fourth digits are not continuous with the ulnar bursa. Usually, the radial bursa and the ulna bursa communicate with one another within the carpal tunnel. Therefore, an infection within the synovial sheath of the flexor tendons in the thumb can spread proximally into the radial bursa and then into the ulnar bursa and into the synovial sheath of the fifth digit.

10. The answer is C.   *(Pathology)*
The most common benign tumor in women, which is also the most common benign tumor in the gastrointestinal tract, is a leiomyoma. These tumors originate from smooth muscle. In women, a leiomyoma is most commonly located in the uterus, where it is frequently called a fibroid. The tumor may obstruct delivery or produce severe menorrhagia, if located just below the endometrial mucosa. In the gastrointestinal tract, the tumors are most frequently found in the stomach, where they are usually asymptomatic. However, in some cases, they may be associated with significant bleeding. Leiomyomas rarely, if ever, transform into leiomyosarcomas.

Regarding the other choices in the question, lipomas are the most common benign tumor of adipose tissue; an osteochondroma is the most common benign tumor of bone; a capillary hemangioma is the most common benign tumor arising from endothelium; and a neurilemmoma, or schwannoma, is the most common benign tumor arising from Schwann cells.

11. The answer is D.   *(Pharmacology)*
Acetaminophen is primarily eliminated by conjugation with glucuronide and sulfate, but a minor metabolite,

N-acetyl-benzoquinone, is toxic to the liver. N-acetyl-benzoquinone accumulates after an acute overdose of acetaminophen because of depletion of sulfhydryl groups required to degrade it. Acetylcysteine provides a source of sulfhydryl groups to enable inactivation of the toxic metabolite and can be life saving after acetaminophen overdose. Acetylcysteine was originally developed as a mucolytic agent, primarily for use in premature infants who lacked lung surfactant. Although it does reduce the viscosity of pulmonary secretions, this effect is not related to its use in treating acetaminophen toxicity.

12. The answer is B. *(Pathology)*
Angiomyolipomas are frequently associated with tuberous sclerosis, an autosomal dominant disease that is also associated with rhabdomyoma, a benign neoplasm in the heart. Angiomyolipomas are hamartomas composed of blood vessels, muscle, and adipose tissue. They are most commonly located in the kidney. In addition to angiomyolipomas and rhabdomyomas of the heart, tuberous sclerosis is also associated with mental retardation; multiple hamartomas composed of abnormal astrocytes, which are located in the brain and around the walls of the ventricles ("candlestick drippings"); intracerebral calcifications; skin nodules (adenoma sebaceum); and periungual fibromas.

Tuberous sclerosis is not associated with lesions in the stomach. Neurofibromatosis, another autosomal dominant disease, is associated with peripheral nerve tumors (neurofibromas); optic nerve gliomas; meningiomas, which may involve the frontal lobe; and acoustic neuromas, which often involve the eighth cranial nerve.

13. The answer is A. *(Physiology)*
The cochlea is the location of the organ of Corti, which contains the receptors for hearing, not for equilibrium (linear or angular acceleration). The base of the cochlea responds to high-frequency sounds. Thus, presbycusis, which occurs with age, is associated with loss of sensitivity to high-frequency sounds.

14. The answer is C. *(Pathology)*
Nail infections and an association with polyendocrinopathy syndromes characterize infection due to *Candida albicans*. The polyendocrinopathy syndromes most

commonly involved with *Candida* are hypoparathyroidism and Addison disease. Nail involvement is called onychomycosis. Diaper rash is another skin disease associated with *Candida*.

Trichophyton species are superficial dermatophytes that commonly involve the hair, skin, and nails.

Microsporum species are superficial dermatophytes that commonly involve the hair and skin.

Staphylococcus aureus is frequently associated with paronychial infections, which develop along the border of the nail.

Herpes simplex may be traumatically implanted into the finger to produce a very painful infection called herpetic whitlow.

15-19. The answers are: 15-C, 16-E, 17-A, 18-D, 19-C. *(Pharmacology)*
Both opiates, such as heroin, and organophosphate cholinesterase inhibitors (parathion) cause pinpoint pupils, but other signs and symptoms can distinguish these compounds. Opiates cause respiratory depression, whereas parathion produces marked salivation, urination, diarrhea, and skeletal muscle fasciculations followed by paralysis. Salicylates cause abdominal distress, vomiting, and respiratory alkalosis followed by metabolic acidosis, and treatment includes appropriate fluids and electrolytes. The ferric chloride test is a qualitative test for the presence of salicylates and does not necessarily indicate overdosage. Acetaminophen overdose causes a delayed hepatic necrosis that can be fatal. Blood acetaminophen levels can determine the need for and dosage of the antidote, acetylcysteine. Both methanol and ethylene glycol cause a metabolic acidosis with an anion gap and an osmolar gap. Methanol causes a visual disturbance leading to blindness, whereas ethylene glycol is associated with oxalate crystals in the urine. Both are treated by administration of ethanol to prevent their conversion to toxic metabolites, and hemodialysis to remove the poisons.

20. The answer is E. *(Pathology)*
Borrelia recurrentis, or relapsing fever, is a spirochetal disease transmitted by ticks or lice and produces high fever, rash, and neurologic abnormalities. It is not associated with bone or joint disease, unlike its close relative *Borrelia burgdorferi,* which is the cause of tick-transmitted Lyme disease.

Treponema pallidum associated with congenital syphilis produces an osteochondritis and periostitis with deposition of new bone around long bones, thus forming the saber shin with forward bowing of the tibia. Tabes dorsalis, which is a manifestation of tertiary syphilis, is associated with the loss of pain and proprioception in the hip, knee, and ankle joints, thus rendering them susceptible to damage, a condition called Charcot's joint (neuropathic joint).

Salmonella species are frequently involved in osteomyelitis in children with sickle cell disease.

The parvovirus may be associated with a chronic arthritis.

Rubella is frequently associated with arthralgias and arthritis, particularly in infected adults.

21. The answer is C.   *(Behavioral science)*
Paranoid schizophrenia is characterized by delusions of persecution, better social functioning, and older age at onset than the other subtypes. The person with disorganized schizophrenia is disinhibited and disorganized and has poor personal appearance and inappropriate emotional responses. The catatonic shows bizarre posturing (waxy flexibility) and stupor. The person with undifferentiated schizophrenia has characteristics of more than one subtype whereas the person with residual schizophrenia has had one psychotic episode and subsequently shows flat affect, odd behavior, and social withdrawal, with no severe psychotic symptoms.

22. The answer is A.   *(Pathology)*
The patient most likely has Lyme disease, which is transmitted by the bite of a tick called *Ixodes dammini*. Lyme disease is caused by the spirochete, *Borrelia burgdorferi*, not to be confused with *Borrelia recurrentis*, the cause of relapsing fever. The early disease is as described in the patient, with the skin lesion representing erythema chronicum migrans. This lesion should not be confused with erythema marginatum, which is associated with rheumatic fever. If left untreated, Lyme disease may progress to a chronic phase characterized by cranial nerve palsies, most commonly of the seventh nerve (bilateral Bell palsy is common); destructive arthritis, most often involving the knee; and cardiac abnormalities, including myocarditis and heart block. The diagnosis is best made with serologic

tests. Tetracycline is used to treat early disease, and ceftriaxone is used to treat chronic disease.

The patient's history and rash are not characteristic of group A streptococcal infections (e.g., sore throat, rheumatic fever), infectious mononucleosis, or rheumatoid arthritis.

23. The answer is D.   *(Physiology)*
Bending the sterocilia toward the kinocilium causes the receptor cell to depolarize; bending the sterocilia away from the kinocilium causes the receptor cell to hyperpolarize. Depolarization increases the release of neurotransmitter from the receptor cell, and hyperpolarization decreases the release of neurotransmitter.

24. The answer is B.   *(Physiology)*
Type I muscle fibers differ from type II muscle fibers in that they are rich in mitochondria.

Type I fibers have the following characteristics:

- Slow-twitch fibers found in red muscle (e.g., postural muscles)
- Rich in mitochondria and myoglobin
- Capable of long, sustained contractions without fatigue (endurance muscles)
- Size unchanged with exercise, but conditioning increases enzymes in aerobic glycolysis
- Increase in oxidative enzymes
- Contain scant glycogen
- Pale even with ATPase staining at an alkaline pH

In contradistinction to type I fibers, type II fibers have the following characteristics:

- Fast-twitch fibers in white muscle (e.g., biceps)
- Poor in mitochondria
- Rich in glycogen
- Faster, shorter, and more powerful contractions than type I fibers
- More enzymes for anaerobic glycolysis than type I
- Reaction to training with hypertrophy
- Dark ATPase staining at an alkaline pH

25. The answer is B.   *(Anatomy)*
The ischiorectal fossa is the fat-filled space below the pelvic diaphragm. The main portion of the fossa is between the pelvic diaphragm and the obturator internus. Anteriorly, the anterior recess of the fossa continues into the region between the pelvic diaphragm

and the urogenital diaphragm. Posteriorly, the posterior recess of the fossa extends into the region deep to the gluteus maximus. The anterior recess of the fossa ends anteriorly where the inferior recess of the pelvic fascia fuses with the superior fascia of the urogenital diaphragm.

26. The answer is C.   *(Pathology)*
The patient has myotonic dystrophy, which is the most common adult muscular dystrophy and has an autosomal dominant inheritance pattern. The pathogenesis relates to an increased number of triplet repeats in an unstable segment of a gene. Muscle biopsies show atrophy of type I fibers and hypertrophy of type II fibers. Additional clinical features include cataracts, testicular atrophy, and cardiac involvement. There is an increase in serum creatine kinase.

Improvement in muscle function after a Tensilon test is characteristic of myasthenia gravis. This disease is associated with autoantibodies against acetylcholine receptors. A dislocated lens is characteristic of Marfan syndrome and homocystinuria.

27. The answer is D.   *(Physiology)*
Spasticity is a condition with increased muscle tone (not hypotonus) in which there is resistance to passive movement of antigravity muscles; this resistance is greater when the velocity of the passive movement is faster. Although there also is resistance to passive movement in rigidity, a condition seen in Parkinson's disease, rigidity differs from spasticity in a number of ways. The resistance in rigidity is found in both flexors and extensors, is not velocity dependent, and does not show the clasp-knife response that occurs in spasticity. The medial lemniscus carries sensory information regarding touch to the thalamus; lesions of the medial lemniscus do not cause spasticity.

28. The answer is C.   *(Pathology)*
Peripheral neuropathy may be due to drugs, toxins, chemicals, infectious agents, infiltrative diseases (e.g., amyloidosis), cancer, or metabolic disease (e.g., diabetes mellitus). The clinical presentation may pursue one or more of the following routes: symmetrical glove-and-stocking distribution of sensory loss due to demyelination; segmental demyelination of the nerve, resulting in conduction failure without evidence of

denervation with muscle fasciculations (like worms under the skin), characteristic of lower motor neuron disease; or degeneration of the axon, resulting in denervation and subsequent muscle fasciculations and atrophy of the muscle. Of the drugs/chemicals/toxins listed, diphtheria toxin is primarily associated with demyelination and not with axonal degeneration. However, axonal degeneration is associated with ethanol abuse, organophosphate poisoning, lead poisoning, and vincristine. Other causes of axonal degeneration include diabetes mellitus (most common peripheral neuropathy); uremic neuropathy; thiamine as well as vitamins B_{12}, B_6, and E deficiencies; and sensorimotor neuropathy associated with small-cell carcinoma of the lung.

29. The answer is D.   *(Anatomy)*
The area of the brain most responsible for visual tasks, in this case, identification of a camouflaged object, is the occipital lobe.

30. The answer is C.   *(Pathology)*
The patient has Guillain-Barré syndrome (GBS). GBS generally follows a viral infection, in this case, an acute influenza-like infection. Herpes, cytomegalovirus, and Epstein-Barr virus are the most common infectious agents associated with GBS. This results in an acute, immune-mediated demyelination of multiple cranial and spinal nerve roots, resulting in lower motor neuron weakness, generally beginning in the lower extremities and extending up the neuraxis to involve the upper extremities and muscles of respiration. The spinal tap reveals (1) a pronounced elevation of spinal fluid protein that has oligoclonal bands on high-resolution electrophoresis; (2) a mild lymphocytosis; (3) normal glucose; (4) normal pressure; and (5) a negative serologic test for syphilis (VDRL). Approximately 85% of patients recover completely.

31. The answer is C.   *(Physiology)*
Gamma motor neurons, which are located in the anterior gray horn of the spinal cord and motor nuclei of cranial nerves, stimulate contraction of intrafusal fibers in muscle spindles to regulate their sensitivity. The gamma motor neurons are controlled primarily by neurons in descending motor tracts from the brain; some are excitatory, but many are inhibitory. Afferents

from the muscle spindles (1a afferents) and the Golgi tendon organ do not synapse with the gamma motor neurons.

32. The answer is A.   *(Pathology)*
A 33-year-old man with neurofibromatosis who, in the absence of vertigo or trauma, has tinnitus and partial nerve deafness in his right ear most likely has an acoustic neuroma involving the right eighth nerve. The Weber test lateralizes to the left ear, which is the normal ear, whereas the Rinne test exhibits air conduction longer than bone conduction in both ears, indicating that the problem is nerve deafness in the right ear. In nerve deafness, air conduction is still longer than bone conduction, whereas in conduction loss, the bone conduction is longer than air conduction and the Weber test lateralizes to the abnormal ear.

Neurofibromatosis, or von Recklinghausen disease, is an autosomal dominant disease with type I (most common) and type II variants. Type I is associated with:

- Multiple neurofibromas, which involve all the elements of a peripheral nerve. There is a 3% chance that these lesions will become malignant.
- Unilateral acoustic neuromas, which produce eighth-nerve deafness
- Pigmented iris hamartomas called Lisch nodules
- Numerous café au lait spots with their long axes parallel to the underlying cutaneous nerve
- Skeletal lesions, such as scoliosis
- An increased incidence of MOP: **m**eningioma, **o**ptic glioma, and **p**heochromocytoma

Neurofibromatosis type II is characterized by bilateral acoustic neuromas, absence of Lisch nodules in the iris, and presence or absence of neurofibromas.

Regarding the other choices:

- Meniere disease is a type of labyrinthitis involving the cochlea. It presents with recurrent episodes of vertigo accompanied by tinnitus and deafness due to fluid accumulation (endolymph) in the labyrinth.
- Otosclerosis refers to sclerosis and fixation of the middle ear ossicles associated with a conductive type of hearing loss and possible deafness. It is the most common cause of conductive hearing loss in adults.
- A glomus jugulare tumor is a type of paraganglioma. Patients often hear the blood rushing through the tumor.

- Presbycusis is the most common cause of nerve deafness in the elderly and is not associated with neurofibromatosis.

33. The answer is B.   *(Anatomy)*
The inguinal ligament is the lower portion of the external oblique aponeurosis. The external oblique aponeurosis attaches to the anterior position of the iliac crest laterally and to the pubic crest medially. The portion of the aponeurosis that is not attached to bone is thickened and reflected on itself. This portion is the inguinal ligament, which extends from the anterior superior iliac spine laterally to the pubic tubercle medially. The inguinal ligament marks the inferior limit of the anterior abdominal wall.

34. The answer is C.   *(Pathology)*
Sequestrum and involucrum describe osteomyelitis. In children, it is primarily located in the metaphysis of bone, the most vascular part of the bone. In neonates, the infection may spread into the joint space, but this situation is uncommon in children and adults. Pyogenic osteomyelitis occurs most frequently in children and young adults and is most commonly due to *Staphylococcus aureus,* which reaches the bone via the hematogenous route. In acute osteomyelitis, the marrow cavity is filled with acute inflammatory cells, which enzymatically destroy bone and leave devitalized portions of bone called sequestra floating in a sea of pus. If not properly treated, it may progress into a chronic osteomyelitis, which is a mixture of both acute and chronic inflammatory cells with extensive reactive bone formation in the periosteum called involucrum.

35. The answer is A.   *(Physiology)*
Phosphodiesterase breaks down cyclic adenosine monophosphate (cAMP), which reduces its concentration and its effect inside the smooth muscle cell. A phosphodiesterase inhibitor prevents this breakdown, allowing the cAMP levels to be higher and cAMP effects to be greater. In smooth muscle, cAMP inhibits myosin light chain kinase from promoting muscle contraction. Therefore, the airway smooth muscle relaxes due to an increase in cAMP.

36. The answer is A.   *(Pathology)*
Langerhans cells are antigen-processing cells located in the epidermis. They contain Birbeck granules,

which are visible with electron microscopy, and are CD1 antigen-positive.

Rete ridge hyperplasia refers to the downward accentuation of the basal cell layer of the epidermis into the underlying superficial dermis. In lichen planus, the rete ridges have a saw-tooth appearance, whereas in psoriasis, they are very regular and club-shaped. Lichen sclerosis et atrophicus is an atrophic vulvar dystrophy with thinning of the epidermis and no rete ridge hyperplasia.

Acanthosis refers to generalized thickening of the epidermis, which most commonly is secondary to hyperkeratosis, or thickening of the stratum corneum. Spongiosis refers to the accumulation of fluid between keratinocytes that may lead to vesicle formation manifested as blisters on the skin.

Acantholysis refers to the separation of epidermal cells, usually because of an immunologic destruction of the intercellular bridges (e.g., pemphigus vulgaris). Ichthyosis has an increased cohesiveness of the keratinocytes.

A macule is a flat, colored lesion on the epidermis. A rash that is described as maculopapular has both flat and raised lesions. A papule is a peaked area of elevation on the epidermis that is less than 5 mm in diameter.

37. The answer is B.   (Behavioral science)
Symptoms of mania include grandiosity, impaired judgment, increased motor behavior, increased energy, and decreased need for sleep. Symptoms of depression include feelings of worthlessness, psychomotor retardation, and lack of energy. Depressed patients may show either decreased or increased sleep.

38. The answer is D.   (Pathology)
The differential list for a malignant small round cell tumor involving bone includes Ewing sarcoma (primary bone disease), Burkitt lymphoma (metastatic bone disease), small cell carcinoma of the lung (metastatic bone disease), acute lymphoblastic leukemia (primary bone disease), and neuroblastoma (metastatic bone disease). A neuroblastoma is the only one of these malignancies that is associated with hypertension. Recall that these malignant tumors originate in the neural crest and are most commonly located in the adrenal medulla. Similar to Ewing sarcoma, Burkitt

lymphoma, and acute lymphoblastic leukemia, neuroblastoma is primarily a childhood disease. Neuroblastomas secrete catecholamines, which produce hypertension. They commonly metastasize to bone, skin, the orbit of the eye, and liver.

39. The answer is B.   (Physiology)
Damage to the upper motor neurons reduces the considerable inhibitory influence these tracts have on the lower motor neurons. As a result, the excitatory influence of reflexes predominates, causing an increase in muscle tone and hyperreflexia (not hyporeflexia). Rarely is there atrophy or fasciculations, and abnormal sensations (paresthesia) do not occur.

40. The answer is D.   (Pathology)
Bone is primarily (90%) composed of type I collagen. Type III collagen is normally present in the initial phases of wound healing before it is replaced by type I collagen. Lamellar bone replaces woven bone, the latter always representing a pathologic type of bone matrix commonly associated with fibrous dysplasia. Lamellar bone is layered, which helps it resist forces equally in all directions. Osteoclasts form Howship's lacunae. Osteoblasts have receptors for parathormone (PTH), vitamin D, estrogen, interleukins 1 and 6, and transforming growth factor (TGF-β). Interleukin-1 released from osteoblasts (PTH-mediated) stimulates osteoclasts, which resorb bone and release TGF-β. TGF-β stimulates osteoblasts to synthesize new bone equivalent to that which was removed. Osteocalcin is an excellent monitor of osteoblastic activity.

41. The answer is E.   (Anatomy)
Normally, during the stance phase of the gait cycle, the knee is kept in a slightly flexed position. This position requires an active quadriceps femoris muscle to prevent the force of gravity from causing the knee to go into full flexion. The quadriceps femoris muscle is innervated by the femoral nerve. If the patient has a lesion of the femoral nerve and therefore does not have an active quadriceps femoris, the knee stays in a fully extended and locked position during the stance phase. This position prevents gravity from causing the knee to "collapse."

42. The answer is E. *(Pathology)*
Osteoblasts play a dominant role in the bone lesions associated with metastatic prostate cancer. Because osteoblasts contain alkaline phosphatase, a patient with metastatic prostatic cancer commonly has an elevation of prostatic acid phosphatase, prostate-specific antigen, and alkaline phosphatase.

Osteoclasts have a primary role in:

- Osteopetrosis, when a defect occurs in osteoclastic resorption of bone
- The early phase of Paget disease, when excessive osteoclastic activity is followed by a later phase of predominantly osteoblastic activity
- Multiple myeloma, when the malignant plasma cells secrete osteoclast-activating factor, which stimulates osteoclasts to produce the lytic lesions in bone that are characteristic of the disease
- Primary hyperparathyroidism, when osteoclasts are responsible for development of the cysts in osteitis fibrosa cystica (commonly located in the jaw)

43. The answer is B. *(Physiology)*
Cholinergic and dopaminergic drugs have antagonistic actions at the basal ganglia. Dopaminergic agonists alleviate hypokinetic disorders such as Parkinsonism and exacerbate hyperkinetic disorders such as Huntington's chorea. Cholinergic agonists have the opposite effects.

44. The answer is B. *(Pathology)*
The lesion that most closely resembles the clinical and microscopic features of Kaposi sarcoma is bacillary angiomatosis. This infectious disease is caused by a *Rochalimaea* species, which is a rickettsia-like bacteria. The disease is associated with a non-neoplastic proliferation of small blood vessels throughout the body, most commonly in patients who are immunocompromised with HIV. When the lesions involve skin, they are raised, erythematous papules and nodules very similar in appearance to Kaposi sarcoma, which is a malignant tumor, most likely of endothelial cell origin. Histologically, the lesions of bacillary angiomatosis have atypical vascular channels, which may be misinterpreted as Kaposi sarcoma or a pyogenic granuloma. The organisms, however, are easily visualized with

silver stains. Erythromycin is used for treatment. *Rochalimaea* species are also the cause of cat-scratch disease.

45. The answer is B. *(Anatomy)*
Normally, during the swing phase of the gait cycle, the foot is kept in a dorsiflexed position by the dorsiflexor muscles of the anterior compartment of the leg. These muscles (tibialis anterior, extensor hallucis longus, extensor digitorum longus, and peroneus tertius) are innervated by the deep peroneal nerve. A lesion of this nerve results in footdrop because of the force of gravity. Therefore, the foot comes through the swing phase of gait and enters the stance phase in a plantar flexed position, and the patient begins the stance phase with a toe strike instead of a heel strike.

46. The answer is D. *(Pathology)*
The patient most likely has Letterer-Siwe disease (LSD), which is part of the malignant histiocytosis X triad of diseases. This disease primarily affects infants and young children. In addition to the findings listed in the history, the lytic bone lesions are also commonly located in the pelvic and long bones. The histiocytes are Langerhan cells, which contain Birbeck granules in the cytoplasm on electron microscopy. These granules look like a tennis racket or a spore of *Clostridium tetani*. Histiocytes are CD1-positive. LSD is the most aggressive histiocytosis X variant and includes eosinophilic granuloma, a benign histiocytic disease involving bone, and Hand-Schüller-Christian disease, a malignant histiocytosis associated with the classic triad of cystic lesions in the skull, diabetes insipidus, and exophthalmos.

47. The answer is C. *(Physiology)*
Both β_1 and β_2 receptors act by increasing cyclic adenosine monophosphate (cAMP) levels. The α_1 receptors act through an increase in intracellular calcium ions via inositol triphosphate. The α_2 receptors act by decreasing levels of cAMP.

48. The answer is A. *(Pathology)*
This patient has mycosis fungoides (MF). MF is a malignant CD4 helper T–cell disease that may also involve lymph nodes and other organs. The malignant

T cells in the epidermis are called Pautrier's microabscesses, which should not be confused with Munro's microabscesses in psoriasis, which are collections of neutrophils in the epidermis. When the T cells enter the bloodstream, the disease is called the Sézary syndrome; the cells are called Sézary cells. These cells are periodic-acid Schiff-positive cells with a prominent fold in the nucleus.

49. The answer is A.   *(Anatomy)*
At heel strike, inertia tends to cause the trunk to flex around the hip joint. Hip extensors normally are active then to prevent this flexion. The gluteus maximus is a strong hip flexor and normally contracts at heel strike. If the gluteus maximus muscle is paralyzed or weak, the patient displaces his upper torso posteriorly to prevent hip flexion at the time of heel strike. This action results in a characteristic "lurching gait" or "gluteus maximus gait."

50. The answer is A.   *(Pathology)*
The pathogen most likely responsible for this patient's condition is the human itch mite, which causes scabies. Tissue injury results when adult female mites bore into the stratum corneum. The burrows are visible as dark lines between the fingers, at the wrists, on the nipples, or on the scrotum. The mites lay their eggs at the end of the tunnel, thus creating an intensely pruritic lesion. In adults, the disease is limited to the intertriginous areas and spares the soles, palms, face, and head, whereas in infants, there are no burrows and the palms, soles, face, and head are affected. Topical benzene hexachloride (lindane) and permethrin dermal cream are the treatments of choice.

A louse (*Pediculosis capitis*) is associated with involvement of the hair and skin and the pubic hair (crabs). Cutaneous *Leishmaniasis* produces ulcers. *Trichinella spiralis* causes trichinosis, which involves the migration of larva into muscle. An *Ancylostoma* species is responsible for cutaneous larva migrans, which produces a pruritic, creeping eruption with pronounced peripheral eosinophilia.

51. The answer is B.   *(Physiology)*
Changing the focus of the eye for close vision (the near response) involves constriction of the pupil, contraction of the ciliary muscles, and convergence of the eyeballs.

52. The answer is D.   *(Pathology)*
A good mnemonic for separating the color sequences of the harmless scarlet kingsnake from the lethal coral snake is "red and yellow kill a fellow" (coral snake), "red and black, friend of Jack" (scarlet kingsnake). Snake venoms (coral snake and cobras in general) are complex and contain neurotoxins, fibrinolytic agents, or coagulants. In general, most pit viper envenomations produce hematologic abnormalities, such as disseminated intravascular coagulation. A copperhead envenomation is the least likely to result in mortality. The key to the treatment of poisonous snake bites is to bring the patient to a hospital. In addition, neither tight tourniquets that stop the blood supply nor ice should be applied. The poison should not be cut or suctioned, and the patient should not be allowed to move around.

53. The answer is B.   *(Anatomy)*
The tenth intercostal nerve is the anterior ramus of the T_{10} spinal nerve. After passing through the tenth intercostal space, the nerve continues forward in the anterolateral abdominal wall, in the plane between the internal oblique muscle and the transversus abdominis muscle. In the abdominal wall, the nerve innervates to the abdominal wall muscles as well as the skin and the parietal peritoneum. The umbilicus is a useful landmark for the region of distribution of the tenth thoracic nerve.

54. The answer is C.   *(Pathology)*
Blurry vision in a child with a recent onset of polyuria, polydipsia, and weight loss strongly suggests type I diabetes mellitus. The hyperglycemia is probably producing an osmotic diuresis and fluid loss, which is stimulating thirst in the patient. Because the lens does not require insulin to absorb glucose, the glucose is being changed into sorbitol by aldolase reductase and water is entering the lens by osmosis, thereby altering the refractive index of the eye. Over time, the osmotic damage could lead to cataract formation.

A retinoblastoma is a rare intraocular tumor that presents as a white-eye reflex. Amblyopia is a complication of strabismus (malalignment of the eyes) and refers to poor vision that is not correctable with lenses. Retinal hemorrhages in diabetes mellitus occur as a late complication of poorly controlled disease and would not be expected in early diabetes.

55. The answer is E. *(Anatomy)*
The obturator internus muscle takes its origin from the ilium, pubis, and ischium surrounding the inner surface of the obturator internus. The tendon of the obturator internus passes through the lesser sciatic foramen to attach to the femur. The obturator internus muscle is covered by the obturator internus fascia. A line of thickening of this fascia, the arcus tendineus, is part of the origin of the levator ani. The levator ani forms part of the muscular layer of the pelvic diaphragm.

56. The answer is D. *(Pathology)*
Almost all patients over 40 years of age with Down syndrome develop neuropathologic changes characteristic of Alzheimer disease. Amyloid β-protein (Aβ) in high concentration is toxic to neurons. The Aβ peptide is derived from amyloid precursor protein (APP), which is coded for on chromosome 21. Down syndrome is most commonly caused by trisomy 21 and is the exception to the rule that Alzheimer disease is rare in young people.

Upper or lower motor neuron disease, stroke secondary to essential hypertension, and ischemic encephalopathy are no more frequent in patients with Down syndrome than in the general population.

57. The answer is C. *(Anatomy)*
The glossopharyngeal nerve provides general sensory innervation to the posterior third of the tongue and to the pharyngeal mucosa; it also provides taste sensation to the posterior third of the tongue. In addition, the glossopharyngeal nerve also carries preganglionic parasympathetic nerves to the otic ganglion. The postganglionic fibers from the otic ganglion innervate the parotid gland. The only skeletal muscle innervated is the stylopharyngeus. The styloglossus is innervated by the hypoglossal nerve, the posterior belly of the digastric and the stylohyoid are innervated by the facial nerve, and the palatoglossus is innervated by the vagus nerve.

58. The answer is D. *(Pathology)*
The patient exhibits symptoms of bacterial meningitis (increased protein, decreased glucose, and increased cell count, predominantly with neutrophils). The Gram stain would most likely reveal gram-negative diplococci consistent with *Neisseria meningitidis*, the most common bacterial meningitis of patients in this age bracket. It is also the most common meningitis in the setting of crowded conditions, such as the military. Furthermore, it is the most common bacterial meningitis associated with a skin rash. The bacteria enters the blood through the posterior nasopharynx and from there, enters the spinal fluid in the subarachnoid space. It may be associated with the Waterhouse-Friderichsen syndrome (disseminated intravascular coagulation [DIC] and bilateral adrenal hemorrhage). If treated quickly, neurologic sequelae are not as common as with other bacterial pathogens.

Thin gram-negative coccobacilli represent *Hemophilus influenzae,* which is the most common overall bacterial cause of meningitis and the most common agent in children less than 6 years of age. Gram-positive diplococci are associated with *Streptococcus pneumoniae* (pneumococcus), the most common bacterial cause of meningitis in people over 30 years of age. Fat gram-negative rods represent *Escherichia coli,* the second most common cause of meningitis in neonates and a common cause of meningitis in the elderly. Gram-positive cocci in chains are consistent with streptococci. Group B streptococcus is the most common pathogen in meningitis of the newborn.

59. The answer is C. *(Anatomy)*
The dorsal nucleus of Clarke within the spinal cord gray matter is the origin of the ascending posterior spinocerebellar tract. Its neurons receive synaptic input from primary afferent neurons (i.e., dorsal root ganglion cells) associated with proprioceptors in the periphery. The axons from the nucleus of Clarke remain ipsilateral and ascend in the lateral funiculus of the spinal cord to end in the ipsilateral cerebellum. This tract is the primary sensory system for unconscious proprioception.

The anterolateral (spinothalamic) tract arises from cells in laminae I, II (substantia gelatinosa) and carries pain and temperature sensation.

The dorsal column-medial lemniscal tract arises from the central processes of primary sensory neurons that ascend the spinal cord and synapse on neurons in the nuclei gracilis and cuneatus. Axons from the neurons in these two nuclei form the medial lemniscus. In addition, this tract carries sensations of two-point touch, vibration, and conscious proprioception are carried in this tract.

The reticulospinal tract arises from neurons in the reticular formation of the brain stem. The axons descend to synapse on interneurons in the spinal cord gray matter. This system serves multiple functions but has a primary effect on spinal cord motor neuron activity. The spino-olivary tract arises from neurons in the dorsal horn gray matter and ascends to synapse on neurons in the inferior olivary nucleus. This tract is part of the complex system coordinating voluntary motor activity and adjustments and maintenance of posture.

60. The answer is A. *(Pathology)*

The lesion is most likely a glioblastoma multiforme (GBM), which is derived from astrocytes. A GBM is the highest grade of astrocytoma and the most common primary brain tumor in adults, with a peak occurrence in 40- to 70-year-old patients. These tumors have a predilection for the frontal lobes, where they commonly cross the corpus callosum to the other hemisphere. Possible predisposing factors include long-term seizure or personality disorder, the presence of scars from previous head trauma, the presence of oncogenes (e.g., sis, myc, src, and n-myc), exposure to petroleum products, and the familial polyposis syndrome (Turcot syndrome). Grossly, the tumors exhibit hemorrhagic necrosis with distortion of the subjacent brain tissue from edema. Prominent histologic features of GBM include hemorrhage, necrosis, palisading of tumor cells around vascular channels, and highly pleomorphic astrocytic cells with frequent atypical mitotic figures. GBMs characteristically seed the neuraxis, but rarely metastasize outside of the central nervous system (CNS). The prognosis for patients is extremely poor and most die within a year.

Oligodendrogliomas derive from oligodendrocytes. These tumors are commonly located in the frontal lobes and are associated with calcifications in more than 90% of cases. Microglial cells are not associated with neoplastic transformation. Ependymomas in adults are usually located in the filum terminale or

the spinal cord. Choroid plexus tumors are rare. The choroid plexus papillomas are most common in the lateral ventricles in children and the fourth ventricle in adults. Hydrocephalus owing to obstruction and increased production of spinal fluid are potential complications.

61. The answer is D. *(Anatomy)*

Damage to the reticular system results in problems with sleep and arousal. Damage to the cerebellum, basal ganglia, or thalamus involves difficulties in coordination, movement, or pain perception, respectively. Damage to the amygdala may result in the Kluver-Bucy syndrome (hypersexuality and docility).

62-63. The answers are: 62-D, 63-A. *(Pathology)*

The patient had a tonic–clonic seizure. These seizures are often associated with a sudden loss of consciousness. The tonic phase is characterized by extended legs, abducted arms, and pronated hands. Snapping of the jaws may occur with possible biting of the tongue, lips, or both. This activity is following by a clonic phase characterized by generalized jerking of the body musculature. Following this jerking is a stage of flaccid coma. On awakening, the patient is frequently confused (postictal state), feels lethargic, and often complains of a headache with muscle aches and pains. Associated manifestations include tongue or lip biting, urinary or fecal incontinence, and other injuries. An aura may precede a generalized seizure and indicates that the seizure began focally.

An electroencephalogram is the gold standard test in working up seizure disorders. A computerized tomography scan is less expensive than a magnetic resonance imaging study, although the latter is more sensitive in identifying epileptogenic foci in the frontal and temporal lobes. Electrolytes, glucose, blood urea nitrogen, liver function tests, and drug screens are frequently ordered to complete the workup. A skull radiograph is unlikely to produce any useful information.

64. The answer is D. *(Anatomy)*

The ligaments of the vertebral column that resist flexion of the column include the supraspinous ligament, interspinous ligament, ligamentum flavum, and posterior longitudinal ligament. The ligament that resists extension is the anterior longitudinal ligament. This longitudinal ligament is very broad and strong. It covers the anterior and anterolateral surfaces of the vertebral bodies and the intervertebral disks. In addition to resisting extension, the anterior longitudinal ligament provides reinforcement to the anterior and anterolateral surfaces of the intervertebral disk. The posterior longitudinal ligament is relatively narrow and covers the posterior surface of the vertebral bodies and the intervertebral disks. This ligament reinforces the posterior surface of the disk. The posterolateral surface of the disk is not reinforced, and it is through this region that herniation of the nucleus pulposus usually occurs.

65. The answer is B.   *(Pathology)*

Neoplasms of peripheral nerves include schwannomas (neurilemoma), neurofibromas, and malignant nerve sheath tumors, designated as either malignant schwannomas or neurofibrosarcomas. Schwannomas, or neurilemomas, are benign tumors arising from the Schwann cell, which is of neural-crest origin. These tumors are typically solitary, well circumscribed, and encapsulated, thereby making their surgical removal easier than other neural tumors. They may involve intracranial nerve roots (acoustic neuroma involving VIIIth nerve), spinal nerve roots, or peripheral nerves. In the autosomal-dominant disease neurofibromatosis, the tumors frequently involve the acoustic nerve. Schwannomas have a classic microscopic appearance, consisting of compact, Antoni type-A areas interspersed with loosely structured myxomatous-appearing areas designated as Antoni type-B. These tumors never undergo malignant transformation.

Neurofibromas are neoplasms of neuroectodermal origin that are composed of Schwann cells and fibroblasts. They are often multiple and nonencapsulated in cases involving small peripheral nerves or large nerve trunks. In the skin, they produce nodular to pedunculated lesions that are frequently pigmented. Tumors with large nerve trunk involvement, which have a small but significant risk for malignant transformation, are more likely to be associated with autosomal-dominant disease. Unlike schwannomas, they are difficult to remove surgically, because they involve the entire nerve.

66. The answer is B.   *(Anatomy)*

Huntington disease is associated most closely with damage to the basal ganglia. Damage to the cerebellum or thalamus involves difficulties in coordination or pain perception, respectively. Damage to the amygdala may result in the Kluver-Bucy syndrome (hypersexuality and docility). Damage to the reticular system results in problems with sleep and arousal.

67. The answer is C.   *(Pathology)*

In analyzing the cerebrospinal fluid (CSF) for a diagnostic spinal tap, three tubes are generally collected: one for microbiologic studies (culture and Gram stain); one for chemistry tests, cytology, and serology; and one for the cell count and differential. Protein studies in the CSF are generally tests for demyelinating diseases or workups for inflammatory diseases of the central nervous system (CNS). Gamma globulins in the CSF, which increase the total protein (range 15–45 mg/dl) come from synthesis of immunoglobulin G (IgG), which should only account for less than 12% of the total on an electrophoresis. Spinal fluid glucose is an ultrafiltrate of plasma (normal 50–75 mg/dl) and is approximately 60% of the plasma sample obtained 30 to 90 minutes before the lumbar puncture. A low CSF glucose, or hypoglycorrhachia, is defined as a glucose less than 40 mg/dl. A normal adult CSF white blood cell count contains 0 to 5 mononuclear cells per μl. Aside from culture, the Gram stain plays a significant role in the early presumptive diagnosis of bacterial meningitis and is best performed on a cytocentrifuge specimen. Acid-fast stains for tuberculosis in suspected tuberculous meningitis are best performed on the protein clot, or pellicle, on top of the CSF when the tube is left in the refrigerator overnight. Direct antigen detection of specific organisms is performed by latex agglutination or coagglutination techniques. These tests are available for most of the pathogenic bacteria and cryptococcus. The limulus test on CSF is used to detect endotoxin from Gram-negative organisms. C-reactive protein is only increased in bacterial infections, so it is very useful in separating bacterial from viral meningitis.

Viral meningitis should not be equated with aseptic meningitis until all other infectious etiologies have been excluded. Enteroviruses (e.g., coxsackievirus, echoviruses, polioviruses) account for approximately 85% of cases of viral meningitis. Viruses may involve the meninges (meningitis), the brain (encephalitis), or both (meningoencephalitis). Viral meningitis usually peaks in the late summer and early autumn and most commonly involves patients under 40 years of age.

Clinical findings are similiar to those of bacterial meningitis, but laboratory findings differ. The following table compares CSF findings in bacterial versus viral meningitis.

	Bacterial	Viral
Total white cell count	1,000 - 20,000 cells/μl	< 1,000 cells/μl
Differential count	> 90% polys	Neutrophils first then lymphocytes/monocytes after 48 hours
CSF glucose	Decreased	Usually normal
CSF protein	Increased	Increased
CSF C-reactive protein	Increased	Normal
Gram stain	Sensitivity 75%	Negative

68. The answer is C. *(Anatomy)*
The top of the iliac crest is at the level of the L_4 vertebra. A line drawn across the back connecting the top of the two iliac crests crosses the spine at L_4. The interspace between L_4 and L_5 or the interspace between L_5 and S_1 is used for a lumbar puncture. This level is below the inferior tip of the spinal cord (which is at the L_1/L_2 level) and above the inferior limit of the subarachnoid space (which is at the S_2 level).

69. The answer is B. *(Behavioral science)*
This patient is probably suffering from dementia. Alzheimer disease is the most common cause of dementia. Whereas normal aging can result in reduced speed of new learning, Alzheimer disease is associated with progressive memory loss and progressive reduction in good judgment. In contrast to delirium, in dementias such as Alzheimer disease, level of consciousness is often normal in the early stages. The memory loss or other cognitive symptoms associated with Alzheimer disease cannot be reversed with pharmacotherapy at present.

70. The answer is B. *(Anatomy)*
The pudendal nerve exits the pelvis through the greater sciatic foramen to enter the gluteal region. After passing behind the ischial spine and the sacrospinous ligament, the pudendal nerve passes through the lesser sciatic foramen to enter the perineum. The pudendal nerve gives rise to the inferior rectal nerve, the perineal nerve, and the dorsal nerve of the clitoris or penis. A

pudendal nerve block is often performed in obstetrics. The ischial spine is used as the landmark because of the very close relationship between the nerve and the spine as the nerve passes from the greater sciatic foramen to the lesser sciatic foramen.

71. The answer is D. *(Physiology)*
The neurotransmitters most closely associated with the development of anxiety are γ-aminobutyric acid (GABA), norepinephrine, and serotonin. Acetylcholine and histamine as well as the endogenous opioids have also been implicated in the development of anxiety.

72. The answer is A. *(Anatomy)*
The spinal accessory nerve passes through the posterior triangle of the neck in a very superficial position immediately deep to the superficial (investing) layer of the deep cervical fascia. The only layers covering the spinal accessory nerve in this position are the skin, superficial fascia, and superficial layer of deep fascia. The spinal accessory nerve innervates two muscles, the sternocleidomastoid and the trapezius. Where the spinal accessory nerve crosses the posterior triangle of the neck, it has already innervated the sternocleidomastoid but has not innervated the trapezius. A lesion at this point results in paralysis of the trapezius muscle.

73. The answer is E. *(Behavioral science)*
Although they frequently have trouble in school, children with attention deficit hyperactivity disorder

(ADHD) commonly have a normal intelligence quotient (IQ). In ADHD, emotional lability and irritability as well as limited attention span are seen. Genetic factors have been implicated, and stimulant drugs such as methylphenidate are the treatment drugs of choice for ADHD.

74. The answer is D.   *(Anatomy)*
The location of the space-occupying mass is near the motor and sensory cortex somatotopically related to distal parts of the lower extremity. Enlargement of the mass would most likely encroach upon the brain tissue in its immediate vicinity and produce related neurologic dysfunction. Precentral and postcentral gyri are primary motor and primary sensory cortex. Therefore, altered neuronal function would most likely produce diminished sensory perception and decreased motor activity, resulting in weakness in the somatotopically related part of the body.

Tremor is related to altered neuronal activity in either basal ganglia or cerebellum neurons.

Behavioral changes and lack of social skills are more likely to be related to dysfunction in the rostral parts of the frontal cortex.

The upper extremity is somatotopically related to lateral aspects of the precentral and postcentral gyri; away from the falx cerebri and closer to the lateral (sylvian) fissure (sulcus).

75. The answer is A.   *(Physiology)*
The electroencephalogram (EEG) during stage 1 sleep (the lightest stage of sleep) is characterized by theta waves. Sleep spindles and K-complexes are seen in stage 2, whereas stages 3 and 4 are characterized by delta waves. In REM sleep, low-voltage, sawtooth waves are seen.

76. The answer is D.   *(Physiology)*
The enkephalins are a neuroactive substance consisting of peptide groups assembled by the rough endoplasmic reticulum. These neuropeptides, which have been shown to affect neuronal activity, now number in the hundreds. They are usually synthesized as large molecules that are cleaved into their active form in time to play their role in cellular communication. Neuropeptides are found in the central and peripheral nervous systems.

Acetylcholine, serotonin, norepinephrine, and glutamate are synthesized enzymatically from specific amino acid precursors. Generally, these substances are molecularly smaller than the neuropeptide family of neurotransmitters. Substances that affect neurons or effector tissue physiologically but do not always fulfill all characteristics of pharmacologically defined neurotransmitters are called putative neurotransmitters.

77. The answer is A.   *(Behavioral science)*
Primary care physicians can handle most of the sexual problems of patients. However, when a wife was raped by her father throughout childhood and has never had a satisfactory sexual experience, the most correct response for the primary physician would be to refer the couple to a professional therapist.

78. The answer is C.   *(Anatomy)*
Neurotubules and neurofilaments are the cellular machinery for transporting substances throughout the cell. In Alzheimer disease, the disruption of tubules and filaments produces characteristic neurofibrillary tangles and prevents the required transport of synthetic and structural proteins, leading to cell dysfunction.

The Golgi complex packages substances into membrane-bound vesicles for transport or secretion.

Inclusion bodies are usually the by-product of cellular metabolisms, or they may become evident in disease or in aging cells.

RNA is found within the cytoplasm associated with rough endoplasmic reticulum or rosette clusters. This RNA is related to protein synthesis within the cytoplasm. Nuclear pores along the membrane of the nucleus provide continuity between the nucleoplasm and the cytoplasm.

79. The answer is C.   *(Anatomy)*
Glial cells react to form the scar tissue of the central nervous system (CNS) in a process called gliosis. The cells that form the scar tissue are described as hypertrophied or reactive astrocytes. These cells can also become phagocytic.

Microglia become reactive and transform into phagocytes in response to CNS damage. They appear to clear away necrotic tissue prior to gliosis.

The CNS does not have a connective tissue component such as fibrocytes or fibroblasts; therefore scar tissue does not consist of collagen.

Ependymal cells are glial cells that line the ventricles of the brain and the central canal of the spinal cord. When ependymal cells cover the choroid plexuses, they constitute the choroid plexus epithelium.

Oligodendroglia are commonly found between the myelinated fibers of white matter. These cells myelinate the fibers of the CNS.

80. The answer is B. *(Anatomy)*
Facial asymmetry leads to suspicion of the facial nerve involvement. The physical examination finding of only the lower half of the facial muscles being affected indicates that the lesion is within the central nervous system and is of an upper motor neuron type. The rationale for this centers on the corticobulbar innervation of the facial nerve motor nucleus in the pons. The facial nucleus is divided in half; the upper neurons innervate the upper muscles of the face, and the lower neurons innervate the muscles in the lower part of the face (buccinator, orbicularis oris, angularis, etc.). Both halves of this nucleus are under control of the opposite cerebral motor cortex for voluntary use of the skeletal muscles of facial expression. The neurons in the upper half also receive an ipsilateral cortical innervation that is capable of exciting these motor neurons, producing muscle contraction in the muscles of the upper half of the face. Therefore, if the lesion is a corticobulbar lesion affecting the facial nucleus/nerve, only the muscles in the lower half of the face completely lose their innervation and are weakened or paralyzed.

A parotid tumor may affect the branches of the facial nerve that pass through it to innervate the muscles of the face. This type of peripheral nerve compression results in a lower motor neuron deficit affecting the muscles.

The deficit resulting from a stroke affecting the tegmentum of the medulla would be seen in the distribution of the cranial nerves arising from this brain stem level. Recall that the facial nerve and nucleus are located at the level of the pons.

An acoustic neuroma is located outside of the brain stem at the cerebellopontine angle, the site of exit of the facial nerve from the pons. Compression of the facial nerve at this site would produce palsy affecting the muscles of facial expression, but all the muscles of the face on the side of entrapment would most likely be affected.

The distribution of the anterior cerebral artery does not have any direct affect on centers involving the function of the neurons in the facial motor nucleus.

81. The answer is D. *(Physiology)*
In hyperopia, the eyeball is too short for the refractive power of the lens, so images tend to come into focus beyond the retina. However, when an unfocused image falls on the retina, it reflexively stimulates contraction of the ciliary muscle, which rounds up the lens (accommodation). This converges the light rays so that they come to focus on the retina. Thus when looking at objects greater than 20 feet away, the images appear in focus because of accommodation. When looking at objects that are closer (3 to 20 feet away), the images are also usually clear as a result of even greater accomodation. The constant and intense use of accommodation, however, produces headaches.

82. The answer is B. *(Anatomy)*
The part of the cerebral cortex around the calcarine fissure is the primary visual cortex. The left half of each visual field is represented on the right cerebral cortex on the "banks" of the calcarine fissure. Formal or informal visual field testing reveals a deficit in function of this part of the cortex.

Testing rapid independent finger movements determines the integrity of the primary motor cortex and corticospinal tract.

A check of cognitive functions in word definition is used to test temporal–parietal cortical areas.

Performing tongue movements can test the orofacial regions of the primary motor cortex of the frontal lobe.

Tests of muscle tone and coordination are used to evaluate deep cortical nuclear groups and the cerebellum.

83. The answer is C. *(Pharmacology)*
Although dobutamine is usually characterized as a selective β_1 adrenoceptor agonist, it also produces significant stimulation of α_1 and β_2 receptors. In the vasculature, the opposing effects of α_1 and β_2 stimulation tend to cancel each other out, and the observed effect of dobutamine appears to be cardiac stimulation. In fact, an α_1 receptor-mediated inotropic effect supplements the β_1-mediated inotropic and chronotropic activity, resulting in a preferential increase in cardiac

force. For this reason, the drug has less effect on heart rate and vascular resistance than other catecholamines. Labetalol would oppose the effects of dobutamine by blocking both α and β adrenoceptors.

84. The answer is E. *(Anatomy)*
The muscles of mastication include the masseter, temporalis, medial pterygoid, and lateral pterygoid. They are all innervated by the mandibular division of the trigeminal nerve. The masseter, temporalis, and medial pterygoid all close the jaw. The lateral pterygoid opens the jaw and is also effective in protruding the jaw. When the right and left muscles contract together, the jaw is protruded. When the lateral pterygoid contracts unilaterally, the jaw deviates to the opposite side.

85. The answer is B. *(Pathology)*
The photomicrograph is an India ink preparation of cerebrospinal fluid (CSF), demonstrating the capsule of *Cryptococcus neoformans*. One of the yeasts exhibits the characteristic narrow-based bud. The India ink preparation has a sensitivity of only 50%, so a negative study does not exclude the diagnosis. A latex agglutination test is available with a higher sensitivity and specificity. *Cryptococcal meningitis* is the most common systemic fungal infection in immunocompromised hosts. It is characterized by numerous budding yeasts (narrow-based bud) with absence of an inflammatory response.

A newborn with a mother who experienced premature rupture of the membranes would most likely have a group B streptococcal meningitis (*Streptococcus agalactiae*—gram-positive coccus). A previously healthy 3-year-old child would most likely have *Hemophilus influenza* meningitis (gram-negative coccobacillus). A previously healthy 20-year-old military recruit would most likely have *Neisseria meningitidis* (gram-negative diplococcus). A patient with infective endocarditis would most likely have a negative CSF, because a cerebral abscess is not usually associated with organisms in the spinal fluid.

86. The answer is C. *(Behavioral science)*
Norepinephrine but not serotonin has been associated with learning. Experimental evidence indicates that serotonin is involved in mood, sexuality, anxiety, and sleep.

87. The answer is E. *(Pathology)*
HIV has various effects on the central and peripheral nervous systems. Cells with CD4 markers, such as T-helper cells, are destroyed by the virus. This process not only reduces the total T-helper cell count, but also diminishes the beneficial effect from cytokines normally released by the cells, such as γ interferon, interleukin-2, and B-cell growth factors. The patient is consequently subject to infections, particularly those requiring cell-mediated immunity for their destruction (e.g., *Mycobacteria, Pneumocystis*, etc.).

The virus enters the central nervous system (CNS) via monocytes/macrophages, which are the reservoir cells of the virus. These cells also have CD4 markers, which interact with the gp120 envelope protein of the virus. Microglial cells derive from monocytes and are the reservoir cells for the virus in the brain. The virus may also directly infect astrocytes, which contain glycolipid residues that bind to the gp120 envelope protein of the virus.

The virus effects all of the cell types in the CNS. In addition, HIV proteins are homologous with proteins in the brain. The antibodies generated against the HIV proteins crossreact with the brain proteins, producing autoimmune neurotoxic damage.

88. The answer is A. *(Pharmacology)*
Most of the adverse effects of β blockers are predictable extensions of their pharmacologic activity, namely bradycardia, precipitation of heart failure, and atrioventricular (AV) block (β_1 blockade) and bronchoconstriction (β_2 blockage). Central nervous system effects include lethargy, depression, and sleep disturbances (nightmares). Sexual impotence is probably also mediated by a central mechanism. The β blockers do not cause hyperglycemia. In fact, β blockers may prolong hypoglycemia in diabetics after insulin overdose by inhibiting β_2-receptor-mediated glycogenolysis that would be physiologically activated by epinephrine in the presence of hypoglycemia. The β blockers may also mask the signs of hypoglycemia, such as tachycardia, nervousness, and sweating.

89. The answer is E. *(Pathology)*
AIDS dementia complex (ADC) is a term that encompasses all of the neuropathologic findings commonly associated with dementia in HIV. It is characterized by a triad of:

- motor impairment, such as tremors, ataxia, hypertonia, and imbalance
- cognitive or neurologic deficits, such as memory loss, poor concentration, and slow thinking
- behavioral or neuropsychologic impairment, such as social withdrawal, apathy, hallucinations, and delusions

The cells involved in the progression of ADC are astrocytes, microglial cells, oligodendrocytes, and multinucleated syncytial cells, which represent the fusion of infected and uninfected microglial cells. T-helper cells are not involved in this progression. Many of the pathologic changes in nerve tissue are associated with cytokines (interleukin-1, interleukin-6, and tumor necrosis factor α) released from activated HIV–infected microglial cells. It is believed that gp120 from the virus and tumor necrosis factor α induce the production of these cytokines from the microglial cells. In addition, HIV proteins are homologous with proteins in the brain. The antibodies generated against the HIV proteins crossreact with brain proteins, producing autoimmune neurotoxic damage.

90. The answer is B. *(Physiology)*
This reflex involves all the structures except the medial geniculate body of the thalamus, which is concerned with the auditory pathway. The lateral geniculate body is involved with the eye and is part of this pupillary reflex.

91. The answer is C. *(Pathology)*
Primary malignant lymphomas of the brain differ from malignant lymphomas that secondarily involve the brain in that they are more likely to be multifocal, whereas metastatic malignant lymphoma is more likely to involve the meninges and spare the parenchyma. The vast majority of malignant lymphomas in the brain are of B-cell origin and are metastatic non-Hodgkin lymphomas. Primary lymphomas are increased in the presence of AIDS, which is the greatest risk factor, and in renal transplant patients. These tumors are aggressive (immunoblastic) and have an association with Epstein-Barr virus, which is a potent polyclonal stimulator of B cells. When tumors metastasize to the meninges, the spinal fluid findings include elevated cell counts, consisting of neoplastic cells intermixed with inflammatory cells, an increase in protein, and low glucose, thereby stimulating meningitis.

92. The answer is E. *(Pharmacology)*
Atropine and other belladonna alkaloids can be highly dangerous in overdose. In children, severe hyperthermia may be lethal, and a few fatalities have even occurred after instillation of atropine solution into the eye. Other drugs that produce hyperthermia in overdose include sympathomimetics and salicylates. Belladonna alkaloids also cause a toxic psychosis consisting of disorientation, delirium, and hallucinations, although lethargy and even coma may occur. Mydriasis and blurred vision, dry mouth, decreased bowel sounds, tachycardia, and other signs of muscarinic blockade are also observed.

93. The answer is C. *(Anatomy)*
The deltoid has its origin on the acromion and the spine of the scapula as well as on the clavicle. The trapezius has its insertion on the same places that the deltoid has its origin. The pectoralis minor has its insertion on the coracoid process of the scapula. The long head of the biceps attaches to the supraglenoid tubercle of the scapula, and the short head attaches to the coracoid process. The pectoralis major has its origin on the sternum, ribs, and clavicle and has its insertion on the humerus.

94. The answer is B. *(Pharmacology)*
Ganglionic blockers such as trimethaphan decrease both parasympathetic and sympathetic tone; the resulting organ effects depend on the predominant neural tone. In the heart, trimethaphan causes decreased contractile force and cardiac output due to sympathetic blockade, but a small increase in heart rate results due to parasympathetic blockade. Other effects of parasympathetic blockade include mydriasis, dry mouth, urinary retention, and decreased gastrointestinal motility.

95. The answer is A. *(Physiology)*
The spinocerebellar tract carries proprioceptive information to the cerebellum and does not synapse in the thalamus. The lateral spinothalamic tract, dorsal column medial lemniscal system, central tract of the

auditory nerve, and optic tract all synapse in the thalamus.

96. The answer is C. *(Pharmacology)*

M_1 receptors are called "neural" receptors and are located on nerve endings in the enteric nervous system and in gastric paracrine cells. The M_3, or "glandular," receptors mediate most of the smooth muscle effects of acetylcholine, including those in bronchial, ocular, and urinary smooth muscle, as well as glandular secretion. The M_2, or "cardiac," receptors mediate effects of acetylcholine on cardiac contraction, conduction, and impulse formation. Full doses of atropine block cardiac M_2 receptors, causing tachycardia; however, small doses activate receptors in the vagal nucleus to increase parasympathetic tone and cause bradycardia.

97. The answer is D. *(Behavioral science)*

Language development is a function of the left hemisphere of the brain in almost all right-handed people and in 70% of left-handed people. Perception of social cues, musical ability, spatial relations, and perceptual ability are functions that primarily involve the right hemisphere of the brain.

98. The answer is D. *(Pharmacology)*

Hemodialysis is of significant benefit in patients who have been poisoned with methanol, ethylene glycol, aspirin, theophylline, and procainamide. However, it is not beneficial in patients who are poisoned with paraquat, a herbicide that may cause extensive toxicity and death due to pulmonary fibrosis after oral ingestion or absorption across abraded skin. Treatment for paraquat poisoning is essentially supportive and palliative. The survival is inversely proportional to the dose ingested.

99. The answer is E. *(Physiology)*

Choices A through D are true and occur in that sequence. However, when the 1a afferents synapse in the spinal cord, they excite rather than inhibit the alpha motor neurons to the muscle.

100. The answer is D. *(Pharmacology)*

Nicotine produces stimulation followed by blockade of nicotinic receptors in autonomic ganglia, skeletal muscle, and the central nervous system. The early effects of acute nicotine poisoning are due to activation of the parasympathetic and sympathetic nervous systems and include stimulated secretions, increased gastrointestinal motility, increased blood pressure, and tachycardia. Later, hypotension and bradycardia may occur. Constipation is not one of the early manifestations of nicotine poisoning.

101. The answer is B. *(Anatomy)*

The vastus intermedius is one of the four heads of the quadriceps femoris. The vastus lateralis, vastus medialis, and vastus intermedius have their origins on the femur and insert as part of the quadriceps tendon on the tibia. These three heads do not cross the hip joint and therefore cannot act on this joint. The rectus femoris is the fourth head of the quadriceps femoris. It has its origin on the ilium and inserts with the quadriceps tendon. Therefore, the rectus femoris crosses both the hip and knee joints and can flex the hip as well as extend the knee. The psoas major and the iliacus join together to form the iliopsoas, which crosses the hip and attaches to the lesser trochanter of the femur.

102. The answer is A. *(Pharmacology)*

Despite their proven efficacy in a variety of other skin conditions, including allergic, eczematous, and seborrheic dermatitis, topical and systemic corticosteroids have no role in the treatment of acne vulgaris. Effective topical agents for acne include a form of vitamin A known as retinoic acid or tretinoin, benzoyl peroxide, and topical formulations of antibiotics such as erythromycin and clindamycin. Systemic therapy for acne includes antibiotics, such as minocycline, and estrogens may be helpful in female patients. The acne medications are believed to act by increasing epithelial cell turnover so as to expel comedones (vitamin A preparations, benzoyl peroxide) and to eradicate bacteria that degrade sebum triglycerides to irritating fatty acids (antibiotics, benzoyl peroxide). Estrogens antagonize androgen stimulation of sebum production.

103. The answer is E. *(Anatomy)*

The structures that pass through the greater sciatic foramen include the piriformis muscle, the superior gluteal nerve and vessels, the inferior gluteal nerve and vessels, the sciatic nerve, the posterior femoral cutaneous nerve, and the pudendal nerve and internal pudendal vessels. The pudendal nerve and internal pudendal vessels also pass through the lesser sciatic foramen. The lateral femoral cutaneous nerve passes from the false pelvis into the thigh by passing under the inguinal ligament.

104. The answer is B. *(Pharmacology)*
Drugs that may cause acneiform skin lesions include beclomethasone ("steroid acne"), androgens such as methyltestosterone, and lithium. Androgens contribute to acne by increasing sebum production, which leads to increased comedo formation. Doxycycline, a tetracycline antibiotic, may be used in the treatment of acne because it eradicates bacteria (*P. acne*) that break down sebum triglycerides to irritating fatty acids. Exposure to oils, fats, or tars in the workplace may contribute to the development of acne vulgaris, as oily skin exacerbates the condition.

105. The answer is C. *(Anatomy)*
The frontal sinus is within the squamous portion and the orbital plate of the frontal bone. The sphenoid sinus is within the body of the sphenoid bone. The tympanic cavity and the mastoid air cells are within the petrous and mastoid portions of the temporal bone. The ethmoid air cells are within the body of the ethmoid bone.

106. The answer is C. *(Pharmacology)*
Benzoyl peroxide is an effective agent for acne, but it has no sunscreen activity. Effective sunscreens include p-aminobenzoic acid (PABA), the benzophenones, and other agents. PABA is the most effective absorber in the ultraviolet B range that causes most erythema, skin aging, and cancer, but it may be sensitizing in some patients. Mupirocin is a highly effective topical agent for the treatment of impetigo due to staphylococci and streptococci. Haloprogin, naftifine, and ciclopirox are newer antifungal agents for treating dermatophyte (tinea) infections. Trioxsalen and methoxsalen are psoralens that can be photoactivated by longwave ultraviolet light to produce pigmentation in patients with vitiligo. Malathion, an organophosphate cholinesterase inhibitor, is an effective pediculicide, as are lindane and permethrin.

107. The answer is D. *(Behavioral science)*
Bruised knees are commonly seen in 6-year-old children. Old healed fractures, bruised buttocks, rupture of the liver, and subdural hematomas are unlikely to occur during a child's normal activities and therefore may be evidence of child abuse.

108. The answer is E. *(Pharmacology)*
Isotretinoin is a vitamin A derivative that is administered systemically in the treatment of severe cystic acne. Although it is quite effective, a number dermatologic and systemic adverse effects may occur. The dermatologic effects resemble hypervitaminosis A and include dry skin and mucous membranes and itching. Other adverse effects include alopecia (not hirsutism), muscle and joint pain, and lipid abnormalities, including hypertriglyceridemia. The drug is highly teratogenic and must be used in conjunction with an effective contraceptive in women of childbearing potential.

109. The answer is E. *(Anatomy)*
Oligodendroglia are glial cells of the central nervous system (CNS). They produce the myelin surrounding nerve processes in a similar fashion to the Schwann cell of the peripheral nervous system. An oligodendrocyte can have segments of several different fibers that lie in its vicinity.

Fibrocytes are found within the connective tissue sheaths of the peripheral nerve. Such cells produce the supportive collagen.

Perineurium surrounds the fascicles of the peripheral nerve. Individual nerve fibers are surrounded by endoneurium and the entire nerve is surrounded by epineurium.

Afferent fibers are a part of the peripheral nerve. They transport information back to the CNS.

Efferent fibers are also found in the peripheral nerve. Afferent and efferent fibers cannot be distinguished by light microscopy.

110. The answer is B. *(Pharmacology)*
Podophyllum resins contain cytotoxic agents that prevent the formation of the mitotic spindle and mitosis. They are used topically to treat condyloma acuminatum, and purified derivatives such as etoposide are used systemically in treating malignancies. Fluorinated corticosteroids are best absorbed from the scrotum,

scalp, and face as compared to the arms, legs, and trunk. Minoxidil is believed to act by an unknown mechanism on hair follicles to partially reverse the effects of testosterone in patients with androgenic alopecia. Topical coal tar preparations are quite effective in treating psoriasis and seborrheic dermatitis and may be used with topical corticosteroids in more severe cases. Salicylic acid is useful as a keratolytic agent in a variety of hyperkeratotic conditions and is believed to work by solubilizing components of the stratum corneum, leading to desquamation of keratotic debris.

111. The answer is E.   *(Pharmacology)*
The benzodiazepines are useful in the treatment of alcohol withdrawal, panic attacks, psychotic agitation, and musculoskeletal problems. They are not commonly used in the treatment of passive–aggressive personality disorder.

112. The answer is C.   *(Anatomy)*
The olfactory nerves arise from neurons imbedded within the nasal mucosa. The axons from these neurons enter the skull through the cribriform plate and enter the olfactory bulb where they synapse. From the olfactory bulb, the neuronal information is carried by the olfactory tract into the frontal and temporal lobes of the cerebral cortex. As a result, olfactory sensory information has direct input to the cerebral cortex without passing through the thalamus. The vagus nerves arise from the medulla; the hypoglossal nerves arise from the low medulla; the optic nerves arise from the diencephalon; and the oculomotor nerves arise from the midbrain.

113. The answer is A.   *(Physiology)*
When light falls on the photoreceptor it stimulates breakdown of photopigment, which decreases the level of cyclic guanosine monophosphate (cGMP). In turn, the decrease in cGMP reduces sodium influx into the cell, which hyperpolarizes the receptor cell. However, hyperpolarization decreases the continuous release of neurotransmitter.

114. The answer is C.   *(Behavioral science)*
The most common indication for electroconvulsive therapy (ECT) is major depression. ECT, which involves induction of a generalized seizure, is a relatively

safe treatment and maximum response is usually seen after 5 to 10 treatments.

115. The answer is A.   *(Pharmacology)*
A number of α and β-receptor antagonists have been developed that have greater affinity for receptor subtypes. Cardioselective, or β_1 selective antagonists include acebutolol, atenolol, and metoprolol. There are no clinically useful β_2-selective antagonists. α_1-selective antagonists include prazosin, terazosin, and doxazosin. These drugs are useful antihypertensives and produce less reflex tachycardia than nonselective α blockers. There is only one drug, labetalol, that blocks both α and β receptors. Labetalol is formulated as a mixture of stereoisomers with differing receptor affinities; it is a selective α_1 antagonist and a nonselective β antagonist.

116. The answer is B.   *(Pathology)*
A muscle biopsy exhibiting atrophy, primarily of type II muscle fibers, signifies a lower motor neuron disease. Parkinson disease produces extrapyramidal findings of muscle rigidity but no evidence of atrophy.

Muscle weakness may be secondary to neurologic diseases involving either the upper or lower motor neuron pathways, diseases involving the neuromuscular synapse (e.g., myasthenia gravis), and primary muscle disease (e.g., Duchenne muscular dystrophy). Upper motor neuron disease produces spasticity and brisk deep-tendon reflexes without significant atrophy, whereas lower motor neuron disease produces muscle atrophy with loss of the deep-tendon reflexes. Studies that are frequently obtained in the evaluation of muscle diseases include electromyography, which measures the action potential of the various muscles; nerve conduction times; measurement of serum creatine kinase and aldolase; and muscle biopsy.

Regarding the other choices in the question, which are lower motor neuron diseases that primarily affect type II fibers:

- In poliomyelitis, the virus destroys the lower motor neurons, particularly the anterior horn cells in the spinal cord.
- Charcot-Marie-Tooth disease is the most common genetic (autosomal dominant) peripheral nerve disease. It involves the peroneal nerve with subsequent muscle wasting in the muscles of the lower leg, thus

causing the patient's legs to look like an inverted bottle.

- Werdnig-Hoffman disease, like amyotrophic lateral sclerosis (ALS), is a degenerative disease involving the motor neuron. Unlike ALS, it is more common in children.

117-120. The answers are: 117-A, 118-D, 119-B, 120-F. *(Pharmacology)*
Lower doses of epinephrine increase heart rate by activating cardiac β_1-receptors, but mean arterial pressure is relatively unchanged due to the opposing effects of α_1- and β_2-receptor activation. Blockade of either α- or β-receptors unmasks the effects of epinephrine on the unaffected receptor type, leading to a depressor or pressor effect, respectively. After propranolol and atropine administration, the only effect of epinephrine is to increase blood pressure.

Injection of acetylcholine causes a profound vasodilation due to activation of noninnervated muscarinic receptors in arterial smooth muscle, while heart rate decreases briefly due to activation of cardiac muscarinic receptors. These effects are blocked by atropine. Isoproterenol increases heart rate and decreases mean arterial pressure by activating β_1- and β_2-receptors in the heart and vascular smooth muscle, respectively. Propranolol blocks both of these effects. Parasympathetic stimulation differs from acetylcholine administration in that parasympathetic stimulation only lowers heart rate because the muscarinic receptors in vascular smooth muscle are not innervated.

121-123. The answers are: 121-C, 122-A, 123-F. *(Pathology)*
The 12-year-old girl has a typical absence (petit mal) seizure, which almost always occurs in children. The seizures usually present with an abrupt onset that stops all activity. The child stares vacantly into space for 5 to 10 seconds. This staring may be accompanied by eye fluttering, mild tonic–clonic symptoms, or both. The patient recovers as abruptly as the seizure began and has either partial or no memory for the event. The classic electroencephalogram finding is a 3-Hz spike-and-wave pattern. As a rule, these seizures terminate by the third decade. Ethosuximide is the drug of choice.

The 38-year-old patient exhibits the key features of a simple partial seizure of the jacksonian type, which is a variant of a simple partial seizure. It is characterized by tonic–clonic concentrations of the extremities, with a march from the hand to the arm and then to the leg, or from the face to the hand or the reverse. Complex partial seizures, unlike simple partial seizures, often have a total or partial loss of memory and consciousness.

The 39-year-old patient shows the classic findings of temporal lobe epilepsy, which is a type of complex partial seizure. Additional stereotypic nonpurposeful movements (automatisms) include constant swallowing, chewing, pacing, fumbling hand movements, humming, or mumbling. These stereotypic automatisms are thought to originate from the anteromedial temporal area near the amygdala nucleus.

124-126. The answers are: 124-C, 125-D, 126-A. *(Pharmacology)*
β_1-receptors mediate cardiac stimulation, resulting in increased heart rate and contractility and accelerated conduction. β_2-receptors mediate vasodilation in some vascular beds, reducing peripheral resistance and blood pressure, whereas activation of α_1-receptors produces vasoconstriction and increased vascular resistance. Dopaminergic receptors activated by dopamine also cause vasodilation in certain vascular beds, particularly renal and splanchnic beds.

127-130. The answers are: 127-I, 128-D, 129-B, 130-H. *(Pathology)*
Mycobacterium leprae (lepromatous type) appears on skin biopsies as a Grentz zone, beneath which are macrophages filled with numerous organisms. *Mycobacterium leprae* (tuberculoid type) is indicated by a positive lepromin skin reaction in a patient with autoamputation of the digits of the hands.

Mycobacterium avium-intracellulare (MAI) can be described as a nonphotochromogen disease associated with a Whipple-like syndrome in a patient with AIDS.

Mycobacterium scrofulaceum produces cervical lymphadenitis (scrofula), most commonly in children, or it colonizes old tuberculosis cavities. In scrofula, patients are afebrile and have nontender, unilateral cervical lymphadenopathy. Both MAI and *Mycobacterium scrofulaceum* are atypical *mycobacteria*.

131-135. The answers are: 131-B, 132-D, 133-A, 134-E, 135-C. *(Pharmacology)*

Oxygen is the primary antidote for the treatment of carbon monoxide poisoning; hyperbaric oxygen is believed to accelerate the breakdown of carboxyhemoglobin and the removal of carbon monoxide from the body. The traditional treatment of cyanide poisoning consists of sodium nitrite to form methemoglobin, which has a higher affinity for cyanide than hemoglobin. In this way, the cyanide is sequestered in the blood and is thereby prevented from inhibiting cellular cytochrome oxidase. Sodium thiosulfate is then administered to react with cyanide to form sodium thiocyanate. Recently, chelators of cyanide, such as hydroxocobalamin, have been introduced. Chelation of cyanide forms cyanocobalamin, which is then excreted in the urine.

Aniline dyes and nitrites are among the oxidizing agents that form methemoglobin and cause methemoglobinemia. The antidote is methylene blue, which reduces the methemoglobin. There is no specific antidote for barbiturates and most other sedatives, except the benzodiazepines, for which flumazanil is a competitive antagonist. Treatment for barbiturates, ethchlorvynol and others, is to support respiration and other vital functions. The same is true of CNS stimulants such as the amphetamines. However, benzodiazepines may be specifically useful to control agitation, delirium, and seizures, and phentolamine may be used to control hypertension caused by amphetamines.

136-143. The answers are: 136-B, 137-A, 138-C, 139-E, 140-D, 141-B, 142-A, 143-E. *(Anatomy)*

Area B corresponds to Broca's speech area, the center for word formation. It is located in the operculum of the frontal lobe in approximately the middle of the inferior frontal gyrus.

The area labeled A is a part of the prefrontal cortex, the part of the brain that provides distinctively human qualities to our behavior. Personality, initiative, and planning and implementing daily activities originate in neural circuits in this part of the brain.

Area C represents the apex of the precentral gyrus on the lateral side of the cortex. The neurons in the lumbosacral spinal cord receive input from this part of the cerebral cortex, driving anterior motor neurons for voluntary motor control of the lower extremity. If this area is destroyed, characteristic features of an upper motor neuron disorder would be present, including Babinski reflex and clonus.

Area E represents a part of the temporal and occipital lobes of the cortex. The posterior cerebral artery distributes to the lateral and inferomedial aspects of the temporal and occipital lobes.

The parieto-occipital cortex represents the associative sensory areas of the brain. Convergence of numerous specific sensory systems at this site allows a person to make "sense" out of sensory stimuli and relate this information to various experiences. Sensory neglect, also referred to as selective inattention or neglect syndrome, is defined as a hemiapraxia with failure to pay attention to bodily grooming and stimuli on one side but not on the other. Because of the lack of sensory perspective, the individuals are often not aware that they are ignoring a significant part of the external environment as it relates to them. An infarct in area D, the posterior part of the parieto-occipital lobe of the right hemisphere, produces a sensory neglect on the opposite side. Recall that, at the cortical level, all sensory systems have crossed to the opposite side from their origin in peripheral receptors.

Area B receives blood supply from branches of the middle cerebral artery, which travels along the lateral surface after passing through the lateral fissure.

The watershed is a clinical term referring to the juxtaposed distribution of the cerebral arteries. The watershed zone, which represents the end-arterial distribution of the major cerebral arteries, is generally an arching line running about 1 to 2 inches lateral of the longitudinal fissure and from the frontal to occipital poles. Because these are end arteries, there is virtually no collateral circulation between the vessels. Therefore, this area is in particular jeopardy with decreasing blood flow due to occlusion of the cerebral arteries. Area A represents an area of juxtaposition between the middle cerebral artery branches on the lateral surface and branches from the anterior cerebral artery coming from the midline onto the lateral surface.

An embolism from a clot, air, or atherosclerotic plaque will travel through blood vessels until it finds a vessel whose diameter is smaller than itself. The tissue beyond this point of occlusion undergoes infarction with irreversible damage. Recall that the posterior cerebral artery, which distributes to the area labeled E, is a branch of the basilar artery. The basilar artery is formed by the junction of the two vertebral arteries, either of which could be the source of the embolism.

144-148. The answers are: 144-E, 145-C, 146-A, 147-D, 148-B. *(Pharmacology)*
Anaphylactic shock, characterized by immediate hypersensitivity reactions, bronchoconstriction, and hypotension, is best treated with epinephrine, which acts as a physiological antagonist of histamine released from mast cells during anaphylaxis. Urinary retention in post-surgical patients can be relieved with a cholinoreceptor agonist such as bethanechol, which increases contraction of the detrusor muscle, leading to micturition. Dyspnea associated with emphysema may be improved with the administration of the muscarinic antagonist ipratropium, which is given as an aerosol and is poorly absorbed from the lungs due to its quaternary ammonium structure. The urinary obstruction due to benign prostatic hypertrophy may be partly relieved with an alpha-adrenergic blocker such as terazosin, because increased sympathetic tone may contribute to the obstruction of contracting prostatic muscle, even though tissue hypertrophy is the primary problem. Patients with frequent migraine headaches may benefit from a course of therapy with the adrenergic beta blocker propranolol, which presumably acts by a central mechanism to prevent the occurrence of such headaches.

149-158. The answers are: 149-B, 150-C, 151-C, 152-E, 153-D, 154-A, 155-A, 156-D, 157-B, 158-C. *(Anatomy)*
Spasticity and hyperreflexia are cardinal signs of an upper motor neuron syndrome. These signs and symptoms are present due to an intact spinal cord reflex that has been released from descending control by the cerebral cortex.

Romberg's sign indicates a loss of conscious proprioception. This sensory modality is carried in the dorsal column-medial lemniscal system. The dorsal column–medial lemniscal system also carries afferent information serving modalities of discriminative two-point touch and vibratory sensations.

The extrapyramidal system consists of all the descending motor pathways except the corticospinal tracts. The extrapyramidal system is facilitatory to postural muscles and groups of muscles used in routine movements such as gait.

The anterolateral system is comprised of second order neurons from dorsal horn, specifically laminae I and II. These neurons process information arising form nociceptors and produce perceptions of pain and temperature. Removing the final common pathway removes the trophic effect of anterior horn motor neurons on skeletal muscle. The result is a loss of skeletal muscle fibers and muscle atrophy.

Flaccid paralysis results from a loss of the motor innervation to skeletal muscle by the anterior motor neurons, which disrupts the spinal reflex.

Paresthesias are abnormal sensations such as tingling, itching, and numbness. These modalities are carried in the spinothalamic tracts.

The axons from cortical neurons that form the corticospinal tract decussate in the lower medulla and form the lateral corticospinal tract.

The nucleus cuneatus receives input from the fasciculus cuneatus. This tract and nucleus are part of the dorsal column–medial lemniscal system. Nucleus cuneatus and fasciculus cuneatus are involved in two-point touch and vibratory sensations from the upper part of the body.

159-161. The answers are: 159-A, B, C; 160-D; 161-A, B. *(Pharmacology)*
The most likely causes of these toxicities are lead (159), iron (160), and mercury (161). The symptoms of acute lead poisoning include colic, irritability, drowsiness, nausea, vomiting, ataxia, and seizures. The treatment of confirmed lead poisoning includes chelation therapy with calcium disodium EDTA, BAL, or succimer (for use in children). Acute iron and mercury intoxication both cause abdominal pain with nausea and hematemesis. Iron toxicity most frequently occurs from ingestion of iron supplement tablets. Acute mercury poisoning may also cause renal toxicity. Serum metal analysis may be required to determine the specific cause of toxicity. Chelation therapy consists of deferoxamine for acute iron poisoning, whereas mercury is treated with dimercaprol (BAL) and succimer (dimercaptosuccinic acid).

162-163. The answers are: 162-C, 163-H. *(Pathology)*

Painful vesicular lesions on the right side of the forehead, dorsum of the nose, upper eyelid, and cornea, producing a keratitis in an immunocompromised patient, are symptoms of herpes zoster involving the ophthalmic division of the trigeminal nerve (cranial nerve V). The virus is most likely dormant in the trigeminal ganglion cells. *Herpes zoster* is associated with a previous varicella infection. The virus travels up the sensory nerves and becomes latent in various sensory ganglia. In this location, reactivation of the virus at a later date allows the virus to spread out through the nerves of the skin, where a painful vesicular eruption occurs that follows the dermatome of the involved nerve. The lesions are most commonly located in the thoracic dermatomes (T5-T10); however, they may also involve the trigeminal nerve, as in this case, or the facial nerve. The incidence of reactivation of the virus increases with age and with the presence of an immunocompromised host.

Meningoencephalitis after swimming in fresh water is associated with *Naegleria fowleri*, which is a protozoan that infects the frontal lobes through the cribriform plate.

Rubeola is associated with subacute sclerosing panencephalitis, which is a demyelinating slow-virus disease. Papovavirus is associated with progressive multifocal leukoencephalopathy (PML), which is a demyelinating disease commonly seen in immunocompromised patients.

Adenovirus may produce encephalitis with Cowdry B intranuclear inclusions. It is also the viral equivalent of "pink eye," which is a viral conjunctivitis. *Hemophilus influenza*, biotype *aegyptius*, is the bacterial counterpart of the disease.

The mumps virus may produce asymptomatic aseptic meningitis in up to 50% of cases. It is the most common extra-salivary manifestation of the disease. The spinal fluid findings often exhibit a low glucose, similar to to that of bacterial meningitis.

Herpes simplex type I is associated with a hemorrhagic necrosis of the temporal lobe. It may also produce a painful keratoconjunctivitis with dendritic ulcers visible after fluorescein staining.

Arthropod-born viruses (arboviruses) have a distinctive geographic distribution. St. Louis encephalitis is the most common type, while Eastern equine encephalitis is associated with the highest mortality.

Acanthamoeba species are associated with a keratoconjunctivitis contracted by patients who use their own lens-cleaning fluids, which become contaminated by the organism.

Taenia solium, the pork tapeworm, can produce cysticercosis. This disease is contracted when an individual ingests food or water contaminated with the feces of a person harboring the eggs of *T. solium*. The eggs only develop into larva (cysticerci) in the tissues, which makes man the intermediate host. In the brain, the cystic lesions frequently calcify and are the foci for seizures.

164-167. The answers are: 164-I, 165-N, 166-B, 167-O. *(Pharmacology)*

The urine sediment in the 3-year-old child with a urinary tract infection reveals an embryonated egg that is flat on one side. This is characteristic of *Enterobius vermicularis* (pinworm), which is a nematode that infests humans who ingest the egg. The larval forms develop within the lumen of the small intestine and the adults develop in the cecum and appendix. When the adult female migrates to the anus and deposits her eggs, intense anal pruritus develops (pruritus ani), resulting in restless sleep with the potential for autoinfection. Acute appendicitis is a rare complication. Urethritis may occur in females. The laboratory diagnosis is best made by noting embryonated eggs similar to the one in the photograph. Peripheral blood eosinophilia is not a feature of the disease, because only the adults have a superficial attachment to the mucosa. Pyrantel pamoate is the treatment of choice.

Hematuria in an Egyptian man whose bladder biopsy reveals squamous metaplasia most likely has schistosomiasis caused by *Schistosoma hematobium*, which is a trematode. Infection is acquired by the penetration of the larvae from infected snails into the skin, where they enter the lymphatics and distribute into subcutaneous tissue and around the body. *S. hematobium* favors development in the urinary venous plexus, where the eggs incite an inflammatory reaction, producing hematuria and squamous metaplasia of the normally transitional epithelium. This disorder predisposes patients to squamous carcinoma of the bladder.

The laboratory diagnosis is made by noting embryonated eggs with a nipple at the end of the egg. Praziquantel is the treatment of choice.

Chronic diarrhea in a patient with immunoglobulin A (IgA) deficiency is most likely associated with *Giardia lamblia,* which is a flagellated protozoan that produces diarrhea and a malabsorptive state after ingestion of cysts in contaminated water. The disease is association with IgA deficiency and other immunodeficiency states. Trophozoites emerge in the duodenum and stick to, or superficially invade, the small intestinal mucosa and damage it, thus producing diarrhea, crampy abdominal pain, flatulence, and steatorrhea (fat in the stool). Organisms sometimes find their way into the biliary tract. Lymphoid polyposis is prominent. Trophozoites encyst and pass in large numbers within the stool, surviving in water for up to 2 months. Recurrences and chronicity frequently occur. The laboratory diagnosis is made by the discovery of trophozoites, which are pear-shaped and have two nuclei that look like eyes, and by the presence of cysts in the stool, a duodenal aspirate, or with the string test. Metronidazole is the treatment of choice.

The most common organism involved in the gay bowel syndrome is *Microsporidia,* a gram-positive protozoan. Chronic diarrhea is the primary disease association, although other species have been associated with keratoconjunctivitis, hepatitis, and myositis. Albendazole is the treatment of choice.

168-180. The answers are: 168-D, 169-K, 170-F, 171-N, 172-H, 173-B, 174-M, 175-C, 176-J, 177-I, 178-A, 179-E, 180-O. *(Pathology)*
A baby with large, red areas of denuded skin and generalized bulla formation has the scalded child syndrome, which is caused by the release of *Staphylococcus aureus* toxin. *S. aureus* is a gram-positive coccus that clusters as a result of coagulase production.

Bilateral adrenal hemorrhage, disseminated intravascular coagulation (DIC), and hemorrhagic vasculitis in a 6-year-old child are characteristic of *Neisseria meningitidis* infection. *Meningitidis* is a gram-negative diplococcus. The patient has the Waterhouse-Friderichsen syndrome.

Bilateral ophthalmia neonatorum in a 4-day-old infant is most commonly caused by *Neisseria gonorrhoeae,* a gram-negative diplococcus. Ophthalmia neonatorum in the first 24 to 48 hours is usually a chemically induced conjunctivitis (e.g., silver nitrate). Bilateral conjunctivitis at 2 to 5 days is most commonly caused by gonococcal conjunctivitis, while unilateral disease is most commonly caused by *S. aureus.*

The infant who died shortly after birth most likely acquired *Listeria monocytogenes* transplacentally. *L. monocytogenes,* a gram-positive rod, often causes stillbirth or abortion in pregnant women. Infants who are born alive often die shortly thereafter as a consequence of septicemia or meningitis.

A common cause of chronic bronchitis, otitis media, and sinusitis is *Branhamella (Moraxella) catarrhalis,* which is a gram-negative diplococcus.

Fish handler disease is caused by *Erysipelothrix rhusiopathiae,* a gram-positive rod. *E. rhusiopathiae* produces a painful, pruritic, creeping violaceous rash most commonly seen on the hands. The diagnosis is best made by culturing a full-thickness aseptic biopsy sample of the lesion. Penicillin is the treatment of choice.

An exudate containing yellow granules in a woman who uses an intrauterine device is most likely caused by *Actinomyces israelii,* an anaerobic gram-positive filamentous bacterium. The yellow granules (sulfur granules) contain the organism. Cervicofacial disease is the most common presentation of actinomycosis, but the disease is also associated with endometritis caused by an intrauterine device.

Yersinia pseudotuberculosis is a gram-negative coccobacillus with a safety pin appearance, and is associated with granulomatous microabscesses in mesenteric lymph nodes. *Y. pseudotuberculosis* and *Y. enterocolitica* produce an enterocolitis primarily in children, who contract the disease by ingesting contaminated food or water. The organisms proliferate and invade the small intestine, producing a watery, bloody diarrhea and mesenteric lymphadenitis. The lymph nodes contain multiple noncaseating granulomatous microabscesses. In young adults, *Yersinia* infections primarily present as mesenteric lymphadenitis, which is clinically indistinguishable from acute appendicitis. *Yersinia* species are sensitive to the aminoglycosides, but most people recommend supportive care because the disease is self-limited.

An infant with ophthalmoplegia, hypotonia, and constipation after drinking milk sweetened with honey most likely has infant botulism caused by *Clostridium botulinum*, a gram-positive, spore-forming anaerobic rod. In infants, the clostridial spores in the honey germinate in the intestine and the toxin is released. Diarrhea is usually noted in adult botulism, whereas constipation is the rule in infants. The diagnosis is made in infants by measuring the toxin in the stool; the toxin is measured in adults in the blood. Because of the danger of infant botulism, honey should not be given to infants during the first year of life. Treatment is supportive.

A malignant pustule characterizes anthrax, which is caused by an aerobic, spore-forming, gram-positive rod. Cutaneous anthrax (90% to 95% of cases) occurs through direct contact with infected or contaminated animals (especially sheep and cattle) or animal products. The cutaneous lesions resemble insect bites, but eventually swell to form a black scab, or eschar, with a central area of necrosis. In untreated cases, death occurs in 20% of patients. The pulmonary form is almost always fatal and is caused by inhalation of spores present in contaminated hides (e.g., wool—Woolsorter disease). It produces a necrotizing pneumonia, pronounced splenomegaly and dissemination throughout the rest of the body (meningitis in 50% of cases). The spores are used in germ warfare, because the "first sign of the disease is death." The laboratory diagnosis is made by demonstrating the toxin products in culture and by standard serologic studies. Parenteral penicillin G is extremely useful in therapy.

Undulant fever is caused by *Brucella melitensis*, a gram-negative rod. *Brucella* species infect animals. Most infections in the United States occur in veterinarians, farmers, or meat packers through direct contact with infected animal hides. Brucellosis in man is usually mild, but severe forms present with disease disseminated throughout the body via the lymphatics, with granulomatous abscesses in the liver, spleen, and bone marrow. Undulant fever is the most severe form of the disease. Serologic tests are the mainstay for diagnosis.

Ludwig angina originates from an infected mandibular molar, where it extends out into the floor of the mouth, and pushes up the posterior tongue, thereby producing problems with respiration and swallowing. It is most commonly caused by an anaerobic streptococcus, which is a gram-positive coccus that forms chains.

Granulomatous inflammation in the lymph nodes of a rabbit hunter is most likely caused by *Francisella tularensis*, a highly infectious organism. Rodents and rabbits are the two main animal carriers of the disease, and tularemia is contracted by arthropod bites, mainly those of deer flies and ticks. The ulceroglandular variant is the most common type and presents with a localized papular lesion on the skin at the point of inoculation (e.g., the bite). The papule ulcerates and regional lymphadenitis (noncaseating granulomatous inflammation) with draining and sepsis occurs, leading to dissemination throughout the body (e.g., to the spleen and liver). The organism is difficult to culture; therefore, serologic tests are the mainstay for diagnosis. Streptomycin is the drug of choice.